Foreword

It has now been 20 years since the book salesman from Mosby walked into my office at Palm Beach Junior College and asked what book I was using for my Introduction to Occupational Therapy class. I replied that, rather than one text, I used sections of many occupational therapy books plus my own lesson plans because I had not found a satisfactory introductory text. He suggested that I submit a book proposal to Mosby for an introductory text. I did so, it was accepted, and for the next year while it was in production, I "test ran" the proposed chapters on my American Association of Occupational Therapy students. That first edition—published in 1989—was titled *Occupational Therapy: Introductory Concepts*. After a successful run, a second edition appeared in 1998 under its present title—*Introduction to Occupational Therapy*. The new expanded edition reflected greater depth of subject matter as well as new directions for occupational therapy. At that time I had recently retired from occupational therapy practice, so Mosby brought in Susan Hussey, OTR, who edited my manuscript and added information about changes that had occurred in the field.

The second edition included format changes that highlighted chapter objectives, key terms, and chapter summaries and that continued to include the suggested learning activities at each chapter's end, which had been enthusiastically received in the first edition.

This third edition comes out under a new publisher, Elsevier, with Sue Hussey at the helm and ably assisted by Jane O'Brien. It is hard to "let go of my baby," but my time for guiding the field is past, and I am grateful for the opportunity to have made a lasting contribution to occupational therapy.

I want to reiterate the thoughts I expressed in the epilogue of the first two editions because they sum up my feelings about occupational therapy's uniqueness in the health field. An occupational therapist is a facilitator of the patient/client's struggle toward independence—of however much or little that person is capable.

Human life is both an external and internal experience. For each of us there is an outer self and an inner spirit. The Eastern approach to health has always been one of body/spirit interaction, whereas the Western approach to health care maintains a focus on the external aspect—the body—with little attention given to the inner spirit. The drive for objective, measurable results has yielded amazing technical advances against disease, trauma, developmental anomalies, and degenerative disorders, but it has left the spirit bereft. In the 1970s, Dr. Elizabeth Kübler-Ross called for medicine to refocus on the spirit in her groundbreaking book, *On Death and Dying*. Since then our awareness of the need for care of the spirit has changed, but the increasingly fast pace of society leaves little room for the time that takes. Where is there a place for "spirit mending"?

As the changes in health care occurred in the twentieth century, the opportunity to address that more inclusive need arose within the realm of rehabilitation. Whereas physical therapy focused upon body functioning, occupational therapy became a prime discipline for a more holistic approach. All occupational therapy students must study psychology as well as physical function and technical skills. This educational emphasis confirms the assertion that occupational therapy is the proper place for a measure of spirit mending. Our discipline functions from a mindset that is different from technical specialties. The concern for the whole person is expected in every individual treatment plan. The therapist is not the repository of some "cure," but the link in assisting a person in finding his or her own abilities or capacities. It has been a conviction of our profession since its beginning that health involves body, mind, and spirit—in total integration. Dysfunction in any part affects the whole person. If a person loses the ability to walk, it is not only his or her legs that are deficient; the entire being is profoundly affected!

When a person is impaired by a disorder, it is not only the physical body that suffers but also the psyche and spirit. When a person is stricken by a catastrophic medical problem, the spirit is wounded and we are called to address that, for it is the spirit that either prevents or enables a person to fight the limitations that threaten and that finds a new way to adapt to life's demands.

To articulate the unique contribution that occupational therapy makes in rehabilitation, I choose to use the term "spirit mending" because it captures an essential, though nebulous, dimension of human needs. Whatever the term, those entering the field should consider and debate the issue—for it can be easily lost in accountability demands that continue to escalate. A profession's strength and respect grow by the profession setting its own parameters.

I unequivocally state that no technical expertise or health-promoting activity is *more* important than spirit mending—the regard for the total humanness of the persons we serve. This in no way devalues the importance of technical expertise, which is of prime importance. Both are needed if we truly are to help gain greater dignity and independence for those whose spirits have been assaulted by life.

Barbara Sabonis-Chafee, MS, OTR/ret

Introduction to Occupational Therapy

evolve

∴ *To access your Student Resources, visit:*

http://evolve.elsevier.com/Hussey/introOT

Evolve® Student Learning Resources for ***Hussey/Sabonis-Chafee/O'Brien: Introduction to Occupational Therapy, ed 3,*** offers the following features:

Student Resources

- **Crossword Puzzles**
  Provide additional classroom activities and exercises.

- **Learning Activities**
  Fill-in-the-blank exercises for each chapter.

- **WebLinks**
  Links to organizations and other helpful resources.

Third Edition

Introduction to Occupational Therapy

Susan M. Hussey, MS, OTR/L
Professor and Coordinator
Sacramento City College
Science and Allied Health Division
Sacramento, California

Barbara Sabonis-Chafee, MS, OTR
Retired

Jane Clifford O'Brien, PhD, OTR/L
Associate Professor
Occupational Therapy Department
College of Health Professions
University of New England
Biddeford, Maine

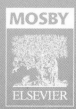
MOSBY
ELSEVIER

11830 Westline Industrial Drive
St. Louis, Missouri 63146

INTRODUCTION TO OCCUPATIONAL THERAPY, THIRD EDITION   ISBN-13: 978-0-323-03369-5
Copyright © 2007, 1998 by Mosby, Inc., an affiliate of Elsevier Inc.   ISBN-10: 0-323-03369-5

Notice

Neither the Publisher nor the Authors assume any responsibility for any loss or injury and/or damage to persons or property arising out of or related to any use of the material contained in this book. It is the responsibility of the treating practitioner, relying on independent expertise and knowledge of the patient, to determine the best treatment and method of application for the patient.

The Publisher

International Standard Book Number 978-0-323-03369-5

Publishing Director: Linda Duncan
Acquisitions Editor: Kathy Falk
Developmental Editor: Melissa Kuster Deutsch
Publishing Services Manager: Deborah L. Vogel
Design Direction: Margaret Reid

Printed in the United States of America

Last digit is the print number: 9   8   7   6   5   4   3   2   1

Preface

Introduction to Occupational Therapy, third edition, is written for those entering the study of the profession of occupational therapy. This text is especially written for those who intend to become practitioners at either the professional level (occupational therapist) or the technical level (occupational therapy assistant) or for those who are exploring the profession to determine whether this is the field for them. *Introduction to Occupational Therapy* gives the reader a solid overview of the important concerns and concepts of occupational therapy, without burdening the student with information and details that he or she may not yet have the background to understand. This edition incorporates the *Occupational Therapy Practice Framework* and the basics of evidence-based practice. Numerous case studies are presented to help illustrate the concepts.

The text is divided into three sections. The first section introduces the reader to the field of occupational therapy, which includes the history and philosophy of occupational therapy, current issues, and future trends in the profession. Section 2 focuses on the occupational therapy practitioner, the educational requirements to practice, roles and responsibilities of practioners, the ethical and legal dimensions of practice, and the national professional organizations. Section 3 concentrates on the practice of occupational therapy and describes the framework and process of occupational therapy practice; the settings in which occupational therapy is practiced; intervention approaches in occupational therapy; and special skills that are needed by the individual practitioner in the field of occupational therapy, including development of therapeutic relationships, selection of therapeutic activities, and development of clinical reasoning.

This edition of *Introduction to Occupational Therapy* has been organized to make learning easy for the reader. Each chapter begins with a testimonial written by an occupational therapist or an occupational therapy assistant about his or her experiences in occupational therapy. These personal accounts highlight the humanistic nature of our profession, and they relate theories and concepts to the real world of occupational therapy. Each chapter is introduced with objectives that outline the main points covered in that chapter; these objectives are followed by a list of key terms, which are typeset in boldface throughout the text. Case studies are interwoven throughout the chapters, and a summary at the end of each chapter provides a synopsis of the material covered. There are also learning activities and review questions at the end of each chapter, which provide ways to apply the information or concepts covered in the chapter.

To the teacher:

To make the best use of this text for occupational therapy students, it is suggested that it be used as the core text in conjunction with three other components:

- Self-paced medical terminology study
- Beginning field research (using suggested activities)
- Individual and group classroom exercises

The student will not only form a coherent picture of occupational therapy and begin to develop problem-solving skills, but he or she will also become an independent active learner.

The suggested activities can be incorporated into class planning by requiring the students to choose one activity from the listed options. Many of the activities require the students to present to the class. The review questions at the end of each chapter may serve as study guides and topics of discussion.

A new Evolve Resources website for the student and instructor and an *Instructor's Resource Manual* have been added as ancillary features to *Introduction to Occupational Therapy*. The website includes a test bank and PowerPoint slides for the instructor, as well as learning activities and vocabulary-building exercises for the student. The *Instructor's Resource Manual* contains a wealth of additional resources, activities, and case studies.

Acknowledgments

This text would not have been possible without the contribution and support of several individuals. First of all, we would like to acknowledge all of the students and faculty who, throughout each of our careers, have provided feedback on our teaching and classroom resources. We would like to thank Bill Croninger, Associate Professor at the University of New England, whose photography was used throughout the text. We would also like to thank the American Occupational Therapy Association for their willingness to provide various materials for this book. Finally, we would like to thank the staff at Elsevier for all of their encouragement and assistance with this project. Kathy Falk, Melissa Kuster, and Leah Bross have been an exceptional team with whom to work.

SMH and JOB

First, I want to thank my husband, Bruce, without whom the completion of this project would not have been possible. He filled so many supportive roles during this project, and I am so grateful for his patience, sense of humor, inspiration, and ability to adapt. I want to thank my parents, Lois and Gary; my sister, Barbara; and my friend, Maureen Paine, for their ongoing encouragement.

Thanks to Mary Turner, Dean of Science and Allied Health, for her wisdom and support and to all the faculty members of the OTA Program at Sacramento City College. Lynette Beadles, Ada Boone Hoerl, Marlene Steele, Suzy Campbell, and Janis Wong—thanks so much for your collaboration, dedication, and especially laughter! To my newest and most geographically distant colleague in occupational therapy, Jane O'Brien—thank you for your collaboration and perseverance.

Finally, to my precious children, Natalie and Cameron, who at the age of 4 didn't quite understand and kept wondering, "When is Mommy going to be done working?" You kept me going throughout this project, and now I'm done, so let's go play!

SMH

I would like to thank my mentors Anita Bundy, Anne Fisher, and Gary Kielhofner for supporting and believing in me early in my career. I would like to thank my husband, Mike, for helping me pursue my interests, encouraging me, and supporting me in many ways. I thank my children, Scott, Alison, and Molly, whose laughter, play, creativity, and interesting stories energize me every day. My parents, Sylvia and Gordon Sherwood, for giving me perspective on occupational changes over time. My sister, Judy, for entertaining me with stories of raising teenagers and life in general. I thank my running friends for keeping me going. My fellow University of New England colleagues deserve recognition for supporting me during this project. A special thanks to Nancy MacRae for reviewing many of the chapters and contributing important content on models of practice. Finally, thank you to my colleague Sue Hussey for sharing this experience with me.

JOB

Contents

Section 1 Occupational Therapy: The Profession

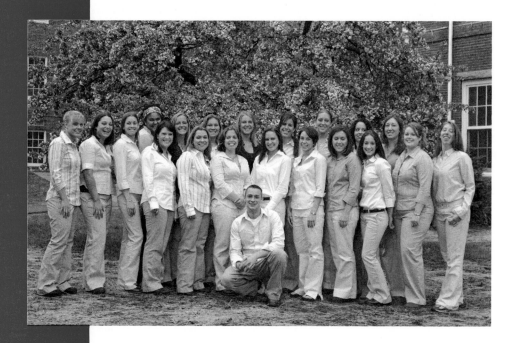

For many years, I believed that I first became interested in occupational therapy when I worked as a research assistant in a psychiatric hospital. The occupational therapy clinic was a few doors from my office, and I had a first-hand view of the patients' responses to creating tie-dyed T-shirts and scented candles. Defeat and uneasiness were replaced by smiles and confidence, all in a matter of hours.

The activities reminded me of my childhood. My mother patiently taught me and my six younger sisters and brothers many different arts and crafts. More importantly, she let us loose in the "playroom," where we spent endless hours with glue, scissors, bits of wire, yarn, plastic lace, found objects, and scraps of paper from my father's office, making whatever we pleased. I learned needle crafts from my mother, and my grandmother taught me cross-stitch embroidery when I was 8 years old. Throughout these formative years, a consistent theme was there—activities are fun and important; they can be life-long companions and sources of joy and self-esteem.

The link between my own childhood experiences of working through activities and the reactions of patients to occupational therapy grew stronger as I watched from my office. It wasn't long before I applied and was accepted into occupational therapy school. In the more than 20 years since I graduated, I never regretted my career decision, and I often look back with some amazement to the coincidences that led me to it. I love teaching people, especially those who fear they cannot learn or cannot do—because, of course, they can learn and can do. To me, it is the greatest pleasure to witness the "ah-hah!" look and the triumphant expression that comes with accomplishment in the face of fear.

It soon became obvious that my ties to occupational therapy predated my research assistant job. It wasn't until after I graduated from school and had been working several years and after one of my younger sisters also graduated from occupational therapy school that my mother revealed that she, too, had also been studying occupational therapy but left school to raise her family after meeting and marrying my father. Now, when I think of the playroom of my childhood, I remember my mother—the almost-occupational therapist—quietly and secretly passing the message and mission to her children.

Mary Beth Early, MS, OTR/L
Professor
Occupational Therapy Assistant Program
LaGuardia Community College
City University of New York
Long Island City, New York

Introductory Questions

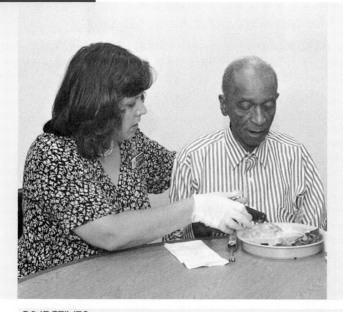

OBJECTIVES

After reading this chapter, the reader will be able to do the following:

- Understand the basic terminology used in occupational therapy (OT)
- Describe the nature and scope of the practice of occupational therapy
- Identify personality traits suitable for a career in occupational therapy
- Describe levels of OT personnel
- Identify types of activities used in occupational therapy intervention

KEY TERMS

Activity
Areas of occupation
Client
Contrived activities
Function
Goal
Independence

Media
Occupation
Occupation-centered activities
Occupational performance
Occupational therapist
Occupational therapy
Occupational therapy assistant

Occupational therapy
   practitioner
Patient
Preparatory activities
Purposeful activity
Therapy

As we consider occupational therapy, we will first look at the broad picture. We will provide an overview of the occupational therapy profession, beginning with answers to questions that someone new to the profession may ask. You may already know bits and pieces of the answers, in which case, compare your knowledge with new insights that may arise by looking at the overall picture.

WHAT IS OCCUPATIONAL THERAPY?

The American Occupational Therapy Association (AOTA) has developed a definition for occupational therapy intended for professional use (Box 1-1).[2] For now, let us take a simplified approach to occupational therapy. Turning to *Merriam-Webster's Collegiate Dictionary*® for an understanding of six commonly used words, we find the following[8]:

Occupation: Activity in which one engages
Therapy: Treatment of an illness or disability
Goal: End toward which effort is directed
Activity: State or condition of being involved
Independence: State or condition of being independent (self-reliant)
Function: Action for which a person is specifically fitted

These terms enable us to build a skeletal definition. **Occupational therapy** is a goal-directed activity that promotes independence in function. The AOTA provides us more specificity in the *Occupational Therapy Practice Framework: Domain and Process* with the following definitions[3]:

Areas of occupation: Various life activities including activities of daily living (ADL), instrumental activities of daily living, education, work, play, leisure, and social participation[3,6]
Occupational performance: The ability to carry out activities of daily life (including activities in the areas of occupation)[3,6]
Purposeful activity: An activity used in treatment that is goal directed and that the client sees as meaningful or purposeful[3,7]

ARE THERE DIFFERENT LEVELS OF THE OCCUPATIONAL THERAPY PRACTITIONER?

Occupational therapy practitioner refers to two different levels of clinicians: an **occupational therapist** (OT) or an **occupational therapy assistant** (OTA). The OT has more extensive education and training in both breadth and depth than the OTA,

---

Box 1-1   AOTA's Definition of Occupational Therapy for the Model Practice Act

"...the therapeutic use of everyday life activities (occupations) with individuals or groups for the purpose of participation in roles and situations in home, school, workplace, community, and other settings. Occupational therapy services are provided for the purpose of promoting health and wellness and to those who have or are at risk for developing an illness, injury, disease, disorder, condition, impairment, disability, activity limitation, or participation restriction. Occupational therapy addresses the physical, cognitive, psychosocial, and other aspects of performance in a variety of contexts to support engagement in everyday life activities that affect health, well-being, and quality of life."

From American Occupational Therapy Association: Definition of occupational therapy practice for the AOTA Model Practice Act, Bethesda, MD, 2004, American Occupational Therapy Association. (Available from the State Affairs Group, American Occupational Therapy Association, 4720 Montgomery Lane, PO Box 31220, Bethesda, MD 20824-1220.)

who works under the supervision of an OT. Often, the OT is referred to as the "professional" level, and the OTA is referred to as the "technical" level of practice. As of 2007, OTs must successfully graduate with a master's degree; OTAs must successfully complete a two-year associate's degree program. Herein, OT practitioner refers to those within the field at either level. These two roles are discussed in greater depth in Chapters 5 and 6.

WHAT DOES AN OCCUPATIONAL THERAPY PRACTITIONER DO?

OT practitioners work with clients of all ages and diagnoses. The goal of occupational therapy intervention is to increase the ability of the client to participate in everyday activities, including feeding, dressing, bathing, leisure, work, education, and social participation. The OT practitioner interacts with a client to assess existing performance, set therapeutic goals, develop a plan, and implement intervention to enable the client to function better in his or her world. OT practitioners may advocate for clients, make or modify equipment, and/or provide hands-on experiences to help people reengage in life. The OT practitioner records progress and communicates treatment specifics to others (i.e., other professionals, families, insurance agencies). However, the OT practitioner does not simply do something to or for the client; the OT practitioner guides the person to actively participate in intervention. Therefore it is important for the OT practitioner to establish rapport (a relationship of mutual trust) with the client. The therapeutic relationship has value and plays a key role in the intervention process. Section III provides a detailed description of the practice of occupational therapy.

DO OCCUPATIONAL THERAPY PRACTITIONERS HELP PEOPLE GET JOBS?

Although the term occupation commonly refers to jobs in which individuals get paid, it also encompasses the many things people do that are meaningful to them. OT practitioners help clients engage in occupations (e.g., activities that have meaning). For example, being a mother is an occupation for many clients. This occupation requires that a person complete many tasks and activities. Mothers shop for food for the family and cook meals. Cooking is an activity associated with the occupation of being a mother. Cooking for another client may be a task or an activity—a chore and not something in which he or she finds meaning. In this case, cooking may be a necessary task for him or her to fulfill, and it may be performed at a much different level than for the mother who finds meaning in cooking for her family. OT practitioners analyze clients' occupations so that they may help them return to those that are of value.

WHY REFER TO BOTH "PATIENT" AND "CLIENT"?

Occupational therapy services are provided to people in many different settings. The term used to refer to those served varies, depending on the setting. For example, in a hospital or rehabilitation setting, the term **patient** is used, but in a mental health facility or training center, professionals often use the term **client.** In some settings individuals may be referred to using terms such as resident, participant, or consumer, and in other places clients are referred to by name. For our purposes, *client* is inclusive.

ARE THERE PERSONALITY CHARACTERISTICS BEST SUITED FOR A CAREER CHOICE IN OCCUPATIONAL THERAPY?

OT practitioners have differing interests, personalities, and backgrounds. All practitioners possess a desire to help others; they genuinely like people, and they are able to relate to both individuals and small groups. OT practitioners appreciate diversity and value people's ability to change. Generally, OT practitioners are creative thinkers who enjoy hands-on work and are skilled problem-solvers. As with any member of the health care professions, those interested in occupational therapy demonstrate the ability to handle their own personal problems and feelings before trying to help others. To support improved engagement in occupation, the OT practitioner empathizes with clients yet expects and demands effort from them. It has been said that a *strong constitution* helps because the OT practitioner is exposed to many medical problems in the field, from open wounds to degenerative disorders. Because OT practitioners must educate and instruct clients and caregivers, an interest in teaching is also desirable. Flexibility is desirable because an OT practitioner needs to both teach *and* display the ability to adapt. Occupational therapy is a lifelong profession; therefore commitment and dedication are important. As in other professions, the OT practitioner is never *finished* with education but must always invest in growing with the field and continually maintaining competency.

WHO ARE THE PEOPLE SERVED AND WHAT KINDS OF PROBLEMS OR DISABILITIES ARE ADDRESSED BY OCCUPATIONAL THERAPY?

The mandate of the occupational therapy profession is to help clients engage in occupations, and the recipients of therapy include people who have problems that interfere with their ability to function. The range of problems includes genetic, neurological, orthopedic, musculoskeletal, immunological, and cardiac dysfunctions, as well as psychological, social, behavioral, or emotional disorders. OT practitioners help clients who have functional disabilities, increasing their abilities to do the everyday things they wish to do.

The recipients of occupational therapy services represent a diverse group of human beings. OT practitioners serve all ages (infants to elders) and clients with physical, cognitive, psychological, and/or psychosocial impairments, which may be the result of an accident or trauma, disease, conflict or stress, social deprivation delays, or congenital anomalies (birth defects).

For example, an OT practitioner working with children may treat a 2-pound newborn infant in a hospital neonatal unit, a preschool child in an early intervention program, or a child who has cerebral palsy and attends public school. An OT practitioner may work with an adolescent in a drug treatment center or an adolescent in a rehabilitation center who has cognitive limitations as a result of a brain injury. Clients may have experienced physical limitations from spinal cord injury after an automobile accident and need to learn to adjust to living with a disability. OT practitioners may teach a homemaker who has had a stroke, resulting in lack of use of one side of her body, how to manage her home and care for her family again. Clients who experience disability or trauma must learn to establish and embrace their new identity. OT practitioners may help with this aspect of disability. Clients with psychological diagnoses, such as schizophrenia, may need help from OT practitioners to learn skills like shopping, keeping a checkbook, and using public transportation or to regain or learn everyday tasks that many take for granted. An OT practitioner might make a splint for a client with a hand injury or work with an elderly person in a skilled nursing facility; an OT practitioner may work in a program that helps an individual learn to use assistive technology and train for a new job after an injury. The common goal of all occupational therapy intervention is to improve the person's ability to participate in daily living. (See the photographic essay at the end of this chapter.)

HOW ARE THESE SERVICES DELIVERED AND IN WHAT KINDS OF SETTINGS?

OT personnel work in hospitals, clinics, schools, clients' homes, community settings, and even prisons. Some practitioners consult or work in the workplace or in specialty settings (e.g., assistive technology centers). OT practitioners may work in inpatient settings (i.e., clients stay in the setting overnight) or outpatient settings (i.e., clients sleep at home and attend during the day). Acute care settings provide care immediately after trauma and typically involve short hospital stays. Rehabilitation settings provide longer-term care and intensive therapy from a variety of professionals. Frequently, OT practitioners consult with other team members, who may include physicians, physical therapists, speech therapists, social workers, nutritionists, case managers, nurses, educators, and family members.

OT practitioners evaluate a client's abilities and areas of weakness to develop an intervention plan, which is based on the client's interests, motivations, and goals. Intervention services may be provided in individual or group sessions, depending upon the specific needs of the clients. Typically, OT practitioners provide home programs for clients and families so that therapy goals may be addressed even when the client is not receiving direct service. Further discussion of the intervention process may be found in Section III.

WHAT KINDS OF ACTIVITIES ARE USED BY THE OCCUPATIONAL THERAPY PRACTITIONER DURING INTERVENTION?

OT practitioners use purposeful activity (e.g., activities that are meaningful to clients) to help clients regain skills and abilities or compensate for changes in abilities. Adaptations or modifications may be used to change the way a certain activity is performed so that the client can be successful. For example, clients may use a built-up–handled spoon to compensate for a weak hand grasp. The goal of therapy sessions is to help clients do the things they wish to do again. Thus OT practitioners analyze the desired occupations and determine the skills and abilities necessary for successful performance.

Intervention may begin with **preparatory activities,** which help get the client ready for the purposeful activity.[3,4] Such things as range of motion (e.g., moving the limbs through a range), exercise, strengthening, or stretching are considered preparatory activities. **Contrived activities** are made-up activities that may include some of the same skills required for the occupation.[4] These activities are used to help simulate the actual activity and may help get the client ready. For example, a client may work on tying shoes by using a doll to simulate this activity before actually tying her own shoes. Or a client may practice the components required to spread jelly before actually preparing a sandwich for lunch. Purposeful activities are generally meaningful to the client but may be one task of the occupation.[3] For example, making a sandwich is only part of making lunch. Purposeful activities have an end product and involve allowing the client to have choice. Fisher advocates that OT practitioners facilitate **occupation-centered activities.**[4] In fact, clients retain skills better and are more motivated when performing the actual occupation. Occupation-centered activities are performed in the natural setting (physical, social, and temporal). For example, preparing lunch at home at noon using one's own kitchen supplies is occupation-centered therapy.

OT practitioners develop goals for each client, based upon the client's strengths and weaknesses. The practitioner selects activities using a variety of therapeutic **media,** the means by which therapeutic effects are transmitted. Media may include games, toys, activities, dressing or self-care activities, work activities, arts, crafts, computers, industrial activities, sports, music and dance, role-playing and theater, yoga, gardening, homemaking activities, magic, clowning, pet care, and creative writing. Activities may also include the use of assistive technology, aquatics, animal-assisted therapy, ergonomics, and community integration. OT practitioners use their creativity and problem-solving skills to design therapy to meet the needs of the client.

WHAT DOES AN OCCUPATIONAL THERAPY EDUCATIONAL PROGRAM COVER?

Because of the broad scope of the profession, the knowledge base for students in occupational therapy represents several scientific areas, including biological and behavioral sciences, sociology, anthropology, and medicine.[1,5] The student gains an understanding of normal human development and pathological conditions that affect normal development and function. With these sciences as a foundation, the student learns the theory and processes related to occupational therapy. Educational programs focus on helping students develop an attitude and awareness that enable the new professional to be sensitive to the various needs of those seeking treatment. Occupational therapy education is aimed not only at developing specific skills, but it also seeks to develop the student's way of thinking. A problem-solving approach that relies on critical thinking is necessary to evaluate function, analyze activities, and design intervention that facilitates engagement in occupations.

Programs provide some specific skills training for those techniques most widely used in the profession, although students continue to learn techniques once engaged in clinical practice. All educational programs include a clinical training phase (referred to as fieldwork). The student's clinical experiences help integrate the elements of theory and practice. Upon completion of the educational and fieldwork programs, students should be prepared to practice in an entry-level position.

WHAT IS THE MAIN EMPHASIS OF OCCUPATIONAL THERAPY CURRICULA?

Both the OT (professional) and OTA (technical) educational programs are accredited by the Accreditation Council for Occupational Therapy Education (ACOTE), which is a part of the AOTA. Programs are designed to conform to a series of guidelines called *standards.* The course of study features general theory, skills training, and the foundation for clinical reasoning. Occupational therapy curricula have a strong science base and include a focus on human development across the lifespan.[1] Curricula promote professionalism and engagement in occupation through a holistic approach to practice (including the psychological, neurological, and musculoskeletal aspects of occupations). Occupational therapy education is designed *not* to give a set of unchanging answers but to teach the student problem-solving techniques and skills.

OCCUPATIONAL THERAPY INTERVENTION ACROSS THE LIFESPAN: A PHOTOGRAPHIC ESSAY

The following photographic essay illustrates the wonderful diversity of occupational therapy and is a visual answer to the question, "What types of people will I work with as an OT practitioner?"

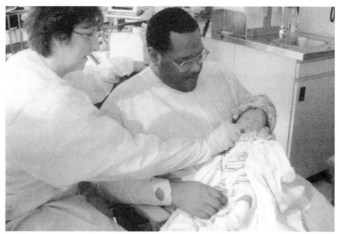

Figure 1-1 Premature and at-risk infants often have problems with feeding. An OT practitioner working in the neonatal intensive care unit (NICU) coaches a father in the application of touch pressure prior to feeding. *(From Case-Smith J:* Occupational Therapy for Children, *ed 5, St. Louis, 2005, Elsevier.)*

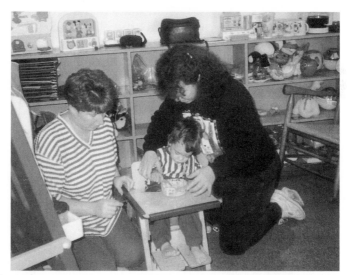

Figure 1-2 An OT practitioner provides a mother with recommendations for improving this child's skills in self-feeding. Supportive positioning equipment and adapted utensils make the task easier for the child and mother. *(From Case-Smith J:* Occupational Therapy for Children, *ed 5, St. Louis, 2005, Elsevier.)*

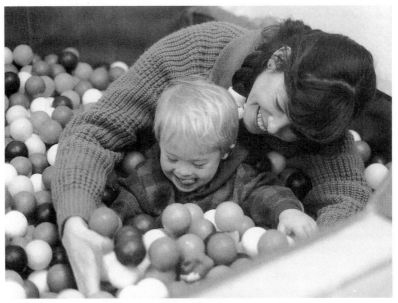

Figure 1-3 An OT practitioner uses sensory integration treatment to provide a variety of sensory experiences. Immersion in a pool of balls presents challenges to a child with a sensory disorder. *(From Case-Smith J:* Occupational Therapy for Children, *ed 5, St. Louis, 2005, Elsevier.)*

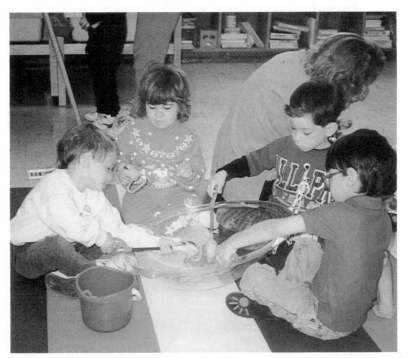

Figure 1-4 The OT practitioner may consult with teachers in the school setting to establish learning centers for sensory exploration. *(From Case-Smith J:* Occupational Therapy for Children, *ed 5, St. Louis, 2005, Elsevier.)*

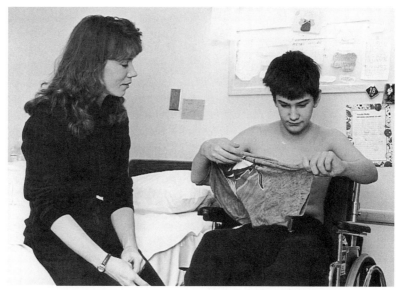

Figure 1-5 Adapted dressing routines are developed to achieve success and ease in learning. To help this adolescent boy, who has perceptual and cognitive deficits resulting from a brain injury, the OT practitioner give cues in a repetitive sequence of steps that accomplish the task. *(From Case-Smith J:* Occupational Therapy for Children, *ed 5, 2005, St. Louis, Elsevier.)*

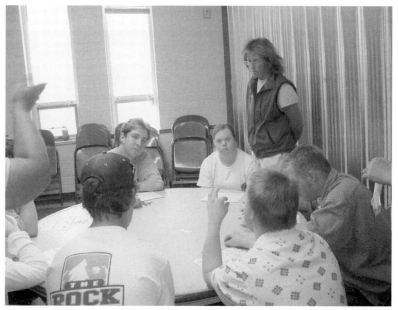

Figure 1-6 Students in a school-to-adult life transition program meet with an OT practitioner to discuss and practice skills needed in a work environment. *(From Case-Smith J:* Occupational Therapy for Children, *ed 5, St. Louis, 2005, Elsevier.)*

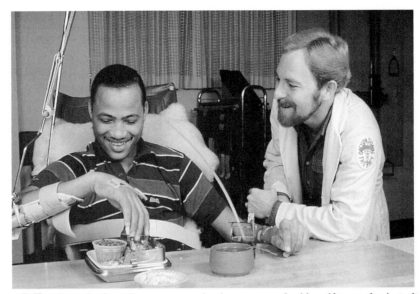

Figure 1-7 Independently performing personal tasks promotes a healthy self-image for the individual with a disability. This OT practitioner has provided a specialized device that allows this client with a spinal cord injury to feed himself. *(Photograph courtesy of AOTA).*

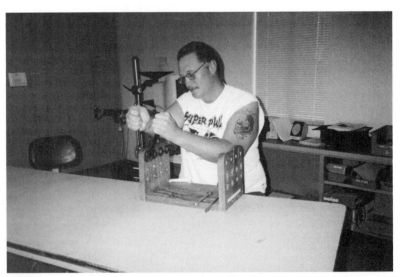

Figure 1-8 OT practitioners use evaluation tools such as the Bennett Hand Tool to evaluate the motor skills of a client. This client is being evaluated to determine if he can use hand tools and return to his job as a carpenter following an injury to his right arm. *(From Pendleton HM, Schultz-Krohn W: Pedretti's Occupational Therapy Practice Skills for Physical Dysfunction, ed 6, St. Louis, 2006, Mosby.)*

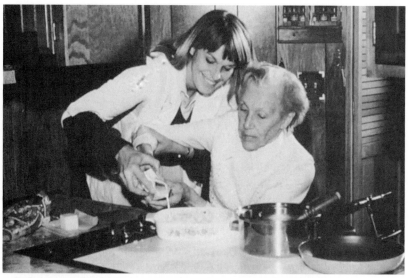

Figure 1-9 Many individuals recovering from a stroke can return to independent living with the aid of occupational therapy. Visiting a client in the home, an OT practitioner provides guidance in safe cooking techniques. *(Photograph by Bob Plunkett. Courtesy of AOTA. Submitted by Myrna Koop Harrington. Central District Home Health, Boise, ID.)*

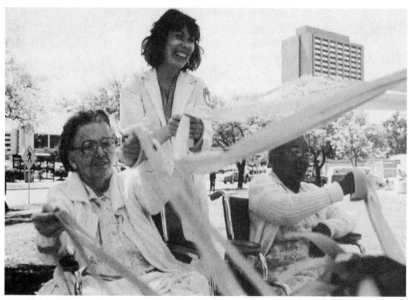

Figure 1-10 A pleasurable group activity stimulates sensory awareness and promotes socialization for these clients. Through occupational therapy, elderly individuals with health problems are more self-sufficient and often require less nursing care. They maintain a higher level of mental alertness, are able to participate more actively in social and recreational activities, and may experience less physical and mental deterioration. *(Photograph by Adam Gillum. Courtesy of AOTA. Submitted by Elise Sulton and Alice Peters. St. Luke's Episcopal Hospital, Houston, TX.)*

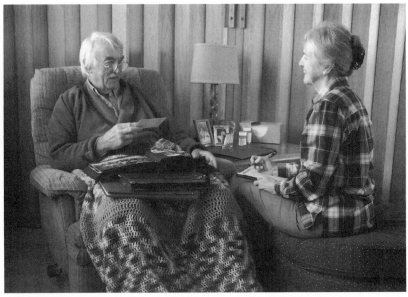

Figure 1-11 An OT practitioner facilitates life review with a client. During this process, the client is guided through open-ended questions to provide a history of his occupations from childhood to the present. *(Photograph by Patricia Smith. Photo courtesy of the American Occupational Therapy Foundation, Bethesda, MD.)*

SUMMARY

These introductory questions show that the person pursuing a career in occupational therapy must be ready to seek solutions to help clients engage in everyday living. OT practitioners work with diverse clients with varying abilities, limitations, and desires. Creative persons who have an interest in science and health care and who like working with clients of all ages and abilities will find the career of occupational therapy rewarding.

Review Questions

1. What is occupational therapy?
2. What type of education is required to become an OT or OTA?
3. What types of things do OT practitioners do?
4. In what kinds of settings do OT practitioners work?
5. What is the difference between preparatory, purposeful, contrived, or occupation-based activity?

REFERENCES

1. Accreditation Council for Occupational Therapy Education: Standards for an accredited master's-level educational program for the occupational therapist and standards for an accredited educational program for the occupational therapy assistant, Bethesda, MD, January 2006, American Occupational Therapy Association.

2. American Occupational Therapy Association: Definition of occupational therapy practice for the AOTA Model Practice Act, Bethesda, MD, 2004, American Occupational Therapy Association. (Available from the State Affairs Group, American Occupational Therapy Association, 4720 Montgomery Lane, PO Box 31220, Bethesda, MD 20824-1220.)

3. American Occupational Therapy Association: Occupational therapy practice framework: domain and process, *Am J Occup Ther* 56(6):609-639, 2002.

4. Fisher AG: Uniting practice and theory in an occupational framework, *Am J Occup Ther* 52(7): 509-521, 1998.

5. Larson E, Wood W, Clark F: Occupational science: building the science and practice of occupation through an academic discipline. In Crepeau EB, Cohn ES, Schell BAB (eds): *Willard and Spackman's Occupational Therapy,* ed 10, pp. 15-26, Philadelphia, 2003, Lippincott Williams & Wilkins.

6. Law M, Cooper B, Strong S, et al: Person-environment-occupation model: A transactive approach to occupational performance, *Canad J Occup Ther* 63:9-23, 1996.

7. Low JE: Historical and social foundations for practice. In Trombly CA, Radomski MV (eds): *Occupational Therapy for Physical Dysfunction,* ed 5, pp. 17-30, Philadelphia, 2002, Lippincott Williams & Wilkins.

8. Mish F (ed): *Merriam-Webster's Collegiate Dictionary*®, ed 10, Springfield, MA, 1994, Merriam-Webster.

Years ago, I chose to become an occupational therapist after observing other therapists at work. I was impressed by their creativity and people orientation. Back then and today, if you were to ask me what I like most about being an occupational therapist, I would list two reasons. Since my education, I have learned to appreciate our holistic roots, which are based on some of the principles of the Moral Treatment Movement. I have also recognized that our profession's meaningful beginning and most of our current literature and research come from this theme. Intrinsic to our field is the emphasis on function and the promotion of client independence. I have tried to incorporate these central themes in my practice over the years, and I could cite many examples of how I have applied them. Although the field continues to grow and change with the times, I have always recognized our roots, which continue to remain inherent to practice.

Helene Lohman, MA, OTR/L
Assistant Professor
Department of Occupational Therapy
School of Pharmacy and Allied Health Professions
Creighton University
Omaha, Nebraska

Looking Back: A History of Occupational Therapy

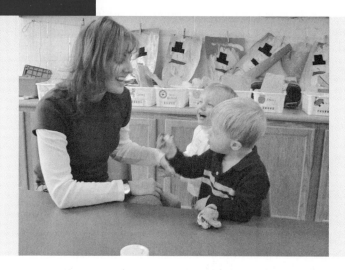

OBJECTIVES

After reading this chapter, the reader will be able to do the following:

- Identify major social influences that preceded and gave rise to the field of occupational therapy
- Name the date of the birth of the profession and the individuals who were involved in its inception
- Recognize how societal influences have helped shape the field of occupational therapy (OT)
- Describe the concepts that have persisted throughout the history of occupational therapy and how these concepts and the profession's history have an effect on the current practice of occupational therapy
- Identify and describe key pieces of federal legislation that have influenced the practice of occupational therapy

KEY TERMS

Adolf Meyer
American Occupational
  Therapy Association
  (AOTA)
Americans with Disabilities
  Act of 1990
Arts and Crafts Movement
Balanced Budget Act of 1997
  (BBA)
Benjamin Rush
Civilian Vocational
  Rehabilitation Act
Education for All Handicapped
  Children Act of 1975

Eleanor Clarke Slagle
George Edward Barton
Habit training
Handicapped Infants and
  Toddlers Act
Herbert Hall
Holistic
Individuals with Disabilities
  Education Act (IDEA)
Medicare
Moral Treatment
National Society for the
  Promotion of Occupational
  Therapy

Phillippe Pinel
Reconstruction aides
Rehabilitation Act of 1973
Rehabilitation Movement
Soldier's Rehabilitation Act
Susan Cox Johnson
Susan Tracy
Technology Related Assistance
  for Individuals with
  Disabilities Act of 1988
Thomas Kidner
William Rush Dunton, Jr.
William Tuke

To characterize the occupational therapy profession as we know it today, it is necessary to examine the past and understand how the profession originated and developed. Robert Bing, an author who has done extensive research on the history of occupational therapy, advises, "We exist in the present, yet are future oriented. To make sense of the present or future, we must have knowledge about and an appreciation of the past."[6] Toward this purpose, Chapter 2 presents an overview of the evolution of the profession of occupational therapy.

When the history of occupational therapy is traced, two threads are intertwined. The social, political, and cultural thread identifies the many currents of human events that have influenced the development of occupational therapy through time. The legislative history that has influenced the delivery of health care services in general and occupational therapy services in particular is part of this thread. The second thread represents the people of the occupational therapy profession and choices that have been made throughout its history. This chapter introduces the individuals who set in motion specific events that identified a new approach to health care—an approach called occupational therapy—and describes courses of action taken by the profession at different times.

EIGHTEENTH AND NINETEENTH CENTURIES

The late 1700s and early 1800s can be distinguished by an awakening of a social consciousness, an awareness that social structures lead to vast inequities. A new sense emerged—a measure of life's goodness should be available to all people. This awakening can be seen in many ways, as in the novels of Charles Dickens or in the founding of various welfare organizations. It was also demonstrated by the Civil War, which eliminated the practice of slavery in America, a previously accepted practice that extended back through all of human history. This social conscience is one thread in the course of human history.

This awakening brought many previously ignored and cruel practices to light, one of which was the treatment of those with mental disorders. Thought to be possessed by the devil, the "insane" were feared by society; locked away like criminals; and often chained, abused, and ignored. With a focus specifically on this group of suffering humanity, the concept of Moral Treatment was initiated.

MORAL TREATMENT

Moral Treatment was grounded in the philosophy that all people, even the most challenged, are entitled to consideration and human compassion. Whereas previously the "insane" were confined and frequently abused, the Moral Treatment Movement sought ways to make the existence of those confined more bearable. One of the ways was involvement in purposeful activity.

Two men from different parts of the world are credited with conceiving the Moral Treatment Movement: **Phillippe Pinel** and **William Tuke**.[5] Phillippe Pinel, a physician in France, introduced "work treatment" for the "insane" in the late 1700s. He used occupation to divert the patients' minds away from their emotional disturbances and toward improving their skills. He used physical exercise, work, music, and literature in his treatment. In addition, an important element was the use of farming as a part of institutional life.[5]

The Society of Friends, also known as Quakers, had a great influence in England. An English Quaker and wealthy merchant, William Tuke, became aware of the terrible conditions in an asylum in York, England, and he suggested establishing the York Retreat.[5] Tuke and

Thomas Fowler, the appointed visiting physician, believed that Moral Treatment methods were preferable to using restraint and drugs. The environment at the York Retreat was like that of a family in which the patients were approached with kindness and consideration.[5]

After the publication of Pinel's work in 1801 and Tuke's work in 1813 on the use of Moral Treatment, many hospitals in both Europe and the United States implemented reforms.[5] In the United States, a Quaker named **Benjamin Rush** was the first physician to institute Moral Treatment practices.

Participants in the Moral Treatment Movement demonstrated that establishing a structure and having the patients engage in simple work tasks promoted better health. Organizing activities for the patients brought order and purpose to unstructured confinement. For these persons, whose day-to-day functioning fell outside the bounds of socially acceptable behavior, there was an individualized routine of personal caretaking and productive involvement.

Though the term "Moral Treatment" began to fade by the mid-1800s, many of the concepts initiated by this movement continued. The practice of occupational therapy eventually emerged from this humanitarian concern for each human being and from the use of structured activity that simulated a more normal life for asylum inmates.

EARLY TWENTIETH CENTURY AND THE BEGINNING OF THE OCCUPATIONAL THERAPY PROFESSION

Looking at the social, political, and cultural thread, changes occurred in science, technology, medicine, and industry toward the end of the nineteenth century and into the beginning of the twentieth century. New modes of communication and transportation accelerated the pace of everyday life. Machines were first used in the production of goods; Henry Ford developed the moving assembly line for the production of automobiles in 1913.

In reaction to the expanding use of tools and machines, a contingency of proponents of the arts and crafts developed. Led by John Ruskin and William Morris, the **Arts and Crafts Movement** was started in England. Ruskin was an English author, poet, artist, and art critic. Morris was an English poet, designer, and socialist reformer. Proponents of the Arts and Crafts Movement in both England and America were opposed to the production of items by machine, believing this alienated people from nature and their own creativity. They sought to restore the ties between beautiful work and the worker, by returning to high standards of design and craftsmanship not to be found in mass-produced items. It was believed that using one's hands to make items connected people to their work, physically and mentally, and thus was healthier.[20] Arts and crafts societies that allowed people to experience the pleasure of making practical and beautiful items for everyday use were set up. These societies had a long-lasting effect on communities.

At the turn of the twentieth century, another issue arose from a slightly different segment of society. There was a concern for those who were taken from the mainstream of life by injury or illness and thereafter expected to sit on the sidelines. Until this time, a person with a disability either "got better" or was denied competitive involvement in life. The time came to look beyond these two alternatives; there was a need and desire for other options. An awareness that a "handicapped" person is still productive was surfacing in sanitariums and hospitals for convalescent individuals. These events would also have an effect on the profession of occupational therapy.

FOUNDERS OF THE PROFESSION

Events at this time brought together several individuals who all had a shared belief in the benefits of occupation as treatment and were influential in the founding of the profession in the United States. These individuals had backgrounds in a variety of disciplines that included psychiatry, medicine, architecture, nursing, arts and crafts, rehabilitation, teaching, and social work. Their backgrounds served to enrich the depth and breadth of the profession of occupational therapy.[20] This fledgling form of treatment was called by various names during this period of development, including *ergotherapy, activity therapy, occupation treatment, moral treatment,* and *the work cure.* The origination of the term *occupation therapy* is ascribed to William Rush Dunton. Later, George Barton recommended that the term be changed to *occupational therapy.*

Herbert Hall

At the turn of the century, chronic illness and disability, such as tuberculosis, neurasthenia, and industrial accidents, were on the rise as people became victims of the urban and industrial life. Adapting the Arts and Crafts Movement for medical purposes was a treatment concept developed by **Herbert Hall,** a physician who graduated from Harvard Medical School. He worked with invalid patients, providing medical supervision of crafts for the purpose of improving their health and financial independence.[20]

In 1904, he established a facility at Marblehead, Massachusetts, where patients with neurasthenia worked on arts and crafts as part of treatment. Neurasthenia, a disorder that was commonly seen in women, caused severe weakness during the performance of work activities. The treatment usually prescribed at the time was total rest. Hall's alternative to the "rest cure" was arts and crafts activities, beginning with participation on a limited basis from bed and gradually increasing the level of activity until the patient went to the workshop, in which she worked on weaving looms, ceramics, and other crafts.[20] He called this approach the "work cure." In 1906, he received a grant of $1000 to study the "treatment of neurasthenia by progressive and graded manual occupation." Hall was also a prolific writer.

Even though Hall was not present at the founding meeting, his work with occupation was widely recognized by the other founders. He also took on a leadership role in the early history of the Society by serving as the President of the National Society for the Promotion of Occupational Therapy from 1920 to 1923.

George Edward Barton

George Edward Barton was a dynamic and resourceful architect who studied in London under William Morris, one of the leaders of Britain's Arts and Crafts Movement. Later, he returned to Boston to incorporate the Boston Society of Arts and Crafts. After personally experiencing a number of disabling conditions—tuberculosis, foot amputation, and paralysis of the left side of his body—Barton was determined to improve the plight of convalescent individuals. In 1914, Barton opened Consolation House for convalescent patients in Clifton Springs, New York, where occupation was used as a method of treatment.

Barton studied rehabilitation courses available at the time and made contact with people dedicated to reforming the conditions in asylums, many of whom were influenced by the Moral Treatment Movement. Among those whom Barton established contact with were Dr. William R. Dunton, Jr., Eleanor Clarke Slagle, Susan Tracy, and Susan Cox Johnson.

Dr. William Rush Dunton, Jr.

William Rush Dunton, Jr., considered the father of occupational therapy, was a psychiatrist who spent his career treating psychiatric patients. In 1891, he was hired as the assistant staff physician at the Sheppard Asylum (later named the Sheppard and Enoch Pratt Hospital) in Towson, Maryland. Having studied the treatment programs of Pinel and Tuke, he was interested in implementing a similar program at the Sheppard Asylum.

In the early 1910s, the hospital introduced a regimen of crafts for its patients. While hospital staff performed necessary medical procedures and provided a structured environment, the patients were expected to actively participate in their rehabilitation by working in the workshop.[20] Dunton was known for his writings on the value of occupation for treatment. In 1915, he published *Occupational Therapy: A Manual for Nurses.*[10] It describes simple activities that the nurse can use or adapt in the treatment of patients. Dunton served as Treasurer and President of the National Society for the Promotion of Occupational Therapy and edited the association's journal for 21 years.

Eleanor Clarke Slagle

Often referred to as the mother of occupational therapy,[20] **Eleanor Clarke Slagle** began her career as a student in social work (Figure 2-1). She attended training courses in curative occupations in 1908 at the Chicago School of Civics and Philanthropy, which was affiliated with Hull House and Jane Addams. After this training, she worked at state hospitals in Michigan and New York. In 1912, she was asked by Adolf Meyer to direct a new occupational therapy

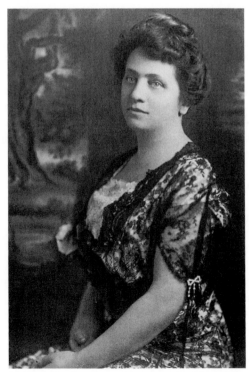

Figure 2-1 Eleanor Clarke Slagle. *(Courtesy of the Archives of the American Occupational Therapy Association, Inc., Bethesda, MD.)*

department at the Henry Phipps Psychiatric Clinic of Johns Hopkins Hospital in Baltimore, Maryland. It was at this time that Slagle developed the area of work for which she is most noted, "habit training." **Habit training** is described as a"re-education program designed to overcome disorganized habits, to modify other habits, and to construct new ones, with the goal of restoring and maintaining health."[6,7] Habit training involved all hospital personnel and took place 24 hours a day. Slagle summarized it as a "directed activity, and [it] differs from all other forms of treatment in that it is given in increasing doses as the patient improves."[14]

In 1914, Slagle returned to Chicago, where she lectured at the Chicago School of Civics and Philanthropy and started a workshop for the chronically unemployed.[20] Soon after, she organized the first professional school for OT practitioners, the Henry B. Flavill School of Occupations.

Slagle's dedication to the profession can be illustrated by the fact that her home was the Association's first unofficial headquarters. During her lifetime, she held each office within the Association and served as Executive Secretary for 14 years. In 1953, the American Occupational Therapy Association (AOTA), formerly known as the National Society for the Promotion of Occupational Therapy, established the Eleanor Clarke Slagle Lectureship Award, named in her honor. Today, the AOTA awards this prestigious honor to occupational therapists (OTs) who have made significant contributions to the profession.

Susan Tracy

Susan Tracy was a nursing instructor involved in the Arts and Crafts Movement and in the training of nurses in the use of occupations. She was hired in 1905 to work at the Adams Nervine Asylum, a small mental institution in Jamaica Plain, Massachusetts. While at this institution, she supervised the nursing school, developed the occupations program, and conducted postgraduate courses for nurses.[20] Tracy's book, *Studies in Invalid Occupations,*[25] is the first-known book written on occupational therapy. In it she describes the selection and practical use of arts and crafts activities for patients. Throughout her career, Tracy was involved in teaching many training courses. She believed only nurses were qualified to practice occupations, and she tried to make patient occupations a nursing specialty. Tracy was involved with her work and not able to attend the first meeting of the National Society for the Promotion of Occupational Therapy, but she actively served as Chair on the Committee of Teaching Methods.

Susan Cox Johnson

Susan Cox Johnson was a designer and arts and crafts teacher from Berkeley, California. She later became the Director of Occupations at the New York State Department of Public Charities. In this position, she sought to demonstrate that occupation could be morally uplifting, that it could improve the mental and physical state of patients and inmates in public hospitals and almshouses, and that these individuals could contribute to their self-support.[16] Following her work in this capacity, she joined the faculty of Teachers College in the Department of Nursing and Health, where she taught occupational therapy. She was an advocate for high educational standards and for the training of competent practitioners versus training large numbers of practitioners.

Thomas Kidner

Thomas Kidner was a friend and fellow architect-teacher of George Barton. He was influential in establishing a presence for occupational therapy in vocational rehabilitation and tuberculosis treatment. In 1915, he was appointed Vocational Secretary of the

Canadian Military Hospitals Commission. In this position, he was responsible for developing a system of vocational rehabilitation for disabled Canadian veterans from World War I. As a Canadian architect, he was recognized for constructing institutions for individuals with physical disabilities. In many of his architectural drawings for these facilities, he included workshops for occupational therapy. When the United States passed the Vocational Rehabilitation Act in 1920 (see the following section), Kidner encouraged OTs to capitalize on this opportunity. He also became very interested in tuberculosis when he realized that large numbers of men disabled in World War I were diagnosed with the disease. He helped promote the movement to hospitalize individuals with the disease and designed hospitals in both Canada and the United States for the treatment of tuberculosis patients.[20] At one point, he served as secretary of the National Tuberculosis Association.

NATIONAL SOCIETY FOR THE PROMOTION OF OCCUPATIONAL THERAPY

The formal "birth" of the profession of occupational therapy can be traced to a specific event. On March 15, 1917, a small group of people from these varied backgrounds convened the initial organizational meeting and produced the Certificate of Incorporation of the **National Society for the Promotion of Occupational Therapy,** in Clifton Springs, New York. Included in this group were George Barton, William Dunton, Eleanor Clark Slagle, Susan Cox Johnson, Thomas Kidner, and Isabel Newton, who attended in the capacity as Barton's secretary (later his wife) and was, in fact, made Secretary of the new organization. Reportedly, George Barton rejected William Rush Dunton's nomination of Hall for inclusion at the founding meeting.[16] Miss Tracy could not attend, but was made a charter member of the Association. The object of the Association as set forth in its Constitution was "to study and advance curative occupations for invalids and convalescents; to gather news of progress in occupational therapy and to use such knowledge to the common good; to encourage original research, to promote cooperation among occupational therapy societies, and with other agencies of rehabilitation."[2]

In September 1917, 26 men and women held the first annual meeting of the organization. Early in these formative years, a set of principles was developed (Box 2-1). Dunton presented the principles in 1918 at the second annual meeting of the National Society for the Promotion of Occupational Therapy.

Box 2-1   Dunton's Principles of Occupational Therapy

1. Any activity should have a cure as its objective.
2. The activity should be interesting.
3. There should be a useful purpose other than to merely gain the patient's attention and interest.
4. The activity should preferably lead to an increase in knowledge on the patient's part.
5. Activity should be carried on with others, such as a group.
6. The occupational therapist should make a careful study of the patient and attempt to meet as many needs as possible through activity.
7. Activity should cease before the onset of fatigue.
9. Genuine encouragement should be given whenever indicated.
10. Work is much to be preferred over idleness, even when the end product of the patient's labor is of poor quality or is useless.

From Dunton WR: The principles of occupational therapy. In Proceedings of the National Society for the Promotion of Occupational Therapy: Second annual meeting, Catonsville, MD, 1918, Spring Grove State Hospital Press.

PHILOSOPHICAL BASE: HOLISTIC PERSPECTIVE

There was another person whose influence helped shape the emerging profession of occupational therapy, though he was not present at the first organizational meeting. **Adolf Meyer,** a Swiss physician who immigrated to the United States in 1892 and later became professor of psychiatry at Johns Hopkins University, expressed a point of view that eventually formed the philosophical base of the profession (Figure 2-2).

Meyer was committed to a **holistic** perspective and developed the psychobiological approach to mental illness. He advocated that each individual should be seen as a complete and unified whole, not merely a series of parts or problems to be managed. He maintained that involvement in meaningful activity was a distinct human characteristic. Further, he believed that providing an individual with the opportunity to participate in purposeful activity promoted health.

In 1921 at the fifth annual meeting of the National Society for the Promotion of Occupational Therapy in Baltimore, Meyer delivered the keynote address. "The Philosophy of Occupational Therapy" was later published in the organization's first journal in 1922. In his keynote address he stated that:

> *There are many . . . rhythms which we must be attuned to: the larger rhythms of night and day, of sleep and waking hours . . . and finally the big four—work and play and rest and sleep, which our organism must be able to balance even under difficulty. The only way to attain balance in all this is*

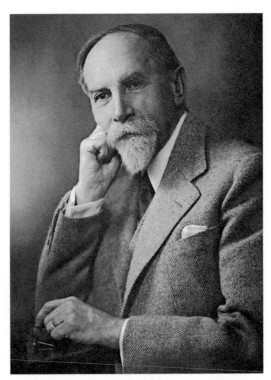

Figure 2-2 Adolf Meyer. *(Courtesy of the Archives of the American Occupational Therapy Association, Inc., Bethesda, MD.)*

actual doing, actual practice, a program of wholesome living as the basis of wholesome feeling and thinking and fancy and interests.[18]

Thus Adolf Meyer provided the initial fundamental philosophical statement of the field and the foundation on which the profession of occupational therapy was built.

Now that the individuals who influenced the founding and formation of the professional organization have been discussed, attention returns to the events that shaped both the world at large and the new profession of occupational therapy.

WORLD WAR I

Beyond the use of occupations for the "insane" and the early sheltered workshops for convalescent individuals, such as Barton's Consolation House, World War I and **reconstruction aides** made up another thread that was woven into the tapestry of the profession's formation.

In May 1917, 1 month following President Woodrow Wilson's declaration of war, the U.S. military initiated a reconstruction program. The purpose of the program was to rehabilitate soldiers who had been injured in the war so that they could either return to active military duty or be employed in a civilian job. The program was placed under the direction of orthopedic professionals and included occupational therapy aides, as well as physiotherapy aides and vocational evaluators. In early 1918 on a trial basis, the program began at Walter Reed Hospital in Washington, D.C., with a group of physiotherapy aides and occupational therapy aides who were civilian women with no military ranking.[12] The physiotherapy aides used techniques such as massage and exercise in their therapy, and they worked primarily with orthopedic patients, whereas the realm of the occupational therapy aides was to use arts and crafts to treat the mind and the body.[20] OTs worked with both orthopedic and psychiatric patients.

Several training programs were implemented, and hundreds of women were trained to be practitioners. The program was implemented overseas when the first group of reconstruction aides was sent to France to assist in the rehabilitation of soldiers. Under appalling working conditions—no rank, no uniforms, no materials or equipment, no prepared working areas—the reconstruction aides demonstrated to the Army that involvement in activities had a beneficial effect on hospitalized soldiers suffering from "shell shock."[17] The approach proved to be beneficial to the Army, and the demand for the aides' services increased throughout the war.

As the need for reconstruction aides increased, so did the need for training. Not only did existing schools and hospitals add quick training courses, but new schools were also started to meet the need. Typically, the programs consisted of instruction in arts and crafts, medical lectures, and hospital etiquette, as well as practical experience in a hospital or clinic. Although only a high school diploma was required, many of the women accepted into these programs had previous training in social work, in teaching, or in the arts.[20] Many supporters of occupational therapy viewed this as an opportunity to expand the field. Others (including Susan Cox Johnson) felt that the training programs were hastily developed in response to the war, and they were concerned about the proficiency of the newly trained practitioners.

The war ended in November 1918, and many of the women who trained to become reconstruction aides left the field. Only a small percentage of the aides were actually OTs. Others eventually became OTs, and some went back to their prior roles (e.g., artist, teacher).[17] Many of the training programs closed.

The historical significance of the reconstruction aides was the validation of the concept of activity as therapy. It was also the means by which occupational therapy became linked with physical disabilities.

POST–WORLD WAR I THROUGH THE 1930s

The attention to rehabilitation given during the war carried over once the war ended. Two pieces of federal legislation provided the impetus for the development or expansion of vocational rehabilitation programs that often included OT practitioners. The Smith-Sears Veterans Rehabilitation Act of 1918, also known as the **Soldier's Rehabilitation Act,** established a program of vocational rehabilitation for soldiers disabled on active duty. Injured soldiers were returning home, and OTs had a role in helping soldiers adjust to their "industrial responsibilities" in civilian life. The focus was on rehabilitating them and returning them to productive living.

In 1920, Congress passed the Smith-Fess Act, also known as the **Civilian Vocational Rehabilitation Act** (PL 66-236). This act provided federal funds to states on a 50-50 matching basis to provide vocational rehabilitation services to civilians with physical disabilities. To be eligible for benefits, applicants for the program had to be unable, because of their disability, to engage "successfully" in "gainful employment." Funds were provided for vocational guidance, training, occupational adjustment, prosthetics, and placement services. The passage of the Smith-Hughes and Smith-Sears Acts was in effect the beginning of the federal government's involvement in funding health care services. Occupational therapy became valued as a provider of some of these prevocational and rehabilitation services.

Another important area of growth for occupational therapy during this time was in treating and caring for patients with tuberculosis. As described earlier, Thomas Kidner was instrumental in promoting occupational therapy services for vocational rehabilitation and tuberculosis treatment. Tuberculosis sanatoriums employed OTs all across the country.

The Great Depression, from 1930 to 1939, affected all aspects of society, including the health care fields. It slowed the development of occupational therapy, bringing department closures and cuts in occupational therapy staff. Schools closed, and membership in the association decreased. Attention to rehabilitative care, which began with World War I, did not reemerge until World War II brought new and similar needs.

PROGRESS OF THE PROFESSION

In 1921, the membership voted to change the name of the National Society for the Promotion of Occupational Therapy to the **American Occupational Therapy Association (AOTA).** The profession continued to grow and evolve under this new name.

Minimum Standards Adopted for Training

Several of the emergency schools set up to provide training during the war remained open in the 1920s and attempted to recruit practitioners to the new profession. The training courses varied considerably from one another. Furthermore, the heterogeneous nature of the existing workforce (arts and crafts instructors, reconstruction aides, and some college-educated practitioners) called for the development of a workforce that was uniform so that occupational therapy could advance as a profession.[20] At the time, there were eight occupational therapy schools in the United States. The first *Minimum Standards for*

Courses of Training in Occupational Therapy was adopted in 1923 by the membership of AOTA. The standards included prerequisites for admission into training programs, length of courses, and content of courses. The standards stipulated that courses of training for OTs needed to be a minimum of 1 year, with 8 or 9 months of medical and craft training and 3 or 4 months of clinical work in hospitals. Lacking any legal ability to close schools that did not meet the standards, the association endorsed those schools that met the standards. These standards were revised twice by AOTA during the 1920s, with each revision requiring more training.

In 1929, AOTA decided to establish a national registry that identified practitioners who had graduated from schools that the association endorsed. The registry was begun on January 1, 1931. In 1935, the American Medical Association (AMA), at the request of AOTA, assumed the inspection and accreditation of occupational therapy schools. Five schools were accredited in 1938. This collaboration with the AMA continued until 1994, when it was determined that the profession of occupational therapy should be responsible for accrediting and monitoring its own educational programs.

Growth Through Publication

An emphasis upon publication greatly shaped the new profession of occupational therapy and continued to mold its emerging character. Within 5 years of the organization's founding, it began to publish a journal devoted to the profession. Credit for the emphasis on publication is given to Dr. Dunton. His articles on the use of occupation for treatment purposes first caught the attention of George Barton, before the plans of an organization had been laid, and he later played a leadership role in journal developments. Dr. Dunton directed publicity and the publications for the newly formed organization. His interest in writing had an early influence upon the nature of the organization.

As reported in Reed and Sanderson's *Concepts of Occupational Therapy,* "In 1921, he [Dunton] proposed that a journal be developed for occupational therapy because the *Maryland Psychiatric Quarterly* and *Modern Hospital* could not devote enough space to the growing profession. The *Archives of Occupational Therapy* began publication in 1922 with Dr. Dunton as editor, a position he held until 1947, when he retired. The name of the journal changed to *Occupational Therapy and Rehabilitation* in 1925 with volume 4." At the time of Dunton's retirement, Reed and Sanderson continued, ". . . the Association had elected to start a journal that would be owned by the Association. This new journal was named the *American Journal of Occupational Therapy*"[21] and began its publication in 1947. Over the years, the journal has become known informally as *AJOT* (pronounced ā-jot).

It should be noted that since 1925, membership in the national organization has automatically included the journal subscription as a membership benefit. Regular distribution of the latest information in the field has been a binding force for occupational therapy's diverse membership.

The significance of this postwar period is that occupational therapy became more closely coupled with medicine and the medical model of education. This led to the beginning of specialization and of a more scientific approach. It also set the stage for attempts by physical medicine to control the developing profession of occupational therapy, which was to be an ongoing dilemma for the next few decades. On one hand, the support occupational therapy had received from physicians was instrumental in the growth of the profession. On the other hand, the profession's unique philosophy based on occupation and a holistic perspective was threatened by the reductionistic views of medicine at the time.

WORLD WAR II: 1940-1947

World War II created a new demand for more OTs. Because they had not achieved military status during World War I, few OTs were employed in the Army or in Army hospitals when World War II broke out.[13] Initially, the War Department required OTs to be graduates of an accredited school. However, the educational requirements took 18 months to complete, and this was too long of a wait for the Army to get trained OTs.[13] Once again, War Emergency Courses were implemented to quickly train needed OTs. As a result, the number of employed practitioners increased significantly. AOTA data indicates that in 1945 there were 2177 members.

Beginning in 1945, successful completion of an examination became a requirement for registering as an OT practitioner. The examination was initially an essay format; in 1947, it adopted the format of an objective test.

POST–WORLD WAR II: 1950s-1960s

After the war, the pace of change accelerated, and the changes that were brought to the profession were vast and rapid. There was a continued shift away from a generalist approach to one of specialization in physical rehabilitation.

NEW DRUGS AND TECHNOLOGY

The discovery of the neuroleptic drugs (tranquilizers and antipsychotics) in the mid-1950s completely changed the course of psychiatric treatment. As psychotic behavior yielded to chemical control, it became possible to discharge many people, eventually leading to a national plan to release clients—the national "Deinstitutionalization Plan." In anticipation of local care needs, community mental health programs were developed.

New technologies were developed, such as splinting materials, wheelchairs, and more advanced prosthetics and orthotics. Special training was required for OT practitioners who would be using this new therapeutic material and equipment.

REHABILITATION MOVEMENT

The time from 1942 to 1960 is often called the period of the **Rehabilitation Movement.**[19] The Veterans Administration (VA) hospitals increased in size and number to handle the casualties of war and continued care of veterans. The VA hospitals, which had employed OTs in psychiatric and tuberculosis units since its beginnings in 1921, developed physical medicine and rehabilitation departments to serve veterans with physical disabilities. OTs were employed in these departments. After the war, in 1947, the U.S. Army established the Women's Medical Specialist Corps. Women in the fields of occupational therapy, physical therapy, and dietetics, who had been classified as civilian employees during the war, were commissioned as officers of the Army. The Corps later became the Army Medical Specialist Corps to allow men and women to serve as commissioned officers in the military. The Korean War that began in 1950 called for the continuation of Army hospitals with active occupational therapy departments.

Growth in health care was not limited to the Veterans Administration. Due to the polio epidemic and new medical procedures and antibiotics that were saving lives, more individuals were living with disabilities. It was recognized that there needed to be facilities and services to meet the needs of individuals with disabilities. The Hill-Burton Act assisted states in determining what hospitals and health care facilities were needed and provided grants to states to construct these facilities. OTs were hired as one type of rehabilitation professional. They were teaching patients in activities of daily living, designing orthotic devices, training patients how to use prosthetics, using progressive resistive exercise, introducing muscle re-education techniques, and evaluating patient's vocational aptitudes and abilities.[19]

FEDERALLY MANDATED HEALTH CARE

Medicare (PL 89-97) was enacted in 1965, and it amplified the demand for occupational therapy services even further. Under Medicare guidelines, those who are 65 years of age or older or those who are permanently and totally disabled receive assistance in paying for their health care. It covers occupational therapy services in the inpatient setting and limited coverage for outpatient services. Initially, this legislation did not provide for services given by OT practitioners in independent, private practice. In 1988, legislation granted OTs the right to Medicare provider numbers, permitting direct reimbursement for occupational therapy services.

CHANGES IN THE PROFESSION

One of the strengths of the field of occupational therapy is its well-run national organization. Throughout its history, AOTA has continued to evolve. The 1950s and 1960s brought organizational changes to AOTA in order to improve both the overall function of and the membership representation in the ever-growing and expanding organization. The American Occupational Therapy Foundation (AOTF) was founded in 1965 to promote research in occupational therapy through financial support. AOTA and AOTF are discussed further in Chapter 8.

As described earlier, there was a shift in practice to physical rehabilitation and working with individuals with severe disabilities. As therapists expanded their knowledge and skills to work with these populations, services that were once based on occupation and arts and crafts changed to a more technical focus, using modalities particular to the area of specialization. There was decreased emphasis in the schools on teaching of arts and crafts. A few leaders of the profession began to speak out against specialization and to encourage the profession to return to its roots of occupation. However, the trend toward the reductionistic model and specialization would continue through the 1960s.

New Level of Practitioner: The Occupational Therapy Assistant

With an increasing number of OTs practicing in medical and rehabilitation facilities, there was a shortage of therapists working in psychiatric settings. Aides and technicians working under OT practitioners in psychiatric settings became knowledgeable in the intervention techniques used. As Shirley Holland Carr reports, "Supportive personnel knew how to do things, but lacked goal-oriented intervention methods necessary to work without immediate supervision."[8] This factor motivated a drive toward organizing courses for occupational therapy assistants. In the late 1950s, a new category of practitioner was initiated—the occupational therapy assistant (OTA). The introduction of this new level of practitioner required many years of experimentation and study by AOTA to determine the appropriate interface and regulation. The first 3-month educational program in psychiatry began in 1958, and a second course for general practice was offered in 1960. Initially, these training programs were based in hospitals. Later, the programs were offered in technical schools and community colleges. The first directory of OTAs was published in 1961 and listed 553 names.[4] Although the introduction of this new level of practitioner was a major milestone for the profession, there was a lack of agreement as to the appropriate roles of the OT and the OTA.

1970s THROUGH 1980s

The social thread during this period included the introduction of personal computers, a substantial increase in drug and alcohol abuse, and the appearance of a new disease with no known cure, acquired immune deficiency syndrome (AIDS). The Deinstitutionalization Plan had gained acceptance and was implemented across the U.S. Individuals who resided in mental hospitals and facilities for the developmentally delayed were transferred from these institutions to smaller community facilities. Many of the large state institutions closed. Some services were developed in communities to support these individuals, but overall there was a lack of services to support these individuals. As a result, many individuals with chronic mental illness and mental retardation ended up homeless. Society is still dealing with this issue today.

Several very important pieces of legislation for persons with disabilities were passed by the United States Congress in the 1970s and 1980s: the Rehabilitation Act of 1973, the Education for All Handicapped Children Act of 1975, the Handicapped Infants and Toddlers Act of 1986, and the Technology Related Assistance for Individuals with Disabilities Act of 1988.

The **Rehabilitation Act of 1973** came during a time of great social change and unrest. Persons with disabilities, inspired by the civil rights movement of the 1960s, became a new force and exerted significant influence on rehabilitation legislation. The Rehabilitation Act of 1973 established several important principles. First, the Act emphasized priority service for persons with the most severe disabilities and mandated that state agencies establish an order of selection that would place the most severely disabled person first for service. Second, under the Act every client accepted for services was to participate with the counselor in the service planning process by completing an Individualized Written Rehabilitation Program (IWRP) that specified the vocational goal and key supporting objectives, such as physical restoration, counseling, educational preparation, work adjustment, and vocational training. Third, the Act called for the development of a set of standards by which the impact of rehabilitation services could be assessed. Fourth, the Rehabilitation Act of 1973 emphasized the need for rehabilitation research. Finally, it included civil rights provisions that gave equal opportunity for people with disabilities. It prohibited discrimination in employment or in admissions criteria to academic programs solely on the basis of a disabling condition.

Pediatrics emerged during this time as another specialty area, aided in part by the passage of the **Education for All Handicapped Children Act of 1975** (PL 94-142). This act establishes the right of all children to a free and appropriate education, regardless of handicapping condition. This law includes occupational therapy as a related service. Before the passage of PL 94-142, many children with disabilities were not in school programs, let alone receiving therapy services. Under the requirements of this law, an individual education plan (IEP) must be written for each student. The IEP describes the student's specialized program and identifies measurable goals. The **Handicapped Infants and Toddlers Act** (PL 99-457) was passed in 1986 as an amendment to the Education for All Handicapped Children Act. The amendment extends the provision of PL 94-142 to include children from 3 to 5 years of age and initiates new early intervention programs for children from birth to 3 years of age.

A primary service included in the amendment is occupational therapy. The result of these two laws has been an increase in occupational therapy services provided to children and an increase in the number of OT personnel employed within the school environment.

The **Technology Related Assistance for Individuals with Disabilities Act of 1988** (PL 100-407) addresses the availability of assistive technology devices and services to individuals with disabilities. Many OT practitioners are involved in providing these services.

These pieces of legislation helped to spur a demand for occupational therapy services. However, the 1970s also saw the beginning of concern for the high cost of health care, and the mid 1980s brought about a great deal of change in the health care system in an attempt to contain health care costs.

PROSPECTIVE PAYMENT SYSTEM

In 1983, President Reagan made a fundamental change to the way in which health care dollars were dispersed by signing the Social Security Amendments into law. Up until this point, hospitals were reimbursed based on the actual cost of services provided. With the implementation of the Medicare Prospective Payment System (PPS) created by these amendments, a nationwide schedule was established that delineated what the government would pay for each inpatient stay of a Medicare beneficiary. The level of payment is set by descriptive categories according to the individual's diagnosis, called diagnosis-related groupings, or DRGs. In this system of fixed payment for DRGs, massive changes in hospital organization and care delivery occurred. Most notably, patient length of stay in acute care hospitals was shortened, and there was an increased use of long-term care facilities and home health services.

ADVANCES AT AOTA

AOTA expended great efforts to ensure that occupational therapy would be appropriately included in the onslaught of new federal governmental legislation directed at the delivery of health care. Lobbying for the interests of occupational therapy became a function of AOTA during the 1970s and 1980s and remains an important aspect of the association's role.

In the 1980s, AOTA moved into its own building, thus signifying a new era that began to yield results of AOTA's long-standing emphasis on research. This decade witnessed a wealth of new books and publications, including a new research journal, the *Occupational Therapy Journal of Research*. There was also growth in the number of educational programs that offered a graduate degree.

In 1986, AOTA separated professional membership and certification procedures by declaring the association no longer responsible for board certification. Instead, on completion of all requirements, an OT practitioner is certified through the National Board for Certification in Occupational Therapy (NBCOT®), subject to certification regulations; AOTA membership is separate and voluntary.

STATE REGULATION OF OCCUPATIONAL THERAPY

State regulatory legislation became a controversial issue of the 1970s. Individual states began to introduce laws requiring that OT practitioners become licensed in order to practice. AOTA's Representative Assembly initially opposed this action, then took a neutral position, and finally in 1975 supported state licensing to ensure quality occupational therapy services. Since these laws are individually determined by each state, licensure of occupational therapy practice has taken place gradually. (Regulation and licensure are discussed in detail in Chapter 7.)

A RETURN TO THE ROOTS OF THE PROFESSION: OCCUPATION

By the 1970s, there was a large contingent of OTs urging the profession to return to its roots in occupation. OTs such as Mary Reilly, Elizabeth Yerxa, Phil Shannon, and Gail Fidler called upon therapists to reject the practices of reductionism and return to the principles of moral treatment and occupation. Shannon described the "derailment of occupational therapy."[24] He observed that there were two philosophies in conflict with each other. One, based on the philosophy of moral treatment, held a holistic and humanistic view of the individual. The other saw the individual as a "mechanistic creature susceptible to manipulation and control via the application of techniques."[24] He further noted that "If OT persists in this direction, what was once and still is one of the great ideas of 20th century medicine will be swept away by the tide of technique philosophy."[24] Fidler described the replacement of occupation with modalities that eliminated the "self as the doer-agent and place[d] the causative agent outside the self."[11]

There was growing realization that something needed to be done. Occupational therapy was lacking a science unique to occupation, theories of practice, and research that demonstrated the effectiveness of occupational therapy. It was during this time that different theories and models for occupational therapy started to emerge. One such model is the Model of Human Occupation that was developed by Kielhofner and his associates.[15] Occupational science, a basic science that supports occupational practice, also emerged.[27]

1990s TO THE PRESENT

As a society in the 1990s to the present day, we are clearly out of the Industrial Age and are in the midst of the Information Age. The Information Age is characterized by information technologies, including cell phones, faxes, personal computer applications, and the networking of computers. Information technology has provided us with immediate access to news and world events, and with the ability to retrieve all kinds of information without leaving the chair. In occupational therapy, computer technology is used to assist in different types of treatment modalities, such as computer software that is used to retrain cognitive skills; moreover, billing and documentation of services are typically done on a computer. The overall effects of the Information Age on society in general, and health care in particular, are yet to be seen.

There are many other societal, cultural, and political threads evident during this period. Two-income families are the norm. The number of individuals living with disabilities is increasing, as is the number of individuals over 65 years of age. The population in the U.S. is becoming ever more culturally diverse, and many individuals and families cannot afford the cost of health care.

One of the most significant pieces of legislation to pass during the 1990s was the **Americans with Disabilities Act of 1990** (ADA) (PL 101-336). The ADA provides civil rights to all individuals with disabilities. It guarantees equal access to and opportunity in employment, transportation, public accommodations, state and local government, and telecommunications for individuals with disabilities. OT personnel provide consultation to private and public agencies to assist them in meeting these guidelines.

The Education for All Handicapped Children Act, Public Law 94-142, (1975) was reauthorized and renamed the **Individuals with Disabilities Education Act (IDEA)** in 1991. IDEA requires school districts to educate students with disabilities in the least restrictive environment (LRE). Specifically, the IDEA requires states to establish procedures assuring that students with disabilities are educated, to the maximum extent appropriate, with students without disabilities. IDEA also mandates that the local school district is responsible for providing assistive technology devices and related services as deemed appropriate to the child's education. In 1997, the president signed Individuals with Disabilities Education Act Amendments of 1997, Public Law 105-17. The Individuals with Disabilities Education Act Amendments of 1997 (IDEA 97) further improves the educational opportunities for children with disabilities. The focus of IDEA 97 is on improving educational results for children with disabilities. The law stipulates that the assistive technology needs of children with disabilities must be considered along with other special factors by the Individualized Education Plan (IEP) team in formulating the child's IEP. IDEA 97 also strengthens the role of parents in educational planning and decision-making on behalf of their children. IDEA defines occupational therapy as a related service that can be provided to a student to enable him or her to participate in and benefit from the educational process.

In the medical arena, occupational therapy services are restricted by what insurance companies will cover, and managed care continues in efforts to contain spiraling health care costs. OTs and OTAs have had to continuously adapt to the regulations and reimbursement limitations affecting the health care environment. Furthermore, health care practitioners struggle on a daily basis with ethical questions related to the allocation of health care services.

The **Balanced Budget Act of 1997 (BBA)** has been a roller coaster ride for the profession, sending the profession and the job market into a tailspin. The intent of the BBA was to reduce Medicare spending, create incentives for the development of managed care plans, encourage enrollment in managed care plans, and limit fee-for-service payment and programs. Though it is not currently implemented, under the Medicare Part B Outpatient Rehabilitation Benefit there is an annual $1,500 cap per person receiving occupational therapy services, and a separate $1,500 cap per person for physical therapy and speech-language pathology services combined. The Balanced Budget Refinement Act of 1999 (BBRA) (PL 106-113) placed a 2-year moratorium on application of the $1,500 caps (for years 2000 and 2001). The Benefits Improvement and Protection Act of 2000 (BIPA) (PL 106-554) extended, by 1 additional year, the 2-year moratorium on the application of the $1,500 caps for outpatient rehabilitation services. This affirmed that the moratorium was in place for dates of service through December 31, 2002. The cap was implemented on September 1, 2003, just prior to another 2-year moratorium that was included in the Medicare Modernization Act of 2003 (PL 108-173). Many beneficiaries reached the cap by the time Congress was trying to pass the Medicare Modernization Act of 2003 in November. Currently, AOTA is working to extend the moratorium.

The uncertainty around the BBA has forced practitioners to broaden their horizons and look beyond traditional areas of practice. More therapists are working in community-based programs, and the job market is on the upswing. The Bureau of Labor Statistics (BLS) predicts that employment for OTs is projected to increase faster than the average for all occupations (21% to 35%). Employment of OTAs is expected to grow much faster than average (increase 36% or more) through 2012. The BLS expects the demand of OT practitioners to rise due to growth in the number of individuals with disabilities or limited function, the baby-boom generation's movement into middle age (when incidence of heart attacks and stroke increases), and growth in the population 75 years of age and older. All of these populations will require therapy services.[26] To help meet the challenges associated with the costs of providing services to an aging population, the Centers for

Disease Control has encouraged community organizations and public health agencies to include health promotion among older adults, prevention of disability, maintenance of capacity, and enhancement of quality of life in their scope.[9] These are all areas in which occupational therapy can have a role.

OCCUPATIONAL THERAPY ENTRY-LEVEL EDUCATION, CONTINUING COMPETENCE, AND RECERTIFICATION

Ongoing issues for the profession include the need to develop scientists in the profession to conduct research, the need for gathering and disseminating occupational therapy research, the application of evidence-based knowledge in practice, and continuing competency of practitioners.

After many years of debate and discussion, the association passed a resolution in 1999 that called for a transition to a post-baccalaureate entry-level requirement for professional occupational therapy practice. This new entry-level requirement will result in the training of OTs who have the knowledge and skills to be competent in today's practice environment and to carry out research. Baccalaureate programs in occupational therapy will be phased out by 2007, and students will be required to have a graduate degree to be eligible to take the certification exam. As of August 2006, the Accreditation Council for Occupational Therapy Education listed 148 accredited occupational therapy programs and 129 accredited OTA programs.

State licensure laws typically require some evidence that the practitioner is keeping current in the field. The Commission on Continuing Competence and Professional Development (CCCPD) was put in place by AOTA in May 2002 to recommend standards for continuing competence and to develop strategies for communicating information to OT practitioners and consumers about issues of continuing competency affecting occupational therapy. NBCOT® also recently implemented recertification, which requires the completion of professional development units to maintain certification as an OT or OTA.

OCCUPATION-BASED PRACTICE

It is an exhilarating time to be practicing in occupational therapy. The richness and complexity of occupation and evidence of its impact on clients is being documented through research. Academic leaders in the profession have been focused on creating a science of occupation, developing theories to guide practice, identifying best practices in treatment by examining evidence-based practice, and generating research that demonstrates the effectiveness of occupational therapy.[23]

In May 2002, the AOTA adopted a revised framework of practice for the profession. The new practice framework, *Occupational Therapy Practice Framework: Domain and Process,*[3] delineates language and concepts that describes the focus of the profession. The document is meant to be used by OT practitioners to examine current practice and to consider emerging practice areas. It was also written to assist external audiences, such as third-party payers, in understanding occupational therapy's unique focus on supporting function and health and the process by which that is achieved. The new practice framework reflects a return to our roots because it is centered on the use of occupation to support participation in life.

As history demonstrates, occupational therapy is a dynamic and ever-evolving profession. Many of the issues that have been identified in this final period will continue to evolve. The profession and practice of occupational therapy will remain responsive to societal, cultural, and political needs.

UNIQUE IDENTITY

Occupational therapy has sought its own separate identity as a health care service, and change has been continual. There are, however, consistent elements throughout its history that confirm the unique identity of occupational therapy. From its beginning, occupational therapy has been based on a holistic point of view. The profession believes that the individual needs to engage in occupations, and that intervention must be based on the use of purposeful activities and on a commitment to support and encourage the independence of the individual. The total function of the person is the focus of treatment, and the interpersonal relationship between the client and OT practitioner is vital to the process. William Rowley, a physician, futurist, and keynote speaker at the 2005 AOTA Annual Conference, cited occupational therapy's holistic approach as unique among health care professions and crucial to addressing the major public health issues of the 21st century.[1]

In the fiftieth anniversary commemorative issue of the *American Journal of Occupational Therapy*, Margaret Rerek states, "Most striking in a historical review of occupational therapy is the dramatic consistency of its basic assumption that man has a need to self-actualize through his work and/or leisure. While techniques have altered considerably over the years, there is an equal consistency in the goals of correcting or ameliorating whatever dysfunction prevents self-actualization . . . occupational therapy has been focused since its birth on health and function."[22]

SUMMARY

By studying the history of occupational therapy, we can gain knowledge that will enhance our current practice. The new profession of occupational therapy officially came into being as the result of a meeting of incorporation in March 1917. It grew out of the rising social consciousness of the early twentieth century, wherein consideration was given to Moral Treatment in psychiatric facilities, rehabilitation in sanitariums, and restoration for soldiers injured in battle; and attention was given to the use of occupation as a course of treatment. The outer or external changes of society have often meant changes in the profession. With the ebb and flow of society's changes, the profession has continued to adapt and meet the demands of the external environment. Occupational therapy has evolved through merging theory and research while focusing on health and function. As a field of practice, occupational therapy's history of a holistic approach and use of occupation makes it unique from other health care services.

Learning Activities

1. Refer to Box 2-1 and Dunton's Principles of Occupational Therapy. How could you update these principles to reflect current occupational therapy practice?
2. Research and write a short paper on the Moral Treatment Movement of the 1800s.
3. Compile short biographies on the founders of occupational therapy by reading three or four sources.
4. Search back volumes of the *American Journal of Occupational Therapy* (and the older *Archives of Occupational Therapy* and *Occupational Therapy & Rehabilitation*, if available). Use lists of article titles to show the changes in emphasis from decade to decade.

5. Research and write a short paper on any single social influence, legislation, or technical development. Elaborate on how the event affected the practice and profession of occupational therapy.

6. Research and make a wall chart with a time line that depicts significant events and changes in AOTA since its inception.

Review Questions

1. What major social influences gave rise to the field of occupational therapy?
2. Who are some of the key people involved in the evolution of the occupational therapy profession?
3. What key concepts have persisted throughout the history of occupational therapy?
4. How has the profession changed over time?
5. What are some key pieces of federal legislation that have influenced the practice of occupational therapy?

REFERENCES

1. American Occupational Therapy Association: 2005 Conference Highlights, June 6, 2005. Retrieved July 29, 2005, from http://www.aota.org/nonmembers/area29/index.asp.
2. American Occupational Therapy Association: History of AOTA accreditation. Retrieved July 25, 2005, from http://www.aota.org/nonmembers/area13/links/link15.asp.
3. American Occupational Therapy Association: Occupational therapy practice framework: domain and process, *Am J Occup Ther* 56(6):609-639, 2002.
4. American Occupational Therapy Association: *Directory Certified Occupational Therapy Assistants for the Year 1961,* New York, 1961, American Occupational Therapy Association.
5. Bing R: Looking back, living forward: Occupational therapy history. In Sladyk K, Ryan SE (eds): *Ryan's Occupational Therapy Assistant: Principles, Practice Issues and Techniques,* ed 4, Thorofare, NJ, 2005, Slack.
6. Bing R: Living forward, understanding backward. In Ryan S (ed): *The Certified Occupational Therapy Assistant: Principles, Concepts, and Techniques,* ed 2, Thorofare, NJ, 1993, Slack.
7. Bing R: Occupational therapy revisited: A paraphrasatic journey, *Am J Occup Ther* 35(8):499, 1981.
8. Carr SH: The COTA heritage: proud, practical, stable, dynamic. In Sladyk K, Ryan SE (eds): *Ryan's Occupational Therapy Assistant: Principles, Practice Issues and Techniques,* ed 4, Thorofare, NJ, 2005, Slack.
9. Centers for Disease Control and Prevention: Public health and aging: trends in aging—United States and worldwide, *Morbidity and Mortality Weekly Report,* February 14, 52(6):101-106, 2003. Retrieved July 29, 2005, from http://www.cdc.gov/mmwr/preview/mmwrhtml/mm5206a2.htm.
10. Dunton WR: *Occupational Therapy: A Manual for Nurses,* Philadelphia, 1915, Saunders.
11. Fidler GS: From crafts to competence, *Am J Occup Ther* 35:567, 1981.
12. Gutman SA: Looking back—influence of the US military and occupational therapy reconstruction aides in World War I on the development of occupational therapy, *Am J Occup Ther* 49:256, 1995.
13. The Historical Unit, U.S. Army Medical Department: Medical Department, United States Army Medical Training in World War II, Washington, D.C., Office of the Surgeon General, Department of the Army, 1974. Retrieved July 24, 2005, from http://history.amedd.army.mil/booksdocs/wwii/medtrain/default.htm.
14. Kidner TJ: Occupational therapy: Its development, scope, and possibilities, *Occup Ther Rehabil* 10:3, 1931.
15. Kielhofner G (ed): *A Model of Human Occupation,* Baltimore, MD, 1985, Williams & Wilkins.
16. Licht S: The founding and founders of the American Occupational Therapy Association, *Am J Occup Ther* 21:269, 1967.
17. Low JF: The reconstruction aides, *Am J Occup Ther* 46:38, 1992.

18. Meyer A: The philosophy of occupation therapy, *Arch Occup Ther* 1:1, 1922. (Reprinted in *Am J Occup Ther* 31:10, 1977.)
19. Punwar AJ, Peloquin SM: *Occupational Therapy Principles and Practice,* ed 3, Baltimore, 2000, Lippincott Williams & Wilkins.
20. Quiroga V: *Occupational Therapy: The First 30 Years 1900 to 1930,* Bethesda, MD, 1995, American Occupational Therapy Association.
21. Reed KL, Sanderson SR: *Concepts of Occupational Therapy,* ed 4, Philadelphia, 1999, Lippincott Williams & Wilkins.
22. Rerek MD: The depression years 1929-1941: Occupational therapy—a historical perspective, *Am J Occup Ther* 25(5):15, 1971.
23. Schwartz KB: History of occupation. In Kramer P, Hinojosa J, Royeen CB (eds): *Perspectives in Human Occupation: Participation in Life,* Baltimore, 2003, Lippincott Williams & Wilkins.
24. Shannon PD: The derailment of OT, *Am J Occup Ther* 31(229), 1977.
25. Tracy SE: *Studies in Invalid Occupation,* Boston, 1910, Whitcomb & Barrows.
26. U.S. Department of Labor, Bureau of Labor Statistics: Occupational outlook handbook, February 2004. Retrieved July 29, 2005, from http://bls.gov/oco/ocos078.htm.
27. Yerxa E: An introduction to occupational science: A foundation for OT in the 21st century, *OT Health Care* 6(4):3, 1989.

The most memorable aspects of my career in occupational therapy education were the wonderful students I had the privilege of knowing, and the opportunity I had to share with them my beliefs and philosophy about the health-giving value of occupation. My students taught me so much about life, teaching, and learning. It was a richly rewarding experience to facilitate and witness the evolution of the occupational therapy student to the professional occupational therapist.

Lorraine Williams Pedretti, MS, OTR/Ret.
Professor Emeritus
Department of Occupational Therapy
San José State University
San José, California

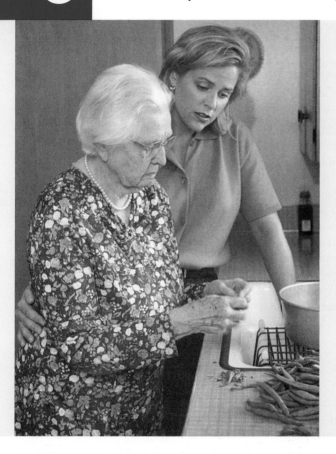

OBJECTIVES

After reading this chapter, the reader will be able to do the following:

- Understand the importance of a profession's philosophical base
- Describe the general components of a philosophy and, more specifically, describe the philosophy of occupational therapy (OT)
- Articulate occupational therapy's view of humankind
- Explain the meaning of *occupation* in the context of the profession and understand its role in occupational performance and well-being
- Explain occupational therapy's view on how humankind knows what it knows
- Name the values of the profession
- Describe adaptation as used in occupational therapy
- Distinguish between occupation as a means and occupation as an end
- Describe the client-centered approach and its relevance to occupational therapy

KEY TERMS

Active being	Freedom	Occupational performance
Activity	Holistic approach	Organismic
Adaptation	Humanism	Mechanistic
Altruism	Justice	Phenomenological
Axiology component	Mechanistic	Professional philosophy
Client-centered approach	Metaphysical component	Prudence
Dignity	Occupation	Quality of life
Epistemology component	Occupation as a means	Role
Equality	Occupation as an end	Task
		Truthfulness

It is essential for the occupational therapist (OT) or occupational therapy assistant (OTA) student to understand and appreciate the philosophical base on which occupational therapy is built. Familiarity with and understanding of the philosophical base of one's profession are important for several reasons. A **professional philosophy** is a set of values, beliefs, truths, and principles that guide the practitioner's actions. It helps define the nature of the existenceof the profession, guides the actions of the practitioners of the profession, and helps practitioners substantiate the reason for existence. Theories, models, frames of reference, and intervention approaches that guide our practice are derived from the profession's philosophy.

Workable philosophies are not imposed from the outside; rather, they unfold through history from within the profession. The roots of occupational therapy can be traced to the moral treatment era. Central themes within the early practice of occupational therapy were identified in Chapter 2. In this chapter, the components of philosophy, in general, are examined first; then the philosophy of occupational therapy along with the central themes of the profession are discussed.

UNDERSTANDING PHILOSOPHY

It is helpful to understand what contributes to philosophy before applying it to a specific profession. In studying philosophy in general and the philosophical basis of a profession in particular, it is necessary to address questions related to three components.[18] The first is the **metaphysical component,** and it concerns questions such as "What is the nature of humankind?" The second is the **epistemology component,** and it is related to the development of a professional philosophy. The epistemology component investigates critically "the nature, origin, and limits of human knowledge."[18] Questions such as "How do we know things?" and "How do we know that we know?" are addressed in the epistemology component. The third is the **axiology component,** and it is concerned with the study of values. There are two types of questions represented in this component—questions of aesthetics (e.g., "What is beautiful or desirable?") and questions of ethics (e.g., "What are the standards and rules of right conduct?").[18] Using these questions as guidelines, the philosophical base of the occupational therapy profession can be examined.

PHILOSOPHICAL BASE OF OCCUPATIONAL THERAPY

The philosophical base of occupational therapy was adopted in 1979 and reaffirmed in 2004 (Box 3-1). Examining occupational therapy in terms of the metaphysical, epistemology and axiology components provides a framework to understand the philosophical base of

---

Box 3-1   The Philosophical Base of Occupational Therapy

Man is an active being whose development is influenced by the use of purposeful activity. Using their capacity for intrinsic motivation, human beings are able to influence their physical and mental health and their social and physical environment through purposeful activity. Human life includes a process of continuous adaptation. Adaptation is a change in function that promotes survival and self-actualization. Biological, psychological, and environmental factors may interrupt the adaptation process at any time throughout the life cycle. Dysfunction may occur when adaptation is impaired. Purposeful activity facilitates the adaptive process.

Occupational therapy is based on the belief that purposeful activity (occupation), including its interpersonal and environmental components, may be used to prevent and mediate dysfunction and to elicit maximum adaptation. Activity as used by the therapist includes both an intrinsic and a therapeutic purpose.

From American Occupational Therapy Association: The philosophical base of occupational therapy, *Am J Occup Ther* 33:785, 1979. (Reprinted in *Am J Occup Ther* 49:1026, 1995). Reviewed by COE and COP in 2004.

---

occupational therapy. Embedded within the philosophical base of the profession are some key concepts that are explored in this chapter (Figure 3-1).

WHAT IS HUMANKIND?

The metaphysical component of philosophy examines the question "What is humankind?" This philosophical question becomes the basis for a profession designed to enhance a person's ability to engage in life.

Occupational Therapy Views Humans Holistically

Historically, much of the health care system in the Western world has been developed from a reductionistic approach, wherein humankind is reduced to separately functioning body parts. Specialties have been designed to treat these body functions independently for greater expediency and efficiency; their purpose is to isolate, define, and treat body functions and to focus on a specific problem. This reductionistic approach has proved valuable in producing many cures and amazing technological developments. In more recent years, however, the trend in medicine has been to move away from the specialist and return to the family practitioner, who addresses all the bodily functions of the client.

In contrast, since its beginning, occupational therapy has viewed humans holistically and has adhered to a **holistic approach.** The holistic perspective can be traced to Adolf Meyer. In *The Philosophy of Occupation Therapy,* he states, "Our body is not merely so many pounds of flesh and bone figuring as a machine, with an abstract mind or soul added to it. [Rather, it is a live organism acting] in harmony with its own nature and the nature about it."[12] The holistic approach emphasizes the organic and functional relationship between the parts and the whole being. This approach maintains that a person is a whole—an interaction of biological, psychological, sociocultural, and spiritual elements. If any element (or subsystem) is negatively affected, a disruption or disturbance will be reflected throughout the whole.

Even though a holistic approach is a fundamental principle of the profession, it is not consistently applied in practice. Unfortunately, some OT practitioners have moved away from a holistic approach to a specialized (reductionistic) approach. For example, some OT practitioners working in the specialized field of hand rehabilitation refer to themselves as hand therapists, or OT practitioners practicing in psychiatry call themselves psychiatric therapists. This presents a contradiction between what the practitioner supposedly believes

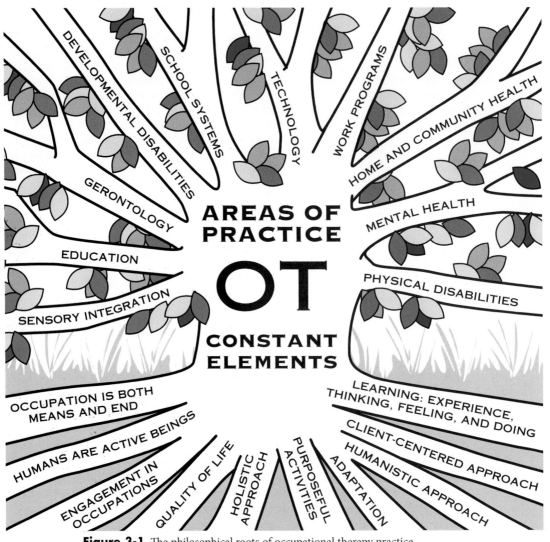

Figure 3-1 The philosophical roots of occupational therapy practice.

(holism) and what the practitioner does. This is also confusing to the student who sees a disparity between the principles being taught in school and what is being applied in practice. First, the student needs to realize that this does not necessarily mean that the "hand therapist" is only treating the hand or the "psychiatric therapist" is only treating the mind. If the student is present for a short observation, he or she may be seeing only a small piece of intervention and not the complete scope of the occupational therapy process. The practitioner may still have a belief in holism, but the particular procedures seen during a brief observation may not have reflected that belief. It is important that this key principle is ingrained in the OT practitioner and that an evaluation and intervention plan that reflects the needs of the whole person is completed. If the OT practitioner is treating only the body (or parts of the body) or only the mind, the commitment to holism has been compromised.[18] In such cases, the consumer is denied one of the unique aspects of occupational therapy: the holistic approach.

Occupational Therapy Views Humans as Active Beings for Whom Occupation Is Critical to Well-Being

Occupational therapy views a human as an **active being.** Again, looking to Meyer, "Our conception of man is that of an organism that maintains and balances itself in the world of reality and actuality by being in active life and active use."[12] Humans are actively involved in controlling and determining their own behavior and are capable of changing behavior as desired.[14] Furthermore, humans are viewed as open systems in which there is continuous interaction between the person and the environment. The person's behaviors influence the physical and social environment; in turn the person is affected by changes in the environment. This view is referred to as **organismic.** A **mechanistic** view, on the other hand, sees the human as passive in nature and controlled by the environment in which he or she lives.[14] Related to the belief that the human is an active being, and at the core of occupational therapy, is the belief that occupation is critical to the existence of human beings. In order to survive, each person must perform certain occupations (such as feeding oneself) or have someone perform the occupations for him or her. Beyond the survival level, occupations also fulfill each individual's need for security, belonging, physiological esteem, and self-actualization.[15]

Those outside the profession often misunderstand the word **occupation.** In contemporary communication, the word *occupation* has been commonly and frequently used to refer to one's job, as in the question, "What is your occupation?" People often overlook its more fundamental meaning from the dictionary, which (as stated earlier) defines the word *occupation* as an activity in which one engages. From the perspective of occupational therapy, occupation refers to "the ordinary and familiar things that people do every day."[1] It is the term used to "capture the breadth and meaning of 'everyday life activity.'"[1]

The *Occupational Therapy Practice Framework: Domain and Process (OTPF)* is a professional document that delineates the unique focus of occupational therapy on occupation. This document identifies the overall concern of occupational therapy as the "engagement in occupation to support participation within context or contexts"[1] and defines occupation as "activities . . . of everyday life, named, organized, and given value and meaning by individuals and a culture. Occupation is everything people do to occupy themselves, including looking after themselves . . . enjoying life . . . and contributing to the social and economic fabric of their communities."[11]

On the surface, it may seem as if the concept of occupation is a simple one; in fact, the nature of occupation contains many dimensions and is rather complex.[2] The various dimensions that comprise occupation and that OT practitioners attend to during service provision include (1) the range of occupations and activities that make up people's lives (performance in areas of occupation); (2) the skills used by people to perform occupations and activities (performance skills); (3) the habits, routines, and roles that are assumed by individuals in carrying out occupations or activities (performance patterns); (4) the internal or external context, or conditions, in which occupation occurs and influences performance (cultural, physical, social, personal, spiritual, temporal, and virtual); (5) the demands of the activity which affect skill and success of performance; and (6) the factors that reside within the client and influence performance such as physiological and psychological body functions and anatomical body structures (organs, and limbs).[1] These various dimensions of occupation all make up occupational therapy's domain of concern and are described in detail in Chapter 9.

At a given time, an individual may be occupied with caring for him or herself by bathing, dressing, or eating. A person may be occupied with productive tasks, such as paid employment or tasks that are necessary for the care of his or her family. At other times, the individual may be involved in activities that he or she simply finds pleasurable, such as playing cards, watching a movie, or exercising. This is referred to as **occupational performance,** or "the ability to carry out activities of daily life."[1] These activities are categorized in the following performance areas of occupation:

- Activities of daily living (e.g., self-care activities such as hygiene and dressing) and instrumental activities of daily living (e.g., activities such as household management, financial management, and child care)
- Education-related activities (e.g., going to school, studying)
- Work-related activities (e.g., activities related to employment and volunteer work)
- Play and leisure activities (e.g., activities that promote pleasure and diversion)
- Participation in social activities (e.g., activities related to interacting with others)

The occupations we perform on a daily basis are also influenced by our individual occupational roles. Christiansen and Townsend define **role** "as a pattern of behavior that involves certain rights and duties that an individual is expected, trained, and often encouraged to perform in a particular social situation."[7] Role has also been defined as "a culturally defined pattern of occupation that reflects particular routines and habits."[6] Expectations of the individual's culture provide subtle messages about which roles to adopt and when.[7] The duration of roles varies, depending upon the role. For example, it may be a long-term role, such as a parent or spouse, or a short-term role, such as a patient in a hospital. A specific occupation may also be carried out in different roles and contexts, which will influence how that occupation is performed. Take, for example, the activity of reading. This activity may be carried out in the role of a parent reading a story to a child at home, in the role of a student reading a textbook in the library, or in the role of a consumer reading food labels in the grocery store. The role in which the activity is being performed gives meaning to it as an occupation.[7]

HOW DOES A PERSON KNOW WHAT HE KNOWS?

Epistemology investigates the nature, origin, and limits of human knowledge.[18] This component of philosophy helps one understand the nature of learning and is key to the field of occupational therapy. Specifically, this component of philosophy provides a base for understanding motivation, change, and learning (Box 3-2).

Human Learning Entails Experience, Thinking, Feeling, and Doing

Occupational therapy believes that humans learn through experience—thinking, feeling, and doing. This principle is found in many of the early writings of the founding members of the profession.[12,17,19] Humans are unique in that they have a sense of time—past, present, and future. This enables humans to remember past experiences and use them for present and future knowing. For example, a child who touches a hot stove and burns himself will learn rather rapidly (and painfully) from this experience not to touch a stove again. Past experiences also play a role in what the person finds meaningful. A child who likes the sound of a toy may be motivated to activate it again.

Box 3-2 Core Concepts of Occupational Therapy

- Occupational therapy views humans holistically.
- Occupational therapy views humans as active beings wherein occupation is critical to well-being.
- Occupational therapy classifies occupations under activities of daily living, instrumental activities of daily living, self care, education, work, play and leisure, and participation in social activities.
- Human learning entails experience, thinking, feeling, and doing.
- Every human being has the potential for adaptation.
- The profession views occupation as both a means and an end.
- Occupational therapy is based on humanism wherein the values of altruism, equality, freedom, justice, dignity, truth, and prudence are central to the profession.
- The client, family, and significant others are active participants throughout the therapeutic process in what is referred to as a client-centered approach.

Occupational therapy emphasizes *doing* as the primary mechanism for learning and relearning various skills. Meyer saw occupational therapy's role as "giving *opportunities* rather than prescriptions." He saw a need for "opportunities to work, opportunities to do and to plan and create, and to learn to use material."[12] The philosophical base mentions the use of purposeful activity (occupation) to improve or maintain health. On a broad level, OT practitioners use both the terms *occupation* and *activity* to describe participation in daily life pursuits. However, there are important differences in these terms. The term **activity** describes a general class of human actions that is goal directed.[13] Goal-directed behavior implies that the person is focused on the goal of the activity rather than the processes involved in achieving the goal.[4] The *OTPF* delineates an activity from an occupation as something an individual may participate in to achieve a goal, but activity may not have importance or meaning in the person's life.[1] **Tasks** are considered the basic units of behavior and are the simplest form of an action (i.e., reaching for a ball).

Through the therapeutic use of occupation and activity, the client is involved on many levels. Coordination between the person's sensorimotor, cognitive, and psychosocial systems is necessary and elicited when an individual engages in occupations and activities.[4] OT practitioners use occupation and activity as a means to help a client learn a new skill, restore a deficient ability, compensate in the presence of a functional disability, maintain health, or prevent dysfunction.[4] Mary Reilly summarizes this concept in her Eleanor Clarke Slagle lectureship when she states, "Man, through the use of his hands as they are energized by mind and will, can influence the state of his own health."[16]

The student may find the use of the term *occupation* confusing at this point. In the previous section, we described the concept of occupation as the individual's occupational performance, or the desired outcome, with an emphasis on the individual's occupational performance, or outcome. Now we discuss doing and the use of occupation as a means of intervention. In the practice of occupational therapy, occupation is seen as both a means and an end. **Occupation as a means** is the use of a specific occupation to bring about a change in the client's performance. When occupation is used as a means, it may be equivalent to activity. **Occupation as an end** is the desired outcome or product of intervention (i.e., the performance of activities or tasks that the person deems as important to life), and it is derived from the person's values, experiences, and culture.[20]

The therapeutic use of occupation and activity requires that the OT practitioner analyze both of these professional tools from multiple perspectives. Analysis of occupation and activity is a skill specific to occupational therapy and is discussed in detail in Chapter 15.

Adaptation: The Potential in Every Human Being

Through this "knowing by doing," a human also learns to adapt. A child who wants a toy on a table may initially cry to obtain it. Eventually, the child will learn to pull up to a standing position to reach for the toy. When he finds that this approach to acquiring objects is successful, the power of this technique is increased, and he will use it more frequently. This is one example of adaptation. As seen in the philosophical base of occupational therapy, individual **adaptation** is defined as "a change in function that promotes survival and self-actualization."[5] The concept of adaptation can also be traced back to Adolph Meyer, who stated that diseases in psychiatry are "largely problems of adaptation" and that "psychiatry was among the first disciplines to recognize the need for adaptation and the value of work as a help in the problems of adaptation."[12] Adaptation takes place as part of the normal developmental process, in the process of adjusting to stress or change.[10]

In occupational therapy, occupation and activity are used to promote adaptation. Through occupation and activity, the individual achieves mastery over the environment, which contributes to the individual's feeling of competency.[8] Gail Fidler and Jay Fidler describe the development of competence. They write, "The ability to adapt, to cope with the problems of everyday living, and to fulfill life roles requires a rich reservoir of experiences gathered from direct engagement with both human and non-human objects in one's environment." They continue, "It is through such action with feedback from both human and non-human objects that an individual comes to know the potential and limitations of self and the environment and achieves a sense of competence and intrinsic worth."[9]

The process of adaptation is viewed as coming from within the individual. The client is actively involved in creating the change. The role of the OT or OTA in this process is to arrange the surroundings, materials, and demands of the environment to facilitate a specific adaptive response.[10] Practitioners of occupational therapy are optimistic that each and every individual has the potential to grow, adapt, and change.[21]

WHAT IS DESIRABLE?

Axiology examines the values of a profession and what is considered just and right in terms of the profession. For occupational therapy, the concepts of quality of life, function, and ethics fall under axiology. As mentioned earlier, occupational therapy works in, around, and with the medical field but belongs to a different model. The purpose of medicine is to treat, medicate, and apply life-saving techniques and technology; its purpose is to fill the needs that a person cannot. Occupational therapy believes that **quality of life** (QOL) is important. Quality of life is relative and depends upon the individual and his or her idea of what constitutes quality of life. What is meaningful and that which provides satisfaction to an individual is **phenomenological;** that is, it is determined by the experience of that individual.[21]

Occupational therapy seeks to improve the quality of life for any person whose functional ability is impaired or limited. This goal is achieved by helping the client develop greater independence in the performance of any area of occupational behavior.

For example, a goal of intervention may be to enable a client to independently brush his or her teeth, or to manage a checkbook, or to become more alert to the body mechanics that help avoid injury on the job. Likewise, the goal of intervention may be to ensure that the client increases the strength in the body part needed to perform a necessary task, or achieve better coordination for all activities, or be better able to enjoy life by developing a hobby, or more fully participate in life by developing social skills. The OT practitioner works with the client to identify those occupations that are meaningful and will improve his or her quality of life. Together, the OT practitioner and client focus intervention on maximizing occupational performance in these areas.

WHAT ARE THE "RULES OF RIGHT CONDUCT"?

As discussed in Chapter 2, the profession of occupational therapy emerged from the era of Moral Treatment, which valued the humanitarian treatment of individuals who were mentally ill. Occupational therapy is still based on **humanism,** a belief that the client should be treated as a person, not an object. The humanistic perspective is one of the pillars of the profession. In today's practice, this belief is encompassed in service delivery through the use of what is called a **client-centered approach.** The profession understands the importance of having the client, family, and significant others as active participants throughout the therapeutic process. The client is actively involved, not only in the modality itself but also in identifying personal goals and preferences for treatment.

From this humanistic perspective, values and attitudes central to the profession have evolved. The paper, *Core Values and Attitudes of Occupational Therapy Practice,*[3] identifies the concepts of altruism, equality, freedom, justice, dignity, truth, and prudence as the core values and attitudes of occupational therapy.

Altruism is the unselfish concern for the welfare of others. It is demonstrated through the commitment of the OT practitioner to the profession and to the client with caring, dedication, responsiveness, and understanding. **Equality** is treating all individuals equally with an attitude of fairness and impartiality and respecting each individual's beliefs, values, and lifestyles in the day-to-day interactions with the OT practitioner. [3]

The OT practitioner also values **freedom,** an individual's right to exercise choice and to "demonstrate independence, initiative, and self-direction."[3] Freedom is demonstrated through nurturing, which is very different from controlling or directing. OT practitioners nurture their clients by providing support and encouragement, enabling the client to develop his or her inherent potential. Nurturing encourages the development of independence in the client, rather than retaining all direction and control in the hands of the practitioner.

Justice is the need for all OT practitioners to abide by the laws that govern the practice and to respect the legal rights of the client. Through the value of **dignity,** the uniqueness of each individual is emphasized. OT practitioners demonstrate this value through empathy and respect for each person. **Truthfulness** is a value demonstrated through behavior that is accountable, honest, and accurate, and that maintains one's professional competence. **Prudence** is the ability to demonstrate sound judgment, care, and discretion.[3] These values and attitudes are reflected in the *Occupational Therapy Code of Ethics* (see Chapter 7).

SUMMARY

This has been a *brief* introduction to the philosophy of occupational therapy and its role in shaping the knowledge base and practice of the profession. The profession has seen a significant increase in the number and breadth of publications that focus on occupation, and the reader is referred to the references listed in this chapter for further information. Individuals in the field have focused on the task of weaving the implications from history and the profession's philosophical base into conceptual models and theoretical approaches. These models and theories have been developed specifically around the concepts of occupation. This has not been the task of one person alone. Some of those involved in this undertaking have included Mary Reilly, Gail Fidler, David Nelson, Elizabeth Yerxa, Gary Kielhofner, Anne Mosey, Janette Schkade, and Sally Schultz. In Chapter 14, we will summarize the body of work of some of these individuals and see how each has added to the profession.

The philosophical base of a profession represents its core beliefs, values, and principles. The history of occupational therapy provides the foundation for the philosophy that represents the current practice of occupational therapy. This history helps address questions such as "What is humankind?" "What is ethical or right conduct?" and "What is desirable?"

When exploring the diversity of the field of occupational therapy, it is important to maintain an awareness of the principles of a holistic approach, occupation, purposeful activity, a humanistic approach, adaptation, and improving the quality of life, for these principles embody the philosophical roots of the field (Figure 3–1).

The common bond between OT practitioners is the importance of occupation and the facilitation of occupational performance. From a holistic perspective, occupational therapy views humans as active beings. Occupation is seen as an essential part of human existence, and it refers to all the daily activities in which people participate. The underlying goal of occupational therapy is to increase the individual's independence in any area of occupational performance; thus the OT practitioner must recognize inhibitors of activity and be able to design an intervention plan.

Humans learn by doing and, through the process of adaptation, develop a mastery of self and competence. Improving a client's quality of life (particularly increasing a person's independence) is the focus of the services provided by OT practitioners. Occupational therapy facilitates the adaptive process by providing the client with opportunities to adapt and improve one's quality of life.

Learning Activities

1. Identify your values and beliefs. Do they relate to the values and beliefs of the occupational therapy profession?
2. Review Chapter 2 and research other historical occupational therapy resources to trace consistencies between the early and current philosophies of the profession.
3. From case study articles (i.e., *OT Practice*), gather examples of quality-of-life changes that result from occupational therapy intervention.
4. In your own words, write a description of occupational therapy.
5. In a small group, identify the various roles within which each person functions. Discuss how your different roles give individual meaning to the activities you perform.

Review Questions

1. What is occupational therapy's view of humans?
2. What are the similarities and differences between occupation, activity, and tasks?
3. What is meant by the terms *occupation as means* and *occupation as an end?*
4. What are the core concepts of occupational therapy practice? Provide examples of each of these.
5. What is the philosophical base of occupational therapy?

REFERENCES

1. American Occupational Therapy Association: Occupational therapy practice framework: domain and process, *Am J Occup Ther* 56(6):609-639, 2002.
2. American Occupational Therapy Association: Position paper: occupation, *Am J Occup Ther* 49:1015, 1995.
3. American Occupational Therapy Association: Core values and attitudes of occupational therapy practice, *Am J Occup Ther* 47:1085, 1993.
4. American Occupational Therapy Association: Position paper: purposeful activity, *Am J Occup Ther* 47:1080, 1993.
5. American Occupational Therapy Association: The philosophical base of occupational therapy, *Am J Occup Ther* 33:785, 1979. (Reprinted in *Am J Occup Ther* 49:1026, 1995). Reviewed by COE and COP in 2004.
6. Canadian Association of Occupational Therapists: *Enabling Occupation: An Occupational Therapy Perspective,* Ottawa, 1997, Canadian Association of Occupational Therapists.
7. Christiansen CH, Townsend EA (eds): *Introduction to Occupation: The Art and Science of Living,* Upper Saddle River, NJ, 2004, Prentice Hall.
8. Fidler GS: From crafts to competence, *Am J Occup Ther* 35:567, 1981.
9. Fidler GS, Fidler JW: Doing and becoming: purposeful action and self actualization, *Am J Occup Ther* 32:305, 1978.
10. King LJ: Toward a science of adaptive responses, *Am J Occup Ther* 32:14, 1978.
11. Law M, Polatajko H, Baptiste W, et al: Core concepts of occupational therapy. In Townsend E (ed): *Enabling Occupation: An Occupational Therapy Perspective,* p. 32, Ottawa, 1997, Canadian Association of Occupational Therapists.
12. Meyer A: The philosophy of occupation therapy, *Arch Occup Ther* 1:1, 1922. (Reprinted in *Am J Occup Ther* 31:10, 1977.)
13. Pierce D: Untangling occupation and activity, *Am J Occup Ther* 22:138-146, 2001.
14. Reed KL: The beginnings of occupational therapy. In Hopkins HL, Smith HD (eds): *Willard and Spackman's Occupational Therapy,* ed 8, Philadelphia, 1993, JB Lippincott.
15. Reed KL, Sanderson SN: *Concepts of Occupational Therapy,* ed 4, Philadelphia, 1999, Lippincott Williams & Wilkins.
16. Reilly M: Occupational therapy can be one of the great ideas of 20th century medicine, *Am J Occup Ther* 16:2, 1962.
17. Robeson HA: How can occupational therapists help the social service worker? *Occup Ther Rehabil* 5:279, 1926.
18. Shannon PD: Philosophy and core values in occupational therapy. In Sladyk K, Ryan SE (eds): *Ryan's Occupational Therapy Assistant: Principles, Practice Issues, and Techniques,* ed 4, Thorofare, NJ, 2005, Slack.
19. Slagle EC: Training aides for mental patients, *Arch Occup Ther* 1:13, 1922.
20. Trombly CA: Occupation: purposefulness and meaningfulness as therapeutic mechanisms. The 1995 Eleanor Clark Slagle lecture, *Am J Occup Ther* 49:960-972, 1995.
21. Yerxa E: The philosophical base of occupational therapy. In *Occupational Therapy 2001 AD,* Bethesda, MD, 1979, American Occupational Therapy Association.

Occupational therapy is by far the most unique of allied health care professions. The delicate balance of art, science, and human interaction on which the profession is based contributes not only to this uniqueness but also to the obvious effectiveness of occupational therapy intervention throughout the life span.

Glen Gillen, EdD, OTR, FAOTA
Assistant Professor in Clinical Occupational Therapy
Columbia University
New York, New York

4 Current Issues and Emerging Practice Areas

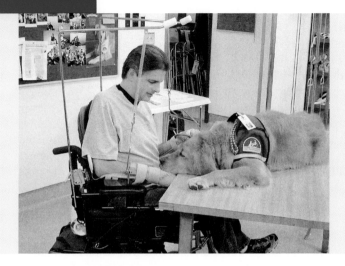

OBJECTIVES

After reading this chapter, the reader will be able to do the following:
- Identify current issues facing the occupational therapy profession
- Describe emerging practice areas
- Discuss the value of evidence-based practice
- Discuss policy impact upon practice

KEY TERMS

Aging in place	Ergonomics	Participatory research
Assistive technology	Evidence-based practice	Vision
Driver rehabilitation specialists	Licensure laws	

The role of the occupational therapy (OT) practitioner has developed significantly since its beginning work in positions such as reconstruction aide and working with injured veterans returning home. OT practitioners provide service to all ages (children to senior citizens) and diagnoses in such settings as hospitals, schools, rehabilitation clinics, private companies, and day treatment centers. With advances in science and technology, the OT practitioner today provides a wide range of technological and occupational-based service supported by current research. The OT practitioner is skilled at problem-solving and clinical reasoning and adept at interpersonal interactions (e.g., therapeutic use of self). OT practitioners today are consumers of research, and this enables them to provide quality evidence-based service to clients. OT practitioners work in a variety of environments and thus understand the legal implications of their services. As such, OT practitioners advocate for the rights of clients and participate in the political process to help generate policy to assist those in need. In general, today's OT practitioner is an informed, active professional whose interest in the client helps to serve the public, the profession, and the individual. This chapter describes the latest trends in occupational therapy practice by providing an overview of the centennial vision and a description of the emerging areas of practice.

CENTENNIAL VISION

A **vision** leads the future direction of a profession or organization. The vision is developed with the members and constituents over time, and it clarifies values, creates a future, and focuses the mission. Visioning helps organizations "stretch the horizon," develop a clear picture for the future,[12] and develop goals and objectives. Thus a vision helps organizations move forward in a clear direction by encouraging all participants to work toward the vision. 2017 will mark the centennial year of the occupational therapy profession. After much discussion and input from members, constituents, and consumers, the American Occupational Therapy Association (AOTA) adopted the centennial vision in 2006.[1]

AOTA's current vision statement is: "We envision that occupational therapy is a powerful, widely recognized, science-driven, and evidence-based profession with a globally connected and diverse workforce meeting society's occupational needs."[1] The vision for the occupational therapy profession continues the emphasis on evidence-based practice and the value of the diversity of clients and practitioners. It highlights the work that OT practitioners do to meet society's needs and articulates the need for science to support practice as well as expand the diversity of clients and practitioners.

OCCUPATION

The centennial vision reflects the trend in occupational therapy practice to return to the roots of the profession: occupation (Box 4-1). Practitioners are encouraged to engage in occupation-based practice, focusing on helping clients re-engage in occupations, as opposed to focusing on specific component skills. The emphasis on occupation-based practice is found in the occupational therapy literature, including the *Occupational Therapy Practice Framework,* standards for accreditation, conference programs, and journal articles. Educational programs have designed programs around the uniqueness of occupation. Therefore the trend to return to occupation remains a focus of research, education, and scholarly work.[1,3,10,15] OT practitioners are embracing the uniqueness of the profession by helping

> **Box 4-1** Definition of Occupation
>
> "Activities . . . of everyday life, named, organized, and given value and meaning by individuals and a culture. Occupation is everything people do to occupy themselves, including looking after themselves . . . enjoying life . . . and contributing to the social and economic fabric of their communities."

From Law M, Polatajko H, Baptiste W, et al: Core concepts of occupational therapy. In Townsend E (ed): Enabling Occupation: An Occupational Therapy Perspective, p. 34, Ottawa, 1997, Canadian Association of Occupational Therapists.

persons do what they wish to do. Furthermore, research supports the premise that engagement in the actual occupation is beneficial and leads to increased physical, psychological, and social benefits.[3,7] Participation in occupations leads to increased motivation, generalization, and improved motor learning.[3,7,10]

EMERGING AREAS OF PRACTICE

As health care and society's needs change, opportunities and new areas of occupational therapy practice emerge. Events such as the aging of baby boomers (those persons born between 1946 and 1964), advancements in technology, and changes in health care policy provide OT practitioners with new opportunities. Former AOTA president Carolyn Baum identified six emerging areas of practice:

1. Aging in place
2. Driver assessments and training programs
3. Community health and wellness
4. Needs of children and youth
5. Ergonomics consulting
6. Technology and assistive-device developing and consulting[6,15]

These areas of practice illustrate the diversity of the profession and the breadth of services that OT practitioners provide. In addition to these areas of practice, OT practitioners continue to provide service in settings such as hospitals, skilled nursing facilities, community agencies, rehabilitation clinics, private clinics, schools, day care centers, and psychiatric facilities. OT practitioners provide services to underprivileged populations, including the homeless, migrant workers, and victims of disaster.

AGING IN PLACE

Occupational therapy has evolved as society's needs change. With advances in medicine and health care, Americans are living longer, and more elderly people wish to remain in their homes and live independently (or with minimal supports). This trend toward staying in the home is termed **aging in place.**[11] The OT practitioner offers a wide range of services to older individuals to allow them to remain at home and continue to be active in their community; these services include home modification, consultation, energy conservation, education, and remediation. Safety in the home includes the ability to manage medications, access emergency numbers, carry through with emergency procedures, show adequate judgment and cognition for daily living (e.g., cooking safety), demonstrate physical safety in the home, and the ability to safely protect oneself from strangers. Not only does the practitioner evaluate the client's skills, abilities, and safety in the home, but the OT practitioner also examines the support systems in place for the client (Box 4-2).

Box 4-2 Questions to Address for Staying in the Home
Is the client able to access emergency numbers?
How far away from emergency personnel does the client live?
How close are family members or support?
What is the disaster plan (e.g., hurricanes, flooding, snow)?
Can the client manage medications?
Is the client able to drive?
Who will be visiting the client on a regular basis?
Is the client able to access financial resources?
How will the client get around the community?
What are the social supports available to the client?
Is the home accessible to the client?
Can the client lock doors at night?

Socializing with others is important to the psychological well-being of individuals living at home. The OT practitioner may direct older persons to new social activities or help clients continue a previous activity with modifications or assistance. OT practitioners can be key players in developing creative programs to address the needs of the elderly. Clark et al. conducted a large, randomized control trial to examine the effectiveness of occupational therapy services on well elders.[7] The results of this study supported occupational therapy intervention as a cost-effective service to improve the health and quality of life of well elders.

DRIVER ASSESSMENTS AND TRAINING PROGRAMS

Safe driving requires many factors (e.g., judgment, reaction time, sequencing, visual perceptual skills). OT practitioners determine a person's ability to drive after a trauma, illness, or decline in function by evaluating cognitive and physical abilities. Intervention is designed to remediate poor abilities or to make adaptations to accommodate dysfunctional skills. The OT practitioner and a team of providers are responsible for assessing whether the client is capable of driving safely; state laws provide driving licensure regulations. Clients may need special modifications to their vehicles in order to drive.

OT practitioners train individuals in the necessary foundation skills to ensure that drivers are safe. Because occupational therapists (OTs) are trained to examine clients in a holistic manner, occupational therapy is well suited to succeed as **driver rehabilitation specialists.** Namely, the OT practitioner evaluates and intervenes in physical, social, cognitive, and psychosocial aspects of functioning that affect driving skills. OT practitioners may consult with technology specialists or mechanics on adapting vehicles to help clients with disabilities.

COMMUNITY HEALTH AND WELLNESS

Because the goal of occupational therapy is to help individuals engage in activities of daily living, work, education, leisure, play, and social participation, OT practitioners may develop programs to keep communities healthy. Such programs focus on wellness and prevention of disability, and they help those with disabilities integrate into the community and contribute to society (e.g., vocational rehabilitation programs).

Advances in health care have enabled individuals to survive many conditions that interfere with functioning. Policy makers and consumers have begun to realize the benefits to helping individuals remain active in their community. OT practitioners facilitate health and wellness in communities through educational programs and services to individuals and groups. Providing services to the community promotes wellness and quality of life. An individual's quality of life is based upon many things, including standard of living, finances, freedom, happiness, and access to goods and services. Therefore, helping senior citizens access health care, social groups, transportation, and daily living activities can increase their quality of life. For example, OTs may consult with a senior citizens' group about the benefits of physical activity, or speak to support groups on a variety of topics, including safety at home, driving tips, cooking modifications, and medication management.

The OT practitioner may design programs to increase wellness in the community or to address a specific concern. Specific areas of concern in the community that OT practitioners might be involved with include addressing the needs of the homeless, migrant workers, or victims of disaster. OT practitioners might also work with communities as consultants to assure accessibility for persons with disabilities (e.g., playgrounds, public buildings).

NEEDS OF CHILDREN AND YOUTH

The needs of children and youth continue to be a growing area for OT practitioners. Childhood obesity is a concern among this population. In fact, *Healthy People 2010* cited childhood obesity in America as one of the leading health issues.[9] Because there are many factors associated with childhood obesity, OT practitioners are becoming involved in developing programs for those children.

OT practitioners serve children in early intervention programs that begin as early as birth. Although federal law mandates these birth–to–3-year-old programs, the states are responsible for the implementation of services. With limited funding and increased need for services, the OT practitioner working in early intervention may need to advocate for the children they serve. There continues to be a need for training and programming in this area.

When children with special needs transition to the public school system, an OT practitioner helps them function in the education environment. OT practitioners provide services within systems with limited funding, despite the vast needs. OT practitioners may be involved in creating after school programs or evening social programs for children and youth. Creative solutions are needed to address the needs of children and youth.

ERGONOMICS CONSULTING

Ergonomics is the science of fitting jobs to people.[17] Ergonomics consulting involves providing recommendations to individuals and companies on workstation set-up to promote safety, efficiency, and comfort to prevent work-related musculoskeletal injury. Examination of seating and positioning, lifting, and other physical requirements falls well within the OT practitioner's expertise. Proper ergonomics may prevent injury to the client. Industries and companies value work evaluations and ergonomic consultation, which may result in fewer missed work days and lower costs to the company and client.

TECHNOLOGY AND ASSISTIVE-DEVICE DEVELOPING AND CONSULTING

Assistive technology, or adaptive technology, commonly refers to "products, devices or equipment, whether acquired commercially, modified, or customized, that are used to maintain, increase, or improve the functional capabilities of individuals with disabilities."[5]

Assistive technology, which includes equipment to assist with communication, computer access, daily living, education and learning, hearing and listening, mobility and transportation, recreation and leisure, seating and position, vision and reading, and prosthetics and orthotics,[16] has improved life for those with disabilities. OT practitioners use technology to help clients function independently in many areas of performance. Because OT practitioners are skilled at analyzing activities including the movement patterns required for success, many practitioners serve as consultants in the development of devices.

Frequently, the OT practitioner consults with the team on the type of assistive device and the physical, cognitive, or psychological skills the client possesses to use the device. The OT practitioner is an important member of the team because he or she determines whether the device helps the client perform in his or her daily occupations in a reasonable amount of time. The OT practitioner and client determine whether the device is practical and helpful to the client after careful analysis.

EDUCATIONAL TRENDS

Educators are consistently evaluating how to teach occupational therapy and occupational therapy assistant (OTA) students to succeed in clinical practice. Educators acknowledge that practitioners entering a diverse workplace with expanding areas of practice need to be lifelong learners and critical consumers of research. Practitioners must be able to support their decisions based upon available research. The trend toward justifying intervention requires practitioners who are able to generate and critically analyze research. Basing practice on the best available research evidence is termed **evidence-based practice.** Insurance companies, consumers, and employers are requiring OT practitioners to provide evidence for what they do. Given so many options for spending one's health care dollar, practitioners must show that therapy is beneficial and cost effective.

This need to become critical consumers of research prompted the move to a master's level degree as the entry-level requirement for therapists. This degree reflects the advanced critical analysis and synthesis required of today's practitioners, especially with regard to the ability to analyze research for practice. The associate's degree is still the educational requirement for OTAs.

The trend to prepare doctoral-trained faculty to teach, advance the research agenda of the profession, and generate evidence for interventions has prompted the development of clinical doctorate programs. Faculty and practitioners may focus on clinical work while pursuing an advanced degree. Another technique to keep occupational therapy faculty in touch with clinical practice while fulfilling faculty commitments is to conduct **participatory research,** which helps close the gap between academia and practice. Participatory research involves the clinician, client, and faculty member in the research process, and it often results in relevant research.

Today's student is well versed in the use of technology. Many occupational therapy programs use distance education (including web-based courses and telecommunication courses) to reach practitioners who might otherwise not have educational opportunities. Educators use new teaching strategies to maximize learning with technology.

In summary, faculty strive to educate occupational therapy clinicians who are critical and innovative thinkers—people who are able to interact therapeutically with clients and peers. Educators hope to bridge the clinical practice and theory gap so that students become practitioners who use current research and judgment to benefit their clients.

STATE REGULATION, POLICY, AND REIMBURSEMENT ISSUES

A discussion of current issues in occupational therapy would not be complete without mention of the influence of state regulation, policy, and reimbursement issues. The practice of occupational therapy is regulated in most states through state licensure laws that safeguard the public and protect the public from unethical, incompetent, or unauthorized practitioners. State **licensure laws,** also called practice acts, give a legal definition of occupational therapy and the domain of occupational therapy practice that differentiates it from other professions. These laws provide important guides for consumers, facilities, and providers, especially with regard to the minimum qualifications for practitioners. AOTA has developed the *AOTA Model Occupational Therapy Practice Act,*[2] which offers states the language for implementing their licensure laws.

The system of regulating health care professionals through state licensure has many opponents who would like to see reforms. For this reason, OT practitioners need to keep up to date on the status of the licensure laws in their state and any proposed changes to the regulations. For example, in Minnesota and Florida, budget cuts that were proposed to streamline government would have resulted in deregulation of occupational therapy practice.[14] The OT practitioners in these states advocated for maintaining licensure to protect consumers, and they were able to defeat these initiatives. State licensure laws may periodically be scheduled for termination unless renewed by the legislature. Again, government leaders and other professional organizations may oppose renewal of the licensure law, unless OT practitioners are actively involved in advocating for their profession. State licensure is discussed in detail in Chapter 7.

OT practitioners also need to be aware of infringement on their scope of practice and be proactive in such situations. Physical therapists, orthotists, and prosthetists have recently challenged the occupational therapy scope of practice. This may be a result of efforts by other disciplines to position themselves as a source for "one-stop shopping" in rehabilitation or for reimbursement purposes.[13] The Federation of State Boards of Physical Therapy (FSBPT) has approved the *Model Practice Act for Physical Therapy,*[4] and states are being encouraged to adopt this act in their licensure laws. In this *Model Practice Act,* physical therapy scope of practice has been expanded to include "functional training in self-care and home management (including activities of daily living and instrumental activities of daily living)."[4] AOTA and state occupational therapy associations are concerned that this definition does not sufficiently speak to the limited scope of practice (i.e., functional skills related to physical movement and mobility) in which physical therapists address client needs in this area.[13] This definition infringes on what is traditionally the domain of occupational therapy and in which OT practitioners have extensive education and training.[13] OT practitioners need to be able to fully articulate their scope of practice so that they can defend it when needed.

Policy affects health services, including occupational therapy. For example, the prospective payment system (PPS) of 1983 resulted in shorter hospital stays, but OT practitioners continued to treat these clients in other settings (such as skilled nursing facilities and home health agencies).[8] Federal laws mandate services, but they require state legislation to determine how the law will be carried out. OT practitioners must become familiar with policies while they are being developed and advocate for services for those with disabilities. Box 4-3 provides a partial listing of some of the laws that have affected occupational therapy services.

OT practitioners advocate for the profession by participating in policy making. Practitioners may advocate on local, regional, or national levels. The first step toward addressing

---

Box 4-3   Laws That Have Affected Occupational Therapy Services

1. *Section 504 of the Rehabilitation Act of 1973:* "No otherwise qualified handicapped individual in the United States . . . shall, solely by reason of . . . handicap, be excluded from participation in, be denied the benefits of, or be subjected to discrimination under any program or activity receiving federal financial assistance."[18] Section 504 provides rights and benefits to persons with disabilities and provides services to children in school systems who may not qualify for services under IDEA. This law requires that programs or activities receiving federal financial assistance provide reasonable accommodations so persons with disabilities may participate.
2. *The Americans with Disabilities Act (ADA) of 1990:* Provides protection from discrimination on the basis of disability. The ADA upholds and extends the standards for compliance set forth in Section 504 of the Rehabilitation Act of 1973 to employment practices, communication, and all policies, procedures, and practices that impact on the treatment of students with disabilities.[18] ADA expanded services to include the work place and public places. This law required that public places be accessible to those with disabilities. For example, occupational therapy professionals work with architects and employers to make work settings accessible to those with disabilities.
3. *Individuals with Disabilities Education Act (formerly PL 94-142 or the Education for All Handicapped Children Act of 1975):* Requires public schools to make available to all eligible children with disabilities a free appropriate public education in the least restrictive environment appropriate to their individual needs.[18] OT practitioners working in school systems work under this act. Thus the role of the OT practitioner is to provide intervention that will allow the child to engage in education. Intervention takes place in the least restrictive environment and is appropriate to the child's needs.
4. *The Balanced Budget Act of 1997:* Set out to contain health care costs by placing caps on therapy services and resulted in a decrease in occupational therapy jobs. Many therapists changed settings during this time or moved on to private practice. Managed care pushed for productivity.[8]
5. *Medicare:* This health insurance program is for people 65 years of age or older and those with certain disabilities. It is a federally funded program that provides limits on spending and reimbursement for occupational therapy services.

---

these challenges is for OT practitioners to be familiar with the scope of practice and the foundations for it. Reading state and local resources including state newsletters, the *Scope of Practice Issues update,* and the *State Affairs Group News* newsletter can increase awareness of the issues that affect the profession. Practitioners can keep up to date on health care policy through active involvement in the state and national occupational therapy associations.

SUMMARY

Occupational therapy is a growing profession. The centennial vision provides a message of growth and support for the profession.[1,6] Continued evidence supporting occupational therapy practice reinforces the work and ensures that the profession will thrive. The diversity of clients, as well as the diversity in practitioners, makes the profession exciting and valuable in a changing health care system. OT practitioners will need to continue to advocate for the profession and be involved in policy and reimbursement issues.

Learning Activities

1. Review five current *OT Practice* magazines and list the current issues. Present your findings to your classmates.
2. Review the AOTA national conference program to identify the current issues.
3. Pick one of the six emerging practice areas. Describe the role of the OT practitioner in the area and how you could develop future programs.
4. Develop a resource list around one of the six emerging practice areas.
5. Examine one health care policy, by discussing the history and intent of the policy. In small groups, describe how the policy has been implemented in practice.

Review Questions

1. What are some current issues facing the occupational therapy profession?
2. What are the emerging practice areas?
3. What is evidence-based practice?
4. How has policy affected occupational therapy practice?
5. What are some current trends in occupational therapy education?

REFERENCES

1. American Occupational Therapy Association: AOTA's centennial vision: shaping the future of occupational therapy. Retrieved July 5, 2006, from http://www.aota.org/nonmembers/area16.
2. American Occupational Therapy Association: *Model Occupational Therapy Practice Act,* Bethesda, MD, 2004, American Occupational Therapy Association. Retrieved August 14, 2006, from http://www.aota.org/members/area4/docs/MPA2004.pdf.
3. American Occupational Therapy Association: Occupational therapy practice framework: domain and process, *Am J Occup Ther* 56(6):609-639, 2002.
4. American Physical Therapy Association: *Guidelines: Physical Therapist Scope of Practice, BOD G03-01-09-29,* Board of Directors Standards, Positions, Guidelines, Policies and Procedures, Alexandria, VA, 2005, American Physical Therapy Association.
5. *Assistive Technology Act of 1998.* Retrieved July 5, 2006, from www.section508.gov/docs/AT1998.html.
6. Brachtesende A: The turnaround is here! *OT Practice* 23(1):13-18, 2005.
7. Clark F, Azen SP, Zemke R, et al: Occupational therapy for independent-living older adults. A randomized controlled trial, *JAMA* 278(16):1321-1326, 1997.
8. Fisher G, Cooksey J: The occupational therapy workforce: part I: context and trends. In Brachtesende A: The turnaround is here! *OT Practice* 23(1):13-18, 2005.
9. Office of Disease Prevention and Healthy Promotion (ODPHP): *Healthy People 2010.* Retrieved July 5, 2006, from www.healthypeople.gov.
10. Law M, Polatajko H, Baptiste W, et al: Core concepts of occupational therapy. In Townsend E (ed): *Enabling Occupation: An Occupational Therapy Perspective,* pp. 29-56, Ottawa, 1997, Canadian Association of Occupational Therapists.
11. Pollak PB, DiGregorio DA: Aging in place, *J Extension* 26(4), 1988. Retrieved July 3, 2006, from www.joe.org/joe/1998winter/a2.html.
12. Scott C, Jaffe D, Tobe G: *Organizational Vision, Values and Mission: Building the Organization of the Tomorrow,* Menlo Park, CA, 1993, Crisp Publishers.
13. Slater DY, Willmarth C: Understanding and asserting the occupational therapy scope of practice, *OT Practice* 10(19):CE-1-CE-8, 2005.
14. Smith KC, Willmarth C: State regulation of occupational therapist and occupational therapy assistants. In McCormack GL, Jaffe EG, Goodman-Lavey M (eds): *The Occupational Therapy Manager,* ed 4, Bethesda, MD, 2003, American Occupational Therapy Association.

15. Strzelecki M: President outlines challenges, opportunities ahead. Retrieved July 5, 2006, from http://www.aota.org/nonmembers/area29.

16. RehabTool LLC: What's assistive technology? Retrieved July 5, 2006, from http://www.rehabtool.com/at.html.

17. UCLA Ergonomics: What is ergonomics and why is it important? Retrieved July 5, 2006, from http://ergonomics.ucla.edu/WhatandWhy.html.

18. United States Department of Justice, Civil Rights Division, Disability Rights Section: A guide to disability rights laws, September 2005. Retrieved July 5, 2006, from http://www.ada.gov/cguide.html.

Section 2

Occupational Therapy: The Practitioner

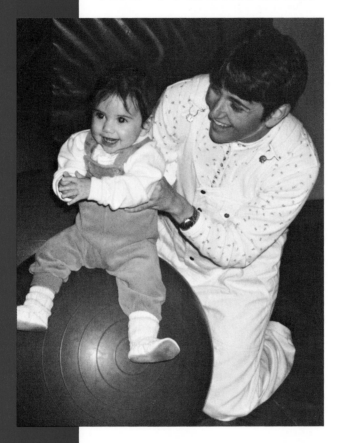

As I transitioned from being an occupational therapy assistant instructor to teaching GED, I realized how much occupational therapy is a part of who I am. We often hear about how transferable our skills are and how we can apply them to many situations. Knowledge of working with persons with learning disabilities, awareness of community resources, valuing the uniqueness of all people and not judging them, and, most of all, empathy have made my transition quite smooth. Working with a student who may need a safe place because his or her home life is in chaos or one who has had substance abuse problems and asks for a resource has provided me with intrinsic rewards that parallel working with a person with disabilities. Occupational therapy is much more than a profession; it is a way of life!

Sue Byers-Connon, MS, COTA/L, ROH
Former Instructor, Occupational Therapy Assistant Program
Instructor, GED Program
Mount Hood Community College
Gresham, Oregon

From Student to Practitioner: Educational Preparation and Certification

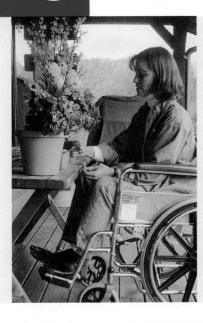

OBJECTIVES

After completing this chapter, the reader will be able to do the following:

- Describe accreditation and the accreditation process for occupational therapy (OT) education programs
- Identify the three categories of occupational therapy personnel
- Delineate the educational and professional requirements for each personnel category
- Describe the purpose of fieldwork and identify the differences between Level I and Level II fieldwork
- Discuss the differences between the Doctor of Occupational Therapy (OTD) and the Doctor of Philosophy (PhD)

KEY TERMS

Accreditation
Accreditation Council for
   Occupational Therapy
   Education
Certification
Doctor of Occupational Therapy

Fieldwork
Level I fieldwork
Level II fieldwork
National Board for
   Certification in
   Occupational Therapy

Occupational therapist
Occupational therapy assistant
Occupational therapy aide
Registered occupational
   therapist
Registration

The personnel who deliver occupational therapy services to consumers can be divided into three categories that vary in the type and amount of training they receive and the duties they perform. The most highly trained at the professional level is the **occupational therapist** (OT). The **occupational therapy assistant** (OTA) is trained at the technical level and works under supervision of the OT. A third category of worker, the **occupational therapy aide,** does not receive specialized training before working in the field; rather, occupational therapy aides receive on-the-job training. In this chapter, the focus is on the educational preparation and certification process for the OT and the OTA.

Consistent with the terminology used by the American Occupational Therapy Association (AOTA), the term *occupational therapy personnel* is used when referring to *any* personnel (including OT students and aides) who deliver occupational therapy services. The term *occupational therapy practitioner* refers to any individual who is "initially certified to practice as either an OT or a OTA, or licensed or regulated by a state, district, commonwealth, or territory of the United States to practice as an OT or OTA and who has not had that certification, license or regulation revoked due to disciplinary action."[5] When it is necessary to distinguish between the three categories of personnel, the respective titles are used.

ACCREDITATION OF EDUCATIONAL PROGRAMS

The **Accreditation Council for Occupational Therapy Education** (ACOTE) of the AOTA regulates entry-level education for both OT and OTA programs in all parts of the United States. Since 1935, AOTA has set standards for educational programs. These standards are reviewed every 5 years by various constituency groups, including bodies within AOTA, educational program directors, and the public at large. The standards are then revised as needed to ensure that they are current. The latest revision of the standards for occupational therapy master's degree programs and OTA programs was completed in 2006. These standards are published in the *Standards for an Accredited Educational Program for the Occupational Therapist*[1] (Box 5-1) and in the *Standards for an Accredited Educational Program for the Occupational Therapy Assistant*[2] (Box 5-2). New accreditation standards for doctoral programs in occupational therapy were adopted by ACOTE in 2006 and become effective on January 1, 2008.

ACOTE evaluates each occupational therapy educational program's compliance with the standards as part of the accreditation process. Each program must follow ACOTE procedures to become accredited and to maintain accreditation. For example, institutions must inform ACOTE of their intention to begin a new program, and they must build a curriculum around the standards. Initial accreditation requires a review of the program design and an on-site inspection after at least 1 year of operation. After passing these requirements, the program becomes fully accredited and is then reviewed on a regular basis. To maintain accreditation, programs must complete a "Report of Self-Study" and undergo a site visit before the end of the period in which accreditation was awarded. The review board has the power to grant or withhold approval. Periodically, programs must make recommended changes in a designated timeframe to become accredited or maintain accreditation.

Accreditation of an occupational therapy educational program means that the minimal educational standards recommended by the profession have been met and the school has received formal approval by ACOTE. This approval ensures that graduates of an

---

Box 5-1 OT Standards

(Effective 1/1/08)

Preamble

The rapidly changing and dynamic nature of contemporary health and human service delivery systems requires the entry-level occupational therapist to possess basic skills as a direct care provider, consultant, educator, manager, researcher, and advocate for the profession and the consumer.

A contemporary entry-level occupational therapist must:

- Have acquired, as a foundation for professional study, a breadth and depth of knowledge in the liberal arts and sciences and an understanding of issues related to diversity.
- Be educated as a generalist with a broad exposure to the delivery models and systems used in settings where occupational therapy is currently practiced and where it is emerging as a service.
- Have achieved entry-level competence through a combination of academic and fieldwork education.
- Be prepared to articulate and apply occupational therapy theory, evidence-based evaluations and interventions to achieve expected outcomes as related to occupation.
- Be prepared to be a lifelong learner and keep current with evidence-based professional practice.
- Uphold the ethical standards, values, and attitudes of the occupational therapy profession.
- Understand the distinct roles and responsibilities of the OT and OTA in the supervisory process.
- Be prepared to advocate as a professional, for the occupational therapy services offered and for the recipients of those services.
- Be prepared to be an effective consumer of the latest research and knowledge bases that support practice and contribute to the growth and dissemination of research and knowledge.

From Accreditation Council for Occupational Therapy Education: *Standards for an Accredited Educational Program for the Occupational Therapist*, Bethesda, MD, August 2006, American Occupational Therapy Association, Inc.

Box 5-2 OTA Standards

(Effective 1/1/08)

Preamble

The rapidly changing and dynamic nature of contemporary health and human service delivery systems requires the entry-level occupational therapy assistant to possess basic skills as a direct care provider, educator, and advocate for the profession and the consumer.

A contemporary entry-level occupational therapy assistant must:

- Have acquired an educational foundation in the liberal arts and sciences, including a focus on issues related to diversity.
- Be educated as a generalist, with a broad exposure to the delivery models and systems used in settings where occupational therapy is currently practiced and where it is emerging as a service.
- Have achieved entry-level competence through a combination of academic and fieldwork education.
- Be prepared to articulate and apply occupational therapy principles and intervention tools to achieve expected outcomes as related to occupation.
- Be prepared to be a lifelong learner and keep current with best practice.
- Uphold the ethical standards, values, and attitudes of the occupational therapy profession.
- Understand the distinct roles and responsibilities of the OT and OTA in the supervisory process.
- Be prepared to advocate as a professional, for the services offered, and for the recipients of those services.

From Accreditation Council for Occupational Therapy Education: *Standards for an Accredited Educational Program for the Occupational Therapy Assistant*, Bethesda, MD, August 2006, American Occupational Therapy Association, Inc.

accredited program will have met the prescribed minimal entry-level standards and that they are qualified to take the national certification examination. As of 2006, there were 148 accredited occupational therapy programs and 129 accredited OTA programs in the United States and Puerto Rico.[3] A current listing of all programs can be found at AOTA's website, www.aota.org.

In selecting a school, prospective students are advised to seek information about the accreditation status, success of program graduates on the national certification examination, job placement rates, mission statement, and philosophy, as well as the emphasis of its educational program. This information enables a student to make an informed choice.

ENTRY-LEVEL EDUCATIONAL PREPARATION

In practice, the roles of the OT and OTA are complementary and collaborative. Therefore the curricula for the entry-level preparation of the OT and the OTA consist of a similar combination of classroom and clinical learning experiences that reflect current practice. Table 5-1 summarizes the characteristics of the different levels of occupational therapy educational preparation. At both levels, students complete anatomy, physiology, medical conditions, kinesiology, and general education courses that lead to a degree awarded by the respective college or university. Courses in the professional areas of the curricula are also similar in content. Students at both levels learn occupational therapy principles, practices, and processes. The difference in the education for the OT is the depth of theory provided in the core and professional curricula as well as a greater emphasis on evaluation and interpretation.

Each level of training requires practical experience, referred to as **fieldwork.** The purpose of fieldwork is to "provide . . . students with the opportunity to apply the knowledge learned in the classroom to practice in the clinical setting."[6] Observation and participation in fieldwork are intended to enhance the academic coursework and to develop competent, entry-level practitioners. Frequently, OT and OTA students are scheduled to complete fieldwork at the same location. This provides students the opportunity to communicate and practice delegation of responsibilities with each other.

Students are expected to increase their technical and critical reasoning skills over time. Therefore both OT and OTA educational programs require two levels of fieldwork. The initial level is referred to as **Level I fieldwork** and is completed concurrently with the academic coursework. The purpose of Level I fieldwork is to introduce the student to the profession and to the various applications of intervention. The amount of time required at this level varies by program.

Level II fieldwork experiences are designed to provide students with supervised, hands-on clinical training. OT students complete full-time fieldwork at a facility for a minimum of 24 weeks, whereas OTA students complete 16 weeks of full-time fieldwork. Students engaged in Level II fieldwork are immersed in occupational therapy practice, and by the end of the experience students are expected to be functioning as entry-level practitioners.

EDUCATIONAL DEMOGRAPHICS OF OCCUPATIONAL THERAPY PRACTITIONERS

Demographic data are listed in Table 5-2, which shows that OT practitioners are primarily women; OTAs hold associate's degrees; and the majority of OTs have baccalaureate degrees. According to AOTA, 26% of OTs hold a master's degree, yet this percentage will increase as educational programs raise requirements to the master's level by 2007 as mandated by the profession.[4]

TABLE 5-1   Characteristics of Levels of Preparation in Occupational Therapy

Degree	Distinctive Curricular Features	Average Program Length	Additional Requirements
Associate AA/AS (required to practice as OTA)	Focus is on technical skills related to the methods and procedures used in occupational therapy.	2 years	16 weeks of Level II fieldwork
Entry-level master's MS/MA/MOT (required to practice as OT)	In depth theory, greater emphasis on evaluation, interpretation, and intervention planning. Emphasis on critically analyzing research for practice. May have a baccalaureate degree in preoccupational therapy/health sciences or another field.	2 years post-baccalaureate degree	24 weeks of Level II fieldwork; basic research project or thesis
Advanced master's MS or MA	Develop advanced research skills and specialization in practice area. Individual has a baccalaureate degree in occupational therapy.	1-3 years post-baccalaureate degree.	Master's thesis or advanced level research project; may require additional fieldwork
PhD	Generate research and knowledge for the profession. Requires completion of master's degree.	3-5 years	Dissertation
OTD	Advanced practice competencies; clinical leadership. Can be earned as entry-level degree or postgraduate.	3 years post-baccalaureate	Clinical research project or practicum required

AA, Associate of Art; *AS,* Associate of Science; *MA,* Master of Arts; *MOT,* Master of Occupational Therapy; *MS,* Master of Science; *OTD,* Doctor of Occupational Therapy; *PhD,* Doctor of Philosophy.

EDUCATIONAL PREPARATION FOR THE OCCUPATIONAL THERAPIST

As of 2007, OTs must complete a postbaccalaureate (master's) degree to practice. Practitioners who obtained a bachelor of sciences or arts degree in occupational therapy prior to 2007 are "grandfathered in"; that is, they may continue to practice. Some universities offer programs to help practitioners with baccalaureate degrees in occupational therapy progress to the advanced master's level. Often, these courses are offered during evenings and week-

TABLE 5-2   Demographic Data on OT Practitioners

	OT	OTA
Men	6%	8%
Women	94%	92%
Associate's	N/A	81%
Baccalaureate	70%	11%
Certificate	2%	6%
Master's	26%	2%
Doctorate	1%	N/A

Data from American Occupational Therapy Association: Membership data: executive summary. Retrieved June 20, 2006, from www.aota.org.

ends to accommodate the working therapist. Students who earned a baccalaureate degree in a related field (i.e., psychology, child development) may enter a basic master's degree occupational therapy program. Students are encouraged to explore the educational options by communicating with local universities and colleges.

DOCTOR OF OCCUPATIONAL THERAPY AND POSTGRADUATE EDUCATION

Students may elect to obtain a **Doctor of Occupational Therapy** (OTD) degree. The OTD is a clinical or practice-based doctorate, also known as a professional doctorate. According to Pierce and Peyton, the OTD focuses on the development of "sophisticated practice competencies rather than research or knowledge production."[8] With these competencies, the individual with the OTD is expected to contribute to outcomes research, program evaluation, and evidenced-based practice. A person may earn an OTD as either an entry-level or as a postgraduate professional degree. For example, the individual may have a Bachelor of Art (BA)/Bachelor of Science (BS) or Master of Art (MA)/Master of Science (MS) in occupational therapy and decide to return to school and get a postprofessional OTD degree.

The Doctor of Philosophy (PhD) is the traditional postgraduate degree and is a research-based degree. Doctorates such as the Doctorate of Education (EdD), Doctorate of Science (ScD), and Doctor of Public Health (DrPH) are also research-based degrees. Some academic institutes offer PhDs in occupational therapy, occupational science, and other related areas, such as psychology, which are appealing to OTs. An individual with a doctoral degree is trained to be an independent researcher, with importance placed on the discovery of knowledge.

EDUCATIONAL PREPARATION FOR THE OCCUPATIONAL THERAPY ASSISTANT

In 1965, AOTA mandated that OTA programs be established in junior or community colleges. Gradually, OTA educational programs were lengthened from to 9 to 12 months and then to 2 years. Beginning in 1977, OTA students were required to take the certification exam. Currently, OTA students must complete at least 2 years of postsecondary education in an accredited program, which may be obtained at a community college, junior college, or technical training school. The OTA student must successfully complete Level I and Level II fieldwork experiences. The type of associate's degree (science or arts) awarded depends on the institution. Students who have completed all the educational requirements and Level II fieldwork are eligible to take the national certification examination for OTAs.

Box 5-2 shows the preamble of the *Standards for an Accredited Educational Program for the Occupational Therapy Assistant,* which describes the foundational requirements for an OTA.[2] Programs for the OTA typically focus less on theory and more on the "doing" aspects of the field, such as methods and procedures used in occupational therapy.[9]

OTA students may elect to further their education by seeking a baccalaureate degree in a related field and then obtain a basic master's degree in occupational therapy. Some universities offer special arrangements so that the OTAs receive credit for the work they have completed toward advanced degrees. Nontraditional programs, such as weekend and on-line formats, are available to help OTAs advance their education. Those wishing to advance their education are urged to communicate with faculty and explore options.

ENTRY-LEVEL CERTIFICATION AND STATE LICENSURE

Certification refers to the acknowledgment that an individual has the qualifications to be an entry-level practitioner, either an OTR or COTA. After completing the educational requirements and fieldwork, candidates at each educational level are eligible to sit for the national certification examination, administered by the **National Board for Certification in Occupational Therapy**. The certification exam is a 4-hour multiple-choice exam that covers evaluation and intervention planning for all areas of practice, ethics, delivery systems, and basic occupational therapy principles. Those candidates who pass the certification exam are then entitled to use the appropriate professional designation after their names—*registered* OT or *certified* OTA. Most states require licensure to practice in occupational therapy. Candidates residing in states that have licensure laws are then eligible to apply for a state license to practice, once they have passed the exam. (See Chapter 7 for further information on licensure.)

Candidates take the exam at a designated site via computer. If the candidate does not pass the examination, he or she may retake it until the test is passed. However, the candidate must pay for each attempt. Typically, persons working under a temporary license who fail the examination may not continue working in the capacity of an OT practitioner. They may work as aides until the test is passed.

Certification and registration have a long history in occupational therapy. In 1931, AOTA began a listing of OTs who had completed approved professional training and 1 year of subsequent work experience. This program for OTs was called **registration.** Those individuals who qualified were placed on the Main Register and granted the designation **registered occupational therapist.**[7] The first National Register, published in 1932, listed 318 OTs. In 1939, the standards for registration included the passage of a written essay examination. In 1947, the essay examination was converted to an objective multiple-choice examination, which is still in use today.

In the late 1950s, certification for OTAs was implemented for those individuals who graduated from an approved educational program. Initially, those individuals who had not graduated from an approved program but had worked a minimum of 2 years in one disability area were "grandfathered" in.[7] This plan was eliminated in 1963. The first OTA certification examination was administered in 1977.

During the 1970s, continued certification based solely on AOTA membership came under criticism. It was argued that each member's certification should come under periodic review rather than be automatically issued with an AOTA membership. As a result of these discussions, a category called "certified only" was created in the 1980s for practitioners who wanted to be certified without being a member of AOTA.[7] Additionally, during this time, state regulatory laws were focusing on the issue of competency in recertification.

The certification process underwent a major administrative change in 1986, when an autonomous certification board was created, separating AOTA membership and certification. This board was initially named the American Occupational Therapy Certification Board (AOTCB). In 1988, the AOTCB was incorporated as a separate entity from AOTA.[7] In 1996, AOTCB changed its name to the National Board for Certification in Occupational Therapy (NBCOT®). NBCOT® consists of a 15-member board of directors composed of 8 OT practitioners and 7 public members. NBCOT® functions independently in all aspects of initial certification. NBCOT® also has established procedures for and implemented a certification renewal program. Certification renewal with NBCOT® is discussed in Chapter 6.

SUMMARY

The OT and OTA are the two official levels of professionals in the field of occupational therapy, and each obtains formal education in occupational therapy theory, philosophy, and process. The formal education of the OT and OTA are similar in content, but a greater investment of time and a greater depth of knowledge are required of the OT. The OTA educational program typically takes 2 years to obtain an associate's degree; the OT degree requires a master's degree (5-6 years of study for a combined bachelor's and master's). Students who complete the required coursework in an OT or OTA program are eligible to sit for the national certification exam.

Learning Activities

1. Prepare a report on the national certification examination (when, where, cost).
2. Write a short paper on the history of occupational therapy education.
3. Interview an OT practitioner. Determine his or her motivation for entering the field. How did he or she learn about occupational therapy? Why did he or she decide to pursue the field? What is his or her educational background? Ask him or her to describe his or her fieldwork experiences.
4. Compare and contrast occupational therapy programs offered at two universities. Describe the levels of education, course requirements, and time.

Review Questions

1. What are the categories of OT personnel?
2. What are the educational requirements for each personnel category?
3. What are the professional requirements for each personnel category?
4. What is the Accreditation Council for Occupational Therapy Education?
5. What is the certification process for OT and OTA personnel?
6. What are the fieldwork requirements for OT and OTA personnel?

REFERENCES

1. Accreditation Council for Occupational Therapy Education of the American Occupational Therapy Association: Draft standards for an accredited educational program for the occupational therapist. Retrieved June 20, 2006, from www.aota.org.
2. Accreditation Council for Occupational Therapy Education of the American Occupational Therapy Association: Draft standards for an accredited educational program for the occupational therapy assistant. Retrieved June 20, 2006, from www.aota.org.
3. American Occupational Therapy Association: ACOTE Summer 2006 accreditation actions. Retrieved September 20, 2006, from www.aota.org.
4. American Occupational Therapy Association: Membership data: executive summary. Retrieved June 20, 2006, from www.aota.org.
5. American Occupational Therapy Association: *The Reference Manual of the Official Documents of the American Occupational Therapy Association, Inc.,* ed 10, Bethesda, MD, 2004, American Occupational Therapy Association.
6. American Occupational Therapy Association: The purpose and value of occupational therapy fieldwork education (2003 statement), *Amer J Occup Ther* 57:644, 2003.

7. American Occupational Therapy Association: Chronology of certification issues dated through January 29, *OT Week,* Feb 13, 1997.
8. Pierce D, Peyton C: A historical cross-disciplinary perspective on the professional doctorate in occupational therapy, *Am J Occup Ther* 53(1):64-71, 1999.
9. Punwar AJ, Peloquin SM: *Occupational Therapy Principles and Practice,* ed 3, Baltimore, 2000, Lippincott Williams & Wilkins.

I like helping people.

Okay, so maybe that sounds a little simplistic, but it is true. I like solving problems, connecting people with resources, working with an individual eye to eye, and setting and meeting goals. I like looking at not only the "forest," but also the "trees," and seeing each "tree" for the individual that he or she is and recognizing the unique and special characteristics that each person has to offer. I like treating a person with respect and dignity, and through the knowledge and skills that I possess as an occupational therapist, helping that person to achieve a life that is purposeful and meaningful to him or her, not by my definitions, but by what he or she defines as important. I like looking at the whole person, not just a body part or specific function, but as a precious asset to society, complex and dynamic. I like the look on someone's face when he or she realizes that he or she can accomplish far more than he or she ever thought he or she would be able to do before working with an occupational therapist. I like when "can't" becomes "can" and "doesn't" becomes "done."

I like helping people; I love being an OT.

Jill J. Page, OTR/L
Industrial Rehabilitation Consultant
ErgoScience, Inc.
Birmingham, Alabama

The Occupational Therapy Practitioner: Roles, Responsibilities, and Relationships

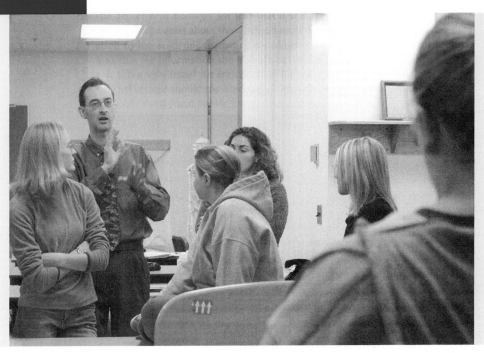

OBJECTIVES

After completing this chapter, the reader will be able to do the following:

- Identify the different roles an occupational therapy (OT) practitioner may assume
- Describe the three levels of performance for OT practitioners
- Explain the role of activity director
- Discuss the minimum responsibilities of the occupational therapist (OT), and the occupational therapy assistant (OTA) in service delivery as described in the *Standards of Practice*
- Understand the levels of supervision and parameters that affect these levels
- Identify the practices that contribute to successful supervisory relationships
- Describe service competency
- Describe the different types of teams in health care and recognize the importance of interdisciplinary teams
- Understand the importance of lifelong learning and professional development.
- Describe tools that can be used to maintain and document continuing competency

KEY TERMS

Activity director	Board certification	Client-related tasks
Advanced-level practitioner	Career development	Close supervision

Continued

When a student graduates from an Accreditation Council for Occupational Therapy Education (ACOTE)–accredited educational program and passes the National Board for Certification in Occupational Therapy (NBCOT®) national certification exam, there is a basic level of competence that is assumed, and a state license (in states that have licensure) is granted. At this point, the practitioner is considered to be an entry-level practitioner. This is an exciting point in time for OTs and OTAs, with many career opportunities and experiences for learning. In this chapter, we first discuss the various roles in which an OT practitioner may function. The responsibilities of the entry-level OT practitioner in service delivery are outlined, along with guidelines for supervision. Next, we describe some of the relationships found in service delivery and how the OT practitioner can work effectively within those relationships. Finally, we discuss how the entry-level practitioner develops knowledge and skills to maintain competency and advance in the profession. By understanding the available roles and responsibilities and their requirements, the entry-level OT practitioner can control the direction of his or her career.

PROFESSIONAL ROLES AND CAREER DEVELOPMENT

As a starting point, the student needs to understand what is meant by professional roles and relationships. As characterized by Crist,[14] **roles** specify positions or sets of stipulated job-related responsibilities. Each role carries with it specific expectations for job performance and responsibilities. An individual's ability to function in a role is based on educational preparation, professional boundaries and responsibilities, and prior experience in the role.[14] As in life, most people working in organizations have multiple roles. The connection of different roles to one another is a **relationship.** Working organizations are made up of many relationships. The combination of roles and relationships defines expectations in the organization and clarifies interactions.[14]

Direct client care is the role most commonly assumed by the OT practitioner who is just entering the field. However, there are an additional 10 roles identified by the profession that can potentially be held by OTs and OTAs. These include consumer educator, fieldwork educator in a practice setting, supervisor, administrator in a practice setting, consultant, academic fieldwork coordinator, faculty, academic program director, researcher/scholar, and entrepreneur. Each of these roles and a description of its major functions are shown in Table 6-1. Often, OT practitioners function in more than one role—at times within the same job. For example, an OT may provide direct client services and perform the functions of an administrator; an OTA may hold positions as both a faculty member and clinician.

As the career of an OT practitioner progresses, he or she may wish to advance within the service delivery path or transition into a role outside of service delivery. This is referred

TABLE 6-1   Occupational Therapy Roles

Role	Major Function
Practitioner—OT	Provides quality occupational therapy services, including evaluation, intervention, program planning and implementation, discharge planning–related documentation, and communication. Service provision may include direct, monitored, and consultative approaches.
Practitioner—OTA	Provides quality occupational therapy services to assigned individuals under the supervision of an OT.
Educator (consumer, peer)	Develops and provides educational offering or training related to occupational therapy to consumer, peer, and community individuals or groups.
Fieldwork Educator (practice setting)	Manages Level I or II fieldwork in a practice setting. Provides OT students with opportunities to practice and carry out practitioner competencies.
Supervisor	Manages the overall daily operation of occupational therapy services in defined practice area(s).
Administrator (practice setting)	Manages department, program, services, or agency providing occupational therapy services.
Consultant	Provides occupational therapy consultation to individuals, groups, or organizations.
Academic Fieldwork Coordinator	Manages student fieldwork program within the academic setting.
Faculty	Provides formal academic education for OT or OTA students.
Academic Program Director	Manages the educational program for OT or OTA students.
Researcher/Scholar	Performs scholarly work of the profession, including examining, developing, refining, and evaluating the profession's body of knowledge, theoretical base, and philosophical foundations.
Entrepreneur	Entrepreneurs are partially or fully self-employed individuals who provide occupational therapy services.

Adapted from American Occupational Therapy Association: Career exploration and development: a companion guide to the occupational therapy roles document. In *COTA Information Packet: A Guide for Supervision,* Bethesda, MD, 1993, AOTA.
Note: Many jobs involve more than one role, and job titles vary by setting.

to as **career development.** How the individual develops in a career will depend upon previous choices about roles and relationships.[14]

There are three ways in which career development occurs in occupational therapy: vertical movement within a setting, lateral movement across settings, and maturation within a role.[14] In vertical movement within a setting, the practitioner moves up in the organization to progressively higher positions. For example, a practitioner may move to the role of fieldwork educator, then department supervisor, and eventually manager of a rehabilitation clinic. A lateral movement across settings might involve an expert clinician transitioning to the role of a clinical instructor in a university setting. The third means of career development is the maturation of the individual within a specific role from entry level, to intermediate level, to an advanced level. For example from entry-level clinician to advanced clinical specialist.

LEVELS OF PERFORMANCE

Beyond entry level, not every practitioner performs at the same level. Three levels of performance can be identified for OT practitioners: entry, intermediate, and advanced. An individual's level of performance is not based on years of experience in the field, because this is not a valid indicator of performance. Instead, the practitioner's level of performance is based on attaining a higher skill level through work experience, education, and professional socialization.[9]

Table 6-2 describes the levels of performance and demonstrates how a practitioner's career may develop as knowledge and skill increase. The **entry-level practitioner** is expected to be responsible for and accountable in professional activities related to the role. In states with licensure laws, entry-level practice is defined by the licensure law and supporting regulations. The **intermediate-level practitioner** has increased responsibility and typically pursues specialization in a particular area of practice. The **advanced-level practitioner** is considered an expert, or a resource, in the respective role.

Each individual progresses along this continuum at a different pace. Some individuals never progress past the entry level in a particular role, or a person may transition to a new role, wherein his or her level of performance is classified at entry level. For example, an individual who has worked as an OT at the advanced level may transfer into an administrative role at the entry level. An OTA at the intermediate level may transition to the role of an entry-level faculty member. Even at the entry level, individuals in both situations may need to acquire additional knowledge and skill to satisfactorily perform the new job functions. It is also possible for an individual to function in two roles at different levels. For example, an OTA intermediate-level practitioner may assume new responsibilities as a fieldwork educator. In the new role, this OTA would initially perform the job function at the entry level.

For any type of role advancement or transition, the OT practitioner must be aware of what the expectations are for the new role and prepare accordingly. Methods to achieve role advancement or transition are discussed later, in the section on professional development.

TABLE 6-2 Levels of Performance

Role	Major Focuses
Entry	• Development of skills • Socialization in the expectations related to the organization, peer, and profession *Acceptance of responsibilities and accountability for role-relevant professional activities is expected.*
Intermediate	• Increased independence • Mastery of basic role functions • Ability to respond to situations based on previous experience • Participation in the education of personnel *Specialization is frequently initiated, along with increased responsibility for collaboration with other disciplines and related organizations. Participation in role-relevant professional activities is increased.*
Advanced	• Refinement of specialized skills • Understanding of complex issues affecting role functions *Contribution to the knowledge base and growth of the profession results in being considered an expert, resource person, or consultant within a role. This expertise is recognized by others inside and outside of the profession through leadership, mentoring, research, education, and volunteerism.*

Adapted from American Occupational Therapy Association: Occupational therapy roles, *Am J Occup Ther* 47:1087, 1993.

SPECIALIZED ROLES

There are specialized roles in which OT practitioners can function; however, these roles are typically outside of the profession. These include roles such as case manager, supervisor of other allied health care professionals, consultant, and activity director. These roles are advanced-level positions for OT practitioners. We discuss the role of activity director in the following section because it is a role that the OTA can function in without supervision.

Activity Director

The role of **activity director** is one for which the OTA is well qualified and can function independently.[22] Activity directors are typically employed in group homes, institutions for people with mental retardation, assisted living facilities, and long-term care facilities for the elderly. In these types of facilities, residents may withdraw and become isolated. The activity director is responsible for planning, implementing, and documenting an ongoing program of activities that meet the needs of the residents. The activity director needs to be aware of and adhere to regulations for activity programs and personnel that have been set forth by Medicare, state health departments, and licensing agencies.

The *Standards of Practice*[19] for the National Association of Activity Professionals classifies activities that are provided to the client as supportive, providing maintenance, or empowering. Supportive activities are commonly provided to individuals who do not have the cognitive or physical ability to participate in a group program. The purpose of these activities is to promote a comfortable environment and to provide stimulation to those individuals. Examples include placing meaningful objects in the person's room and providing background music. Maintenance activities are those that provide opportunities for the individual to maintain physical, cognitive, social, emotional, and spiritual health. Examples of maintenance activities are exercise groups, games such as shuffleboard, creative writing, and choir. Empowering activities are geared toward promoting self-respect, and they offer opportunities for self-expression, personal responsibility, and social responsibility. Writing a facility newsletter or forming a council dedicated to resolving residents' issues are examples of empowering activities.[19] In-depth information on the role of the OTA as an activity director can be found in *Ryan's Occupational Therapy Assistant*.[22]

ROLES AND RESPONSIBILITIES DURING SERVICE DELIVERY

The *Standards of Practice for Occupational Therapy*[6] defines the minimum requirements for OT practitioners working in service delivery. The standards are delineated into four areas: (1) professional standing and responsibility; (2) screening, evaluation, and re-evaluation; (3) intervention; and (4) outcomes. These standards are summarized in Table 6-3 and printed in full in Appendix B.

It is important to remember that these standards are guidelines developed by the American Occupational Therapy Association (AOTA) that support the *Scope of Practice for Occupational Therapy*.[8] They are often used by states in the formation of licensure laws and supporting regulations for occupational therapy practice. State licensure laws provide a legal definition of practice for that state and may delineate specific responsibilities for the OT and OTA related to role delineation, supervision, documentation, and advanced practice (see Chapter 7). The OT practitioner must provide services in accordance with the laws or regulations of the state in which he or she practices. Other regulatory agencies,

TABLE 6-3 Responsibilities of the Occupational Therapist and Occupational Therapy Assistant during the Delivery of Occupational Therapy Services

Service	Occupational Therapist	Occupational Therapy Assistant
Evaluation	Directing the evaluation process. Directing all aspects of the initial contact during the evaluation, including need for service, defining the problems within the domain of occupational therapy; determining client goals and priorities, establishing intervention priorities, determining further assessment needs, and determining assessment tasks that can be delegated to the OTA. Initiating and directing the evaluation, interpreting the data, and developing the intervention plan.	Contributing to the evaluation process by implementing delegated assessments. Providing verbal and written reports of observations and client capacities to the OT.
Intervention planning	Overall development of the occupational therapy intervention plan. Collaborating with the client to develop the plan.	Collaborating with the client to develop the plan. Being knowledgeable about evaluation results and for providing input into the intervention plan, based on client needs and priorities.
Intervention implementation	The overall implementation of the intervention. Providing appropriate supervision when delegating aspects of intervention to the OTA.	Being knowledgeable about the client's occupational therapy goals. Selecting, implementing, and modifying therapeutic activities and interventions that are consistent with demonstrated competency levels, client goals, and the requirements of the practice setting.
Intervention review	Determining the need for continuing, modifying, or discontinuing occupational therapy services.	Contributing to this process by exchanging information with and providing documentation to the OT about the client's responses to and communications during intervention.
Outcome evaluation	Selecting, measuring, and interpreting outcomes that are related to the client's ability to engage in occupations.	Being knowledgeable about the client's targeted occupational therapy outcomes and providing information and documentation related to outcome achievement. Implementing outcome measurements and providing needed client discharge resources.

Adapted from American Occupational Therapy Association: Standards of practice for occupational therapy, *Am J Occup Ther* 59(6):663–665, 2005, and from American Occupational Therapy Association: Guidelines for supervision, roles, and responsibilities during the delivery of occupational therapy services, *Am J Occup Ther* 58(6):663-667, 2004.

such as the Centers for Medicare and Medicaid Services (CMS), also have regulations that supersede these guidelines.

The first standard delineates requirements related to professional standing and responsibility for all OT practitioners. Key points related to Standard I are that the OT practitioner: (1) deliver services that reflect the philosophical base of occupational therapy; (2) be knowledgeable about and deliver services in accordance with AOTA standards, policies, and guidelines, and state and federal regulations; (3) maintain current licensure, registration, or certification as required; (4) abide by the AOTA *Occupational Therapy Code of Ethics*,[4] and *Standards for Continuing Competence*[5]; (5) maintain current knowledge of legislative, political, social, cultural, and reimbursement issues; and (6) be knowledgeable about evidence-based research.[6]

The second standard outlines the practitioner's responsibilities during screening, evaluation, and re-evaluation. An OT accepts and responds to referrals and initiates the screening, evaluation, and re-evaluation process. The OT is responsible for analyzing and interpreting the evaluation data. The OTA contributes to the process by performing assessments that have been delegated by the OT. The OTA communicates verbally or in writing to the OT his or her observations of the assessment and the client's abilities. The OT then completes and documents the evaluation results. The OTA contributes to the documentation of the evaluation results. The OT recommends additional consultations or refers client to appropriate sources as needed.[6]

Practitioner responsibilities during the intervention stage of service delivery are described in Standard III. The OT has the overall responsibility for documentation and implementation of the intervention, based on the evaluation, client goals, current best evidence, and clinical reasoning. The OTA can select, implement, and modify therapeutic activities (consistent with his or her demonstrated competency, delegated responsibilities, and intervention plan). The OT, with contributions from the OTA, modifies the intervention plan throughout the process and documents the client's responses and any changes to treatment.[6]

Requirements and responsibilities related to outcomes are delineated in Standard IV. The OT selects, measures, documents, and interprets outcomes that are related to the client's ability to engage in occupations. The OT is responsible for documenting changes in the client's performance and for discontinuing services. A discontinuation plan or transition plan is prepared by the OT, with contributions from the OTA regarding the client's needs, goals, performance, and follow-up services. Either practitioner facilitates the transition process in collaboration with the client, family members, and significant others. The OT evaluates the safety and effectiveness of the occupational therapy processes and interventions; the OTA contributes to this evaluation of safety and effectiveness.[6]

SUPERVISION

After initial certification and applicable state licensure, the entry-level OT functions independently in delivering occupational therapy services. It is recommended that he or she seek supervision and mentoring from a more experienced OT to grow professionally and to develop best approaches to practice. OTAs require supervision from an OT to deliver occupational therapy services. The OT is ultimately responsible for all aspects of the services provided by the OTA, the occupational therapy aide, and the OT student.

The document *Guidelines for Supervision, Roles, and Responsibilities During the Delivery of Occupational Therapy Services*[7] provides a definition of supervision and parameters for supervision. However, it is important for the OT practitioner to adhere to state and federal regulations, the *Occupational Therapy Code of Ethics*[4] (see Chapter 7), and the policies of the workplace. The regulations that delineate the specific responsibilities and supervisory requirements for the OT and OTA vary considerably from state to state. Each OT practitioner needs to be responsible for familiarizing him or herself with the appropriate state regulations. The AOTA website (www.aota.org) provides a summary of the supervision requirements for each state. Outside accreditation bodies (see Chapter 7) and third-party payers also have specific requirements related to supervision. For example, CMS specifies requirements regarding provision of services by students. Any facility that is reimbursed by Medicare needs to abide by these requirements.

Supervision is defined by AOTA as a "cooperative process in which two or more people participate in a joint effort to establish, maintain, and or elevate a level of competence and performance."[7] The supervisor is an individual "who has some official responsibility to direct, guide, and monitor the supervisee's practice."[12] It is important that the OT and OTA work collaboratively to develop and implement a plan for supervision that ensures safe and effective service delivery and promotes professional competence and development.[7]

LEVELS OF SUPERVISION AND PARAMETERS THAT AFFECT SUPERVISION LEVELS

Supervision can be quantified by the number of hours and the level, or intensity, of supervision that is provided. State and federal regulations specify requirements for levels of supervision. The OT student needs to be aware of terminology that may be used to describe the different levels of supervision.

It is helpful for the student to conceptualize supervision along a continuum as shown in Figure 6-1.[9,14] Supervision ranges from a level of being in direct contact at all times with the supervisee to a level wherein face-to-face contact occurs on a monthly basis. At the high end of the continuum is **direct supervision** (or continuous supervision), wherein the supervising OT is on site and available to provide immediate assistance to the client or supervisee if needed. **Close supervision** is the need for direct, daily contact. **Routine supervision** follows, in which there is direct contact at least every 2 weeks, with interim supervision as needed. **General supervision** is described as at least monthly face-to-face contact.[9]

Contact between a supervisor and supervisee can be face-to-face or via telecommunication. Some state regulations are very specific about the amount of face-to-face contact that is to take place at the different levels. For example, descriptors such as "daily," "once every seventh treatment," "one hour per 40 occupational therapy work hours," or "every 21 calendar

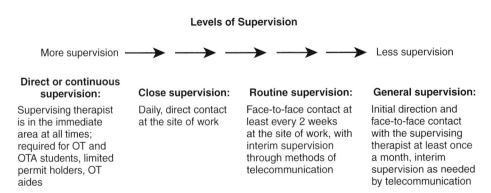

Levels of Supervision

More supervision ⟶ ⟶ ⟶ ⟶ ⟶ Less supervision

Direct or continuous supervision:	Close supervision:	Routine supervision:	General supervision:
Supervising therapist is in the immediate area at all times; required for OT and OTA students, limited permit holders, OT aides	Daily, direct contact at the site of work	Face-to-face contact at least every 2 weeks at the site of work, with interim supervision through methods of telecommunication	Initial direction and face-to-face contact with the supervising therapist at least once a month, interim supervision as needed by telecommunication

Figure 6-1 Levels of supervision in occupational therapy.

days" may be used by states to regulate the amount of face-to-face contact. Many state regulations specify that when the OT is not providing direct supervision, he or she must be available via methods of telecommunication at all times while the OTA is treating clients. These methods include the use of mobile phones, pagers, voice mail, and laptops with the capability of sharing client data and emailing each other.

Elaine is an OTA with over 10 years of experience in home health. She works under the supervision of an OT, but only sees her face-to-face once a month. She takes a mobile phone, a pager, and a laptop with her to every home visit. After her first visit of the day is complete, she checks her email using her laptop computer. She has an email message from her supervising OT that there is a new client whose evaluation has recently been completed, and the client needs to be scheduled for therapy. Elaine then goes into the agency database on her laptop and searches for the new client. In the client's electronic file, Elaine finds and reads the OT's evaluation report and treatment plan. Elaine locates the client's phone number and schedules an appointment for later that afternoon.

Most state regulations specify the number of OTAs whom an OT can supervise at any one time. For example, current regulations in California stipulate that an OT may supervise up to two OTAs; in Delaware, the maximum number of OTAs who can be supervised is three.[2] In some cases, states also stipulate how many years of experience the supervising OT needs to have before he or she can supervise an OTA.

The process of supervision is an ongoing one that changes with the setting and the individuals involved. Given the definitions of the levels described above, let us discuss the parameters that help determine the frequency, method, and content of supervision. The frequency, method, and content of supervision are dependent on several parameters. First, it is important to determine the regulatory requirements and requirements of the practice setting that pertain to supervision. The supervisor and supervisee also need to understand each other's level of competence, experience, education, and credentials. After these parameters have been established, supervision is based on the following:

- The complexity of client needs
- The number and diversity of clients
- The skills of the OT and OTA
- The type of practice setting

A level of supervision that is *more frequent* than the minimum level required by the practice setting and regulatory agencies may be required if (1) the needs of the client and the occupational therapy process are complex and fluctuating; (2) a large number of clients with diverse needs are served by occupational therapy in the practice setting; and (3) it is determined by the OT and OTA that additional supervision is necessary for the delivery of safe and effective occupational therapy services.[7] Based on all of these factors, the OT working with the OTA determines how much and what type of supervision is appropriate. Collaboratively, they develop and document a plan for supervision.

Once the plan is put in place, the supervisory contacts should be documented as well. This documentation may include the frequency of supervisory contact, the methods(s) or types(s) of supervision, content areas addressed during the contact, evidence to support areas and levels of competency, and signatures and credentials of the individuals participating in the supervisory process.[7] Keeping such records will meet regulatory requirements and also allow both the supervisor and supervisee to observe the progress made, to adjust job expectations as needed, and to provide evidence for both individuals of the completion of professional development activities.[11]

A co-signature of the supervising OT on treatment notes completed by the supervisee is another way of documenting that supervision has taken place. As a rule of thumb, documentation written by either an OT or OTA student always needs to have a signature by the supervisor. Individuals (OTs and OTAs) holding a temporary license or limited permit must also have a co-signature on documentation until the permanent license is received. OTAs do not necessarily have to have their documentation co-signed. Whether documentation by the OTA is co-signed depends on state and federal regulations, third-party reimbursement policies, and the policies of the practice setting. However, keep in mind that the supervisory process is an interactive one; it requires more than paper review and the execution of a co-signature on documentation.

Service Competency

Because the OT is responsible for the performance level of the OTA, he or she must have confidence that the OTA will obtain the same results when providing occupational therapy services. **Service competency** is a useful mechanism to ensure that services are provided with the same high level of confidence. Service competency is defined as "the determination, made by various methods, that two people performing the same or equivalent procedures will obtain the same or equivalent results. In test development, this is known as interrater reliability. The same concept can be applied to professionals working together in the service provision process. It stems from the assumption that the OT employs currently acceptable practices."[10]

The methods and standards to establish service competency vary, depending on the task or procedure involved. Methods such as independent scoring of standardized tests, observation, videotaping, and co-treatment can be used. For frequently used procedures, service competency is more easily established; procedures that are used less frequently may take longer to establish service competency and may require closer supervision in the meantime. Before service competency is established for a particular procedure, it is recommended that the acceptable standard of performance be met on three successive occasions between the OT and OTA.[10] It is important for each procedure that service competency is established to document the process used and the outcome.

SUPERVISION OF THE OCCUPATIONAL THERAPY AIDE

An occupational therapy aide is an individual who supports the OT and OTA by performing specifically delegated tasks.[7] Occupational therapy aides may also be referred to as restorative aides, service extenders, or rehabilitation aides/technicians. Depending on state law, either an OT or an OTA may supervise the occupational therapy aide; however, the OT remains the individual ultimately responsible for the actions of the aide. He or she directs the development, documentation, and implementation of a supervisory plan. The person working as an aide is not required to have any special training; typically, he or she receives on-the-job training from the OT practitioners. Because the level of training is limited, it is important that supervision remain close.

The aide is assigned to perform delegated, selected, client-related and non–client-related tasks for which the aide has demonstrated competency.[7] **Non–client-related tasks** include the preparation of the work area and equipment, clerical tasks, and maintenance activities. Examples of these types of tasks include setting up for a group activity in an outpatient mental health setting, making the daily schedule in an inpatient rehabilitation setting, and cleaning equipment in an outpatient hand clinic. The aide may provide **client-related tasks** that are routine tasks in which the aide may interact with the client but not as the primary service provider of occupational therapy.[7] These tasks must have (1) a predictable outcome; (2) a situation in which the client and environment are stable and that does not require judgments, interpretations or adaptations to be made by the aide; (3) a client who has demonstrated prior ability to perform the task; and (4) a clearly established task routine and process.[7] When assigning such tasks, the supervisor needs to ensure that the aide is competent in carrying out the selected task and in using related equipment; has been instructed in how to perform the task with the specific client; and is aware of any precautions, signs, or symptoms the particular client may demonstrate that would be an indication that assistance is needed.[7] The supervision of the aide needs to be documented as described earlier for the OTA.

OCCUPATIONAL THERAPIST–OCCUPATIONAL THERAPY ASSISTANT PARTNERSHIP: STRATEGIES FOR A SUCCESSFUL SUPERVISORY RELATIONSHIP

Beyond the practical need to determine appropriate duties and supervision, each OT practitioner needs to be aware that the roles of the OT and OTA are intentionally interrelated. The relationship is a partnership. For that partnership to be effective, there needs to be mutual respect and trust.

There are many factors that contribute to a successful supervisory relationship. The supervisor should have a solid knowledge base related to the practice of occupational therapy and guidelines for supervision. It is also important that the supervisor have an understanding of the different ways in which individuals learn, and an awareness of his or her own learning style as well as that of the supervisee. A key element in successful supervisory relationships is communication. Especially important is the ability to listen actively, to give and receive constructive feedback, to be assertive and tactful, and to resolve conflicts.[11] Instead of providing quick and easy answers to concerns brought up by the supervisee, the supervisor should be able to provide resources and direction that facilitate problem solving and clinical reasoning. Communication is discussed in Chapter 16.

Berger identifies some helpful practices to increase the likelihood for success in the supervisory process.[11] Setting a designated and prioritized time for supervision meetings will save time and make it more likely that the process will take place. Having a written agenda so that both the supervisor and supervisee know the issues and the priority in which they will be discussed will ensure that the time allotted is used most efficiently. As supervisory topics come up during the course of a week, it is helpful to jot these down on a running list of topics for supervisory meetings. Active participation by both supervisor and supervisee is critical to the success of the supervision process. Both parties should be involved in actively evaluating and discussing levels of competency, seeking feedback on performance, setting goals for the future, and maintaining records of professional development.[11]

HEALTH CARE TEAMS AND TEAMWORK

Another type of relationship that the practitioner will need to navigate is that of a health care team. Common disciplines that may be on a team with the OT practitioner are shown in Box 6-1. In health care today, working as a member of an interdisciplinary team is the norm. Entry-level practitioners need to first establish a solid identity with their own profession and its uniqueness.[15] The OT practitioner needs to have knowledge of the roles and responsibilities of other health professionals and good interpersonal, communication, and team-building skills.[21] Once this foundation is established, the practitioner is capable of building productive relationships with members of other disciplines.[15] An experienced OT

Box 6-1 Professionals Who Team with Occupational Therapy Practitioners

Adapted physical educator
Audiologist
Biomedical/rehabilitation engineer
Case manager
Dietician
Durable medical equipment provider
Nurse
Orthotist and prosthetist
Physical therapist
Physicians (primary care provider, physiatrist, neurologist, psychiatrist, ophthalmologist,
    orthopedist, cardiologist)
Psychologist
Rehabilitation counselor
Respiratory therapist
Recreation therapist
Social worker
Special educator
Speech-language pathologist
Vocational counselor

Adapted from Cohn ES: Interdisciplinary communication and supervision of personnel. In Crepeau EB, Cohn ES, Schell BAB
(eds): *Willard and Spackman's Occupational Therapy,* ed 10, Philadelphia, 2003, Lippincott Williams & Wilkins.

practitioner may in time have the responsibility for coordinating the interdisciplinary treatment team and supervising team members. Responsibilities of this role include organizing and leading team meetings, managing client data, and communicating results to doctors and administrators.

There are three different types of teams: multidisciplinary, interdisciplinary, and transdisciplinary. In a **multidisciplinary team,** there is a mix of multiple disciplines that work together in a common setting. However, the relationship between the team members is not interactive. At the other extreme is the **transdisciplinary team,** in which members cross over professional boundaries and share roles and functions.[13] In this approach, there is a blurring of traditional practitioner roles. The **interdisciplinary team** is somewhere in the middle of these two and is the one most commonly found in health care today. Members of an interdisciplinary team maintain their own professional roles and use a cooperative approach that is very interactive and centered on a common problem to solve.

In the interdisciplinary team approach, various disciplines meet and plan the overall care of the client, maintaining an awareness of his or her needs, responses, and goals. Team members become mutual sources of information and support in treatment. It is not uncommon for team members using this approach to co-treat (treatment provided by each team member at the same time) a client. For example, the team OT and speech-language pathologist may both treat a client with a swallowing disorder at mealtime. The OT will focus treatment on the client's skill of bringing the food to his mouth and chewing it, whereas the speech-language pathologist may be focused on producing an effective swallow. In this case, the common problem the therapists are working to remediate is the client's swallowing disorder. Each member focuses on what he or she does best and supports the other during the treatment.

There are many similarities between the working partnership of the OT and the OTA and interdisciplinary teams of professionals that work in health care. Similarities include the need to have an understanding about the roles of team members, knowledge of professional boundaries, knowledge of the group process (see Chapter 16), and good communication skills. Teams whose members are open minded, willing to hear and try new things, and tolerant of change are the most effective.[15]

LIFELONG LEARNING AND PROFESSIONAL DEVELOPMENT

The focus of this chapter has been on the roles and responsibilities of the entry-level practitioner who has a minimum skill base. But what about the OT practitioner who has been in practice 5, 10, or 15 years? The environment in today's world is dynamic and changes rapidly. In health care, changes in technology, research evidence, best practices, delivery mechanisms, and regulations occur constantly. A practitioner who does not keep up with these changes is opening himself or herself up to consequences ranging from self-dissatisfaction with one's performance to employer or client dissatisfaction and potential client harm.[17] How do the employer, third-party payers, and consumer know that the practitioner has kept abreast of these changes and continues to be competent to practice? Who is responsible for making certain that a practitioner is competent?

To keep pace with these changes, the OT practitioner needs to continually acquire new knowledge, skills, and other assets. The *Code of Ethics* states that the OT practitioner is responsible for achieving and maintaining competence in order to practice.[4] Thus, OT practitioners are obligated by the profession's *Code of Ethics* to commit to lifelong learning to ensure that they are competent to practice. Organizing and personally managing a cumulative series of work experiences to add to one's knowledge, motivation, perspectives, skills, and job performance is referred to as career development or **professional development.**[21]

An element of lifelong learning and professional development is continuing competence.[17] **Continuing competence** is defined as "a dynamic, multidimensional process in which the professional develops and maintains the knowledge, performance skills, interpersonal abilities, critical reasoning skills, and ethical reasoning skills necessary to perform his or her professional responsibilities."[16] The *Standards for Continuing Competence* establishes criteria in each of these areas by which the practitioner should examine his or her own competence (Table 6-4). The practitioner can use these standards as a guide for assessing the

TABLE 6-4 Standards of Continuing Competence

Standard	Description
Standard 1: Knowledge	OTs and OTAs shall demonstrate understanding and comprehension of the information required for the multiple roles and responsibilities they assume. The individual must demonstrate the following: • Mastery of the core of occupational therapy as it is applied in the multiple responsibilities assumed • Expertise associated with primary responsibilities • Integration of relevant evidence, literature, and epidemiological data related to primary responsibilities and to the consumer population(s) served • Integration of current Association documents and legislative, legal, and regulatory issues into practice

Continued

TABLE 6-4 Standards of Continuing Competence—cont'd

Standard	Description
Standard 2: Critical reasoning	OTs and OTAs shall employ reasoning processes to make sound judgments and decisions. The individual must demonstrate the following: • Deductive and inductive reasoning in making decisions specific to roles and responsibilities • Problem-solving skills necessary to carry out responsibilities • The ability to analyze occupational performance as influenced by environmental factors • The ability to reflect on one's own practice • Management and synthesis of information from a variety of sources in support of making decisions • Application of evidence, research findings, and outcome data in making decisions
Standard 3: Interpersonal abilities	OTs and OTAs shall develop and maintain their professional relationships with others within the context of their roles and responsibilities. The individual must demonstrate the following: • Use of effective communication methods that match the abilities, personal factors, learning styles, and therapeutic needs of consumers and others • Effective interaction with people from diverse backgrounds • Use of feedback from consumers, families, supervisors, and colleagues to modify one's professional behavior • Collaboration with consumers, families, and professionals to attain optimal consumer outcomes • The ability to develop and sustain team relationships to meet identified outcomes
Standard 4: Performance skills	OTs and OTAs shall demonstrate the expertise, aptitudes, proficiencies, and abilities to competently fulfill their roles and responsibilities. The individual must demonstrate expertise in the following: • Practice grounded in the core of occupational therapy • Therapeutic use of self, the therapeutic use of occupations and activities, the consultation process, and the education process to bring about change • Integration of current practice techniques and technologies • Updating performance, based on current research and literature • Quality improvement processes that prevent practice error and maximize client outcomes
Standard 5: Ethical reasoning	OTs and OTAs shall identify, analyze, and clarify ethical issues or dilemmas to make responsible decisions within the changing context of their roles and responsibilities. The individual must demonstrate the following: • Understanding and adherence to the profession's Code of Ethics, other relevant codes of ethics, and applicable laws and regulations • The use of ethical principles and the profession's core values to understand complex situations • The integrity to make and defend decisions based on ethical reasoning

Adapted from American Occupational Therapy Association: Standards for continuing competence, *Am J Occup Ther* 59(6):661-662, 2005.

current level of competence, developing capacity for the future, and documenting continuing competence.[5] The standards also serve as a foundational element in the development of AOTA's board certifications and specialty certifications (see following section).

The mission of AOTA, the National Board for Certification in Occupational Therapy (NBCOT®), and state regulatory boards is to protect the public and ensure quality services. Therefore they have a vested interest as well in the continuing competency of OT practitioners. Many states with licensure regulations require demonstration of continuing competence in order for the individual to renew his or her license. The OT practitioner demonstrates continuing competence through participation in various continuing education activities. The practitioner earns a certain number of contact hours or continuing education units. The number of contact hours required varies from stateto state and is specified in each state's licensure regulations. There are many avenues and resources available to practitioners for professional development. It is the practitioner's responsibility to determine what to do and which resources to use.

STRATEGIES FOR PROFESSIONAL DEVELOPMENT AND CONTINUING COMPETENCE

Each OT practitioner needs to accept personal ownership of his or her career and manage his or her own process for professional development and continuing competency. The key is for the OT practitioner to develop an idea of the direction he or she wants his or her career to take and set goals and activities to get there. Many activities are available for professional development and continuing competency. For example, the individual can participate in professional development activities at work, at conferences, at universities, in courses, or online. Practitioners are advised to develop a habit of reading a wide range of literature and attend as many state, regional, and national occupational therapy conferences as possible.[15] Attending conferences allows one to network with other practitioners and learn about the latest practices and research in the profession. A summary of typical professional development activities is listed in Box 6-2.

Tools, such as the Professional Development Tool (PDT), assist practitioners in the professional development process. The PDT, developed by AOTA, is available on the AOTA website. The objectives for the use of the PDT are the following[1]:
- Assess learning needs and organized professional growth activities toward self-identified professional or career outcomes
- Identify and pursue professional development opportunities that will improve practice and career opportunities
- Promote quality in the profession and contribute to the growth of the profession
- Fulfill one's responsibility for continuing competence

Using the PDT, the practitioner completes steps to identify personal and professional development interests and needs, create a professional plan, and document completion of activities in a professional development portfolio. Aside from AOTA's PDT, there are other resources that can assist practitioners in developing a professional portfolio.[18] Many students learn about professional portfolios and start the development of a portfolio during their educational process.

Certification renewal with NBCOT® is another mechanism that can be used to facilitate the process of professional development and continuing competency. When a practitioner is initially certified with NBCOT®, he or she can use the credential Registered Occupational Therapist® (OTR®) or Certified Occupational Therapy Assistant® (COTA®). This initial certification is in effect for 3 years. Every 3 years, the practitioner must complete NBCOT®'s

---

Box 6-2 Examples of Professional Development Unit Activities

These are examples of professional development activities that qualify for PDUs by NBCOT®. Professional development activity requirements for state licensing boards may be different.

- Attend outside workshops, seminars, lectures, professional conferences
- Complete self-assessment and professional development plan
- Develop instructional materials such as training manual
- Complete external self-study series or telecommunication course
- Find fellowship training in specific area
- Teach academic courses in occupational therapy or occupational therapy assistant program as a guest lecturer
- Complete independent learning/study with and without assessment component (e.g., continuing education article, video, audio, and/or online courses)
- Present at state, national, or international workshops, seminars, and conferences
- Make presentations for local organizations/associations
- Make peer presentations on specific treatment approaches or case studies
- Become a primary investigator in scholarly research
- Review a professional manuscript for journals or textbooks
- Join a professional study group/online study group
- Provide professional inservice training
- Publish an occupational therapy article in non–peer-reviewed publication (e.g., *OT Practice, SIS Quarterly, Advance, Community Newsletters,* etc.)
- Publish chapter(s) in occupational therapy or related professional textbook
- Do reflective OT practice in collaboration with an advanced-certified OT colleague
- Volunteer services to organizations, populations, or individuals

Refer to the NBCOT® website for complete and updated information: www.nbcot.org.
NBCOT®, National Board for Certification in Occupational Therapy; *PDU,* personal development unit.

---

requirements for certification renewal to continue to use the OTR® or COTA® credential. Renewal of certification with NBCOT® is voluntary, yet may be required by employers or for state licensure. To renew, practitioners submit proof of having completed a minimum of 36 professional development units (PDUs) within each 3-year certification renewal cycle. At least 50% of those units must be directly related to the delivery of occupational therapy services.[20] PDUs can be earned through a number of methods. Box 6-2 lists professional development activities that may apply to NBCOT® renewal.

Obtaining an advanced practice credential or specialty certification is another avenue for pursuing and documenting competency. Many OT practitioners gain advanced knowledge, skill, and experience in a specialized area of practice. The OT practitioner who completes the requirements for an advanced practice credential or specialized certification can represent himself or herself to employers, payers, and consumers as having a certain level of expertise and the qualifications to practice in the specialized area. Table 6-5 shows examples of credentials for advanced practice or specialty certification that OT practitioners may obtain.

AOTA currently provides **specialty certification** for both OTs and OTAs in driving and community mobility; environmental modification; feeding, eating, and swallowing; and low vision.[3] Competencies unique to each of these areas of practice have been defined. Practitioners must document a minimum of 2000 hours of experience as an OT or OTA and 600 hours of delivering occupational therapy services in the certification area to clients

TABLE 6-5   Specialty Certification/Advance Practice Credentials

Examples of Advanced Practice and Specialty Certification Credentials	Credential Awarded	Granting Organization*
Advanced Practitioner (for OTAs)	AP	AOTA
Board Certified in Pediatrics (for OTs)	BCP	AOTA
Board Certified in Mental Health (for OTs)	BCMH	AOTA
Board Certified in Gerontology (for OTs)	BCG	AOTA
Board Certified in Rehabilitation (for OTs)	BCR	AOTA
Assistive Technology Practitioner	ATP	RESNA
Certified Case Manager	CCM	CCMC
Certified Driving Rehabilitation Practitioner	CDRS	ADED
Certified Hand Therapist	CHT	ASHT
Certified Professional Ergonomist	CPE	BCPE
Certified Vocational Evaluation Specialist	CVE	CCWAVES
Trained in Neuro-developmental Therapy	NDT	NDTA
Certified to administer the Sensory Integration and Praxis Tests	SIPT	WSP/USC; SII

Adapted from Schell BAB, Crepeau EB, Cohn ES: Professional development. In Crepeau EB, Cohn ES, Schell BAB (eds): *Willard and Spackman's Occupational Therapy*, ed 10, Philadelphia, 2003, Lippincott Williams & Wilkins.
ADED, Association for Driver Rehabilitation Specialists; *AOTA,* American Occupational Therapy Association; *ASHT,* American Society of Hand Therapists; *BCPE,* Board of Certification in Professional Ergonomics; *CCMC,* Commission for Case Manager Certification; *CCWAVES,* Commission on Certification of Work Adjustment and Vocational Evaluation Specialist; *NDTA,* Neuro-developmental Training Association; *RESNA,* Rehabilitation Engineering and Assistive Technology Society of North America; *SII,* Sensory Integration International; *WSP/USC,* Western Psychological Service/University of Southern California.

over the last 3 calendar years. After these requirements are met, the applicant submits an application, verification of employment, and a reflective portfolio demonstrating achievement of defined competencies.

Board certification, which incorporates more generalized areas of practice that have an established knowledge base in occupational therapy, is also offered by AOTA. Board certification is targeted specifically for OTs and is offered in gerontology, mental health, pediatrics, and physical rehabilitation.[3] Certification is based on the completion and peer review of a portfolio, a professional development plan, and a rigorous self-assessment that is grounded in the *Standards for Continuing Competence*[5] instead of an exam. To apply for board certification, the practitioner needs to have a minimum of 5000 hours of experience as an OT in the certification area in the last 7 calendar years and a minimum of 500 hours of experience delivering occupational therapy services (paid or voluntary) in the certification area to clients in the last 5 calendar years.

Several other organizations offer voluntary certification based on the passage of an examination, evidence of experience, or both (see Table 6-5). Sensory Integration International offers a specialty certification in sensory integration (SI). The American Society of Hand Therapists certifies individuals in hand therapy, and those who pass the examination are allowed to use the designation of certified hand therapist (CHT) after their names. The Rehabilitation Engineering and Assistive Technology Society of North America (RESNA) offers a specialty certification in assistive technology. Those who submit verification of a certain amount of work experience and pass the examination are allowed to use the designation of assistive technology provider (ATP) after their name. These are just a few examples of the many specialty certifications currently available.

SUMMARY

The primary role for the entry-level OT practitioner is in service delivery. Once a practitioner increases his or her level of expertise and knowledge, he or she can assume or transition to various other roles within and outside of occupational therapy. The *Standards of Practice* delineates the responsibilities of OT practitioners in service delivery. The OT and OTA have a collaborative partnership in which they plan, implement, and document frequency and methods of supervision. For health care professionals, involvement in lifelong learning and professional development is important to maintain competency for practice.

Learning Activities

1. Develop a career plan based on your education. In what role(s) and at what level of performance do you want to be functioning in 5 years? 10 years? 15 years?
2. AOTA has published papers that describe the specialized knowledge and skills needed to practice in specific areas. Find these documents online or in your library, and identify the areas of practice that have developed special knowledge base and skills. Why have these been developed? How are these different from the minimum standards of practice?
3. Some states licensure laws delineate advanced areas of practice in which the OT practitioner is required to have specialized knowledge and skills. Research the regulations for the state in which you live, and identify any areas requiring advanced knowledge and skills.
4. Box 6-1 lists a number of professionals with whom OT practitioners may team. Are you familiar with the roles of each of these professionals? If there are professional roles that are not familiar to you, research them online, and write down their primary functions.
5. Interview an OT practitioner. Write a paper describing his or her job, requirements, supervision, and role within the team. Provide examples of the level of performance the practitioner functions.
6. Observe an OT and OTA working together. Describe the relationship and the type of supervision the OTA receives from the OT. Interview each practitioner to gain insight on how this relationship works or could be improved. Write a summary of your findings, and present to class.
7. Compare and contrast in a short paper the role of the OT practitioner when working in a multidisciplinary, transdisciplinary, or interdisciplinary team.
8. Develop a presentation on professional development opportunities in your state. Complete the AOTA Professional Development Tool.[1] Provide a summary of your findings.

Review Questions

1. Describe the three levels of performance that OT practitioners progress through as they obtain experience.
2. What are the minimum requirements (hint: standards) for OT and OTA working in service delivery?
3. What is meant by service competency, and how may it be achieved?
4. Describe the OT/OTA relationship.
5. Describe the OT practitioner's role in multidisciplinary, transdisciplinary, and interdisciplinary teams.

REFERENCES

1. American Occupational Therapy Association: Professional Development Tool, Bethesda, MD, 2003, AOTA. Retrieved July 25, 2006, from http://www.aota.org/pdt.

2. American Occupational Therapy Association: Occupational therapy assistant supervision requirements, June, 2003. Retrieved July 29, 2006, from http://www.aota.org/ members/ area4/docs/otachart.pdf.

3. American Occupational Therapy Association: AOTA board and specialty certification programs. Retrieved July 17, 2006, from www.aota.org/nonmember/area 15.

4. American Occupational Therapy Association: Occupational therapy code of ethics (2005), *Am J Occup Ther* 59(6):639-642, 2005.

5. American Occupational Therapy Association: Standards for continuing competence, *Am J Occup Ther* 59(6):661-662, 2005.

6. American Occupational Therapy Association: Standards of practice for occupational therapy, *Am J Occup Ther* 59(6):663-665, 2005.

7. American Occupational Therapy Association: Guidelines for supervision, roles, and responsibilities, *Am J Occup Ther* 58(6):663-667, 2004.

8. American Occupational Therapy Association: Scope of practice, *Am J Occup Ther* 58:673-677, 2004.

9. American Occupational Therapy Association: Occupational therapy roles, *Am J Occup Ther* 47: 1087, 1993.

10. American Occupational Therapy Association: Entry-level role delineation for registered occupational therapists (OTRs) and certified occupational therapists (COTAs), *Am J Occup Ther* 44:1091, 1990.

11. Berger S: Personnel considerations and supervision. In Solomon A, Jacobs K (eds): *Management Skills for the Occupational Therapy Assistant,* Thorofare, NJ, 2003, Slack Inc.

12. Cohn ES: Interdisciplinary communication and supervision of personnel. In Crepeau EB, Cohn ES, Schell BAB (eds): *Willard and Spackman's Occupational Therapy,* ed 10, Philadelphia, 2003, Lippincott Williams & Wilkins.

13. Cook AM, Hussey SM: *Assistive Technologies: Principles and Practice,* ed 2, St. Louis, 2002, Mosby.

14. Crist P: Roles, relationships, and career development. In Johnson M (ed): *The Occupational Therapy Manager,* rev. ed, Bethesda MD, 1996, American Occupational Therapy Association.

15. Gilkeson GE: *Occupational Therapy Leadership: Marketing Yourself, Your Profession, and Your Organization,* Philadelphia, 1997, FA Davis.

16. Hinojosa J, Bowen R, Case-Smith J, et al: Standards for continuing competence for occupational therapy practitioners, *OT Practice* 5(20):CE-1–CE-7, 2000.

17. Moyers PA, Hinojosa J: Continuing competence. In McCormack GL, Jaffe EG, Goodman-Lavey M (eds): *The Occupational Therapy Manager,* ed 4, Baltimore, 2003, American Occupational Therapy Association Press.

18. Nagayda J, Schindehette S, Richardson J: *The Professional Portfolio in Occupational Therapy: Career Development and Continuing Competence,* Thorofare, NJ, 2005, Slack Inc.

19. National Association of Activity Professionals: *Standards of Practice: Section A-Standards of Care,* Washington, DC, 1991, National Association of Activity Professionals.

20. National Board for Certification in Occupational Therapy: PDU activities chart. Retrieved August 1, 2006, from www.nbcot.org.

21. Punwar AJ: Roles and functions of the occupational therapist and occupational therapy assistant. In Punwar AJ, Peloquin SM: *Occupational Therapy: Principles and Practice,* Baltimore, 2000, Lippincott Williams & Wilkins.

22. Ryan SE, Sladyk K: The occupational therapy assistant as activity director. In Sladyk K, Ryan SE, (eds): *Ryan's Occupational Therapy Assistant: Principles, Practice Issues and Techniques,* Thorofare, NJ, 2005, Slack Inc.

I chose the field of occupational therapy because the profession seemed limited only by the individual professional. As an occupational therapist, I have had numerous choices of work settings and ages of clients with whom I have interacted. I have worked in acute care hospitals, comprehensive outpatient and adult day care settings, public school settings, regular day care settings, preschool settings for children with special needs, as well as home environments. I have had the pleasure of working with clients of all ages from diverse cultural backgrounds. I am currently teaching in a community college. Our typical OTA student is nontraditional in age and historical background.

While working in the direct service arena, I was rewarded on a regular basis as my clients progressed, gaining more active interaction with others and control of themselves and their environment. I believe I have been able to significantly impact the quality of life of my clients. In essence, it is not how long we live (quantity) but rather how we live (quality). Occupational therapists are in a unique position to assist in improving the quality of life of the persons whom we serve.

Jean W. Solomon, MHS, OTR/L
Clinical Coordinator and Instructor
Occupational Therapy Assistant Program
Department of Rehabilitative Services
Trident Technical College
Charleston, South Carolina

Practicing Legally and Ethically

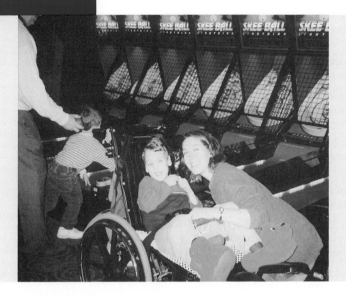

OBJECTIVES

After reading this chapter, the reader will be able to do the following:
- Understand the purpose of a code of ethics
- Identify the seven principles in the *Occupational Therapy Code of Ethics*
- Describe the function of the Ethics Commission
- Outline the steps to ethical decision-making
- Distinguish between ethical and legal behavior
- Explain the purpose and implementation of state laws regulating occupational therapy (OT)
- Describe the disciplinary processes developed by state regulatory boards and the professional association
- Discuss the similarities and differences of morals, ethics, and laws and their connection to the practice of occupational therapy

KEY TERMS

Autonomy	Ethics	Morals
Beneficence	Fidelity	Nonmaleficence
Clinical reasoning	Informed consent	Regulations
Code of ethics	Law	Statutes
Confidentiality	Licensure	Veracity
Ethical dilemma	Locus of authority	
Ethical distress	Mandatory reporting	

Health care today is very complicated, and systems often place the practitioner in a position to deal with ethical dilemmas. The need for increased productivity, managed care policies, and an increase in consumer activism have placed extra burden on practitioners for decision-making. On a daily basis, occupational therapy practitioners are confronted with situations that require decisions. Morals, ethics, and laws have the potential to affect the clinician's decision-making in practice.

Morals are related to character and behavior from the point of view of right and wrong. Morals develop as a result of background, values, religious beliefs, and the society in which a person lives. Thus, OT practitioners bring their individual morals to a given situation, and those morals may or may not be in agreement with the client's morals. Professional decisions may or may not be based on the practitioner's morals; rather, decisions are based upon ethics. In other words, practitioners must rely on more than "this is what I believe or was raised to believe." No practitioner should be obligated to abide by another person's morality; however, practitioners are required to comply with professional ethics and legal mandates.[13]

Ethics is the study and philosophy of human conduct. Ethics is "a systematic reflection on and an analysis of morals."[12] Ethics guide how a person behaves and makes decisions so that the best or "right" conduct is carried out. **Law** is defined as "a binding custom or practice of a community: a rule of conduct or action prescribed or formally recognized as binding or enforced by a controlling authority."[11] Laws are established by an act of the federal or state legislature. Laws are intended to protect citizens from unsafe practice, whereas ethics compel the professional to provide the highest level of care.

Ethics and laws are closely intertwined. However, ethics differ from laws and rules in that ethical standards are more general, and their intent is to give positive guidance rather than impose binding and negative limits to specific situations. However, because ethics today have been blended with laws to form professional standards, ethical misconduct may also constitute a violation of the law.[13]

In this chapter, the *Occupational Therapy Code of Ethics* and an approach to ethical decision-making are described. State licensure laws and regulations of the profession are also discussed, including potential sanctions when a practitioner violates the regulations.

PRACTICING ETHICALLY

Frequently, OT practitioners encounter situations in which they must weigh alternatives and make decisions about a course of action. Some situations are easy to resolve whereas others may challenge one's decision-making abilities. Clinicians frequently rely on their own values and morals when deciding a course of action. However, professional decision-making relies on a systematic ethical problem-solving process.

Clinical reasoning involves understanding the client's diagnoses, strengths, weaknesses, prognosis, and goals. Practitioners use clinical reasoning to develop and provide intervention to address goals and make necessary adaptations. Clinical reasoning requires problem-solving and professional judgment; therefore, it improves with experience, reflection, and critical analysis. Practitioners use clinical reasoning along with morals and ethics when making professional decisions.

A professional **code of ethics** provides direction to members of a profession for mandatory behavior and protects the rights of clients, subjects, their significant others, and the general public.[13] For example, the code of ethics dictating that OT practitioners treat each client equitably describes a basic principle of the occupational therapy profession. Ethical codes provide guidelines for making correct or proper choices and decisions of health care practice in the field.[4,12] These guidelines are usually stated in the form of principles.

AMERICAN OCCUPATIONAL THERAPY ASSOCIATION CODE OF ETHICS

The American Occupational Therapy Association (AOTA) *Occupational Therapy Code of Ethics*[4] was initially adopted by AOTA's Representative Assembly in April, 1977. This code provides guidelines to practitioners to help them recognize and resolve ethical dilemmas, to practice at the expected standard using guiding principles, and to educate the public (see Appendix A). The *Code of Ethics* is meant to inspire professional conduct for quality and empathetic occupational therapy while respecting the diversity of clients. The *Code of Ethics* is based upon the core values of the profession.[9]

The *Occupational Therapy Code of Ethics* consists of seven principles, each addressing a different aspect of professional behavior.[4] Following is a brief description of each principle and an example to illustrate professional application.

PRINCIPLE 1: BENEFICENCE

In general terms, the principle of **beneficence** means that the OT practitioner will contribute to the good health and welfare of the client. Principle 1 of the *Occupational Therapy Code of Ethics* has four parts, each of which is related to the well-being of the recipient of services. This principle highlights the need for OT practitioners to (1) treat each client fair and equitably, (2) advocate for recipients to obtain needed services, (3) promote public health and safety and well-being, and (4) charge fees that are reasonable and commensurate with the services provided.[4]

> Mr. Parker can no longer pay for occupational therapy services. The occupational therapist (OT) (Karen) started a daily self-feeding program for Mr. Parker prior to his funds running out. The therapist visits Mr. Parker at mealtime and explains the proper use of the adaptive equipment to the aide. Karen discusses how to work on independence and what assistance may still be needed upon discharge. The therapist does not bill for this instructive visit, knowing that Mr. Parker will receive better care after she has personally addressed the issues.

This example illustrates the principle of beneficence in that the OT practitioner shows concern for the client by ensuring that the aide is properly trained in feeding techniques. The OT practitioner advocates that the client receive the services he needs.

> When serving as a consultant to a residence facility for individuals who have severe mental retardation, Judy, the OT, becomes aware that another therapist, Sam, is billing for one-half-hour individual intervention sessions. In reality, Sam only passes through the unit and briefly talks with the clients and does not provide treatment. After observing the pattern for several weeks, Judy speaks with Sam, who brushes off the inquiry, "Look, we all have plans on file, but these kids aren't going to progress no matter what we do." Judy documents the situation and brings the matter to the attention of the administrator.

In this case, Judy must address the breech of ethical conduct by Sam. Sam is financially exploiting the client by charging for intervention services that do not take place.

PRINCIPLE 2: NONMALEFICENCE

The principle of **nonmaleficence** means that the practitioner should not inflict harm on the client. This principle ensures that OT practitioners maintain therapeutic relationships that do not exploit clients physically, emotionally, psychologically, socially, sexually, or financially. Furthermore, the OT practitioner is obligated to identify and address problems that may impact professional duties and bring concerns regarding professional skills of colleagues to the appropriate authority.[4] In that OT practitioners work with a variety of clients, it is the practitioner's responsibility to address concerns and foresee possible harmful situations so that harm can be avoided. The principle of nonmaleficence requires practitioners to avoid any relationships, activities, or undue influences that may interfere with services.[4]

> Tonya, a 15-year-old teen attending an outpatient group for eating disorders, becomes exceptionally attached to the OT practitioner, Mark. The teen calls Mark at home to discuss her intervention plan, telling Mark she got his phone number from her cousin, whom Mark knows from school. Mark limits the call and speaks to Tonya the next day at group, explaining to Tonya that it is inappropriate to call him at home and reiterating the professional nature of their relationship. Tonya is upset, but agrees that she will not call him. Mark asks a colleague to work with Tonya. He does not completely stop working with Tonya because he does not want her to feel rejected, but rather reinforces professional boundaries.

This example illustrates nonmaleficence (i.e., do no harm). Mark believes the relationship between himself and the teen may be harmful to the teen's intervention plan. Tonya has become too attached and is unsure of the boundaries. Mark is truthful with the teen and brings the situation up with the team so that no emotional harm will come to Tonya. The team supports him in continuing to serve on the team so that he does not completely reject Tonya. The team fears that complete rejection may harm Tonya emotionally and result in slower progress or regression in her treatment.

PRINCIPLE 3: AUTONOMY AND CONFIDENTIALITY

Principle 3 protects the client's right of **autonomy** and **confidentiality**. Autonomy is the freedom to decide and the freedom to act.[11] Confidentiality refers to the expectation that information shared by the client with the OT practitioner, either directly or through written or electronic forms, will be kept private and shared only with those directly involved with the intervention (under conditions expected by the client).[2,12] Confidentiality also stipulates that the client will determine how and to whom information may be shared. This principle requires OT practitioners to respect a client's right to refusal of treatment, and it protects all privileged communication.[12]

According to Principle 3, the OT practitioner (1) collaborates with clients and caregivers to determine goals; (2) informs clients of the nature, possible risks, and outcomes of services; (3) receives informed consent for services; (4) respects a client's decision to refuse treatment; and (5) maintains confidentiality concerning information.[4]

Informed consent refers to the "knowledgeable and voluntary agreement by which a client undergoes intervention that is in accord with the patient's values and preferences."[12] Thus clients have the right to refuse intervention and the right to be made aware of the risks, benefits, and cost of occupational therapy intervention.

Mrs. Jones, who is indigent and lives in a nursing home, resists going to occupational therapy but rather constantly asks to return to her room. The therapist, Andrea, learns that Mrs. Jones is afraid someone will steal her things. Andrea deals with the issue by making an intervention plan to address Mrs. Jones's fear that she will lose her hairbrush, an old mirrored compact, a brocade change purse, a bottle of toilet water, and a pair of underpants. Mrs. Jones does not want to tell anyone, but with her consent Andrea obtains a wheelchair carrier. Part of Mrs. Jones's intervention plan is the use of a checklist to pack her carrier with these treasured belongings each morning and to unpack it at the end of each day. The staff is informed that using a daily checklist is part of her occupational therapy program. Now Mrs. Jones goes to activities and therapy without protest.

This example illustrates a respect for the rights of both autonomy and confidentiality. The therapist allowed Mrs. Jones the freedom to choose to keep her treasures with her. This autonomy gave Mrs. Jones the assurance and comfort to participate in occupational therapy activities. The therapist respected her confidences by being careful to only discuss the contents of the carrier with Mrs. Jones, but informing the team of the intervention plan. The therapist respected Mrs. Jones's right to decide if and how she will participate in therapy and allowed her to contribute to the intervention planning process. The practitioner respected Mrs. Jones's right to confidentiality by not discussing with others the reasons she refused to go to therapy.

PRINCIPLE 4: DUTY

Principle 4 stipulates that all OT practitioners must maintain a high standard of competence, that is, one's standard of practice. It is the OT practitioner's duty to have the appropriate credentials, participate in continuing education and professional activities, and take responsibility for lifelong learning. Competent practitioners follow AOTA's *Standards of Practice,* use procedures that are accurate and current, receive appropriate levels of supervision, perform duties appropriate to their qualifications and experience, and know when to consult or refer to other service providers.[5] Remaining competent requires that practitioners read and critique current literature, evaluate evidence concerning practice, reflect upon practical skills, and seek feedback and mentoring. The principle of duty also requires that OT practitioners refer to or consult with other services as needed.

Ricardo, an OT, accepted a new job in a school system that occasionally uses sensory integration (SI) therapy. Ricardo's only exposure to SI was in school several years earlier, and thus he does not feel qualified to use SI therapy. He plans to take an SI workshop. Furthermore, he requests guidance and mentoring from his supervisor (who is SI trained) on SI intervention programs.

In this example, the therapist asked a qualified OT practitioner to closely supervise an area in which he does not have the level of competence required. The therapist is aware that he needs further education and experience before he is competent to practice in this area.

PRINCIPLE 5: PROCEDURAL JUSTICE

OT practitioners are obligated to comply with the laws and regulations that guide the profession. The OT practitioner must be aware of and follow federal, state, and local laws, as well as institutional policies. The practitioner may also need to inform employers, employees, and colleagues about these laws and policies. OT practitioners must accurately report and document information related to professional activities.[4]

> Before Kaitlin, an occupational therapy assistant (OTA), moves to a new state, she requests a copy of the licensure law and notes that the new state limits some treatment modalities. Once employed, she reads the employer's policies and procedures manual regarding facility records and acquaints herself with the department's style of record-keeping. The facility uses a specific style for documenting intervention. Although not familiar with the style of charting, Kaitlin refreshes her understanding with the format and implements it in her documentation.

The OT practitioner in this example is in compliance with state laws related to intervention procedures and with the documentation policies delineated by the facility where she works.

PRINCIPLE 6: VERACITY

Veracity refers to the duty of the health care professional to tell the truth. OT practitioners must accurately represent their qualifications, education, training, and competence.[2,4] Practitioners may not use any form of false advertising or exaggerated claims. The OT practitioner must disclose instances that pose actual or potential conflicts of interest. Furthermore, the OT practitioner must accept responsibility for actions that reduce the public's trust in occupational therapy services.

> Kevin, a therapist who is opening a private practice, makes certain that the advertising circulars promoting his private practice center do not the make any exaggerated claims about the center's ability to "cure" or make unrealistic promises of creating a "new life."

This example illustrates the principle of veracity because the clinician assures that advertisements for his private practice are truthful while promoting its services.

PRINCIPLE 7: FIDELITY

Fidelity, or faithfulness, in professional relationships describes the interactions between an OT practitioner and his or her colleagues and other professionals. Such aspects as the importance of maintaining confidentiality in matters related to colleagues and staff; accurately representing qualifications, views, and findings of colleagues; and reporting any misconduct to the appropriate entity are considered part of fidelity.[4] This principle includes statements concerning taking measures to discourage, prevent, expose, or correct any breeches of the code.[4]

Lindsay, an OT student, just completed her thesis for her master's degree, and her faculty advisor wants to present the results at national conference. The faculty advisor asks Lindsay for permission to submit a conference proposal describing the results of her thesis with the understanding that Lindsay will be listed as the principal author. Lindsay is also encouraged to present the paper with the faculty advisor, if the proposal is accepted.

In this example, the professor demonstrates the principle of fidelity to her student colleague. By ensuring that both the faculty advisor's name and the student's name are on the paper, she is accurately reporting who has been involved in both gathering the data and reporting the findings.

SOLVING ETHICAL PROBLEMS

Ethical problems may be divided into three categories: ethical distress, ethical dilemma, or locus of authority problems. **Ethical distress** situations challenge how a practitioner maintains his or her integrity or the integrity of the profession.[12] An **ethical dilemma** is a situation in which two or more ethical principles collide with one another, making it difficult to determine the best action. Problems with **locus of authority** require decisions about who should be the primary decision-maker.[12] These situations rely on the ethical decision-making process.

Generally, six steps are used to resolve an ethical problem:[11,12]

1. Gather all the relevant facts about the situation. Describe the clinical, contextual, individual, and personal preferences concerning the situation.
2. Identify the type of ethical problem (e.g., distress, dilemma, locus of authority). Determine the ethical principles involved (e.g., beneficence, nonmaleficence, justice, veracity, autonomy, confidentiality, fidelity).
3. Clarify professional duties in this situation that may be outlined in the *Code of Ethics* (e.g., do no harm, tell the truth, keep promises, and be faithful to colleagues). What is the conduct required of each professional (including yourself)?
4. Explore alternatives, including the desired outcome and consequences of actions.
   a. Describe features that are pertinent to this situation, including facts, laws, wishes of others, resources, risks, *Code of Ethics,* degree of certainty of the facts on which a decision is based, predominant values of the others involved.[3,12]
   b. Who are the other people involved? What are the consequences of the actions for the interested parties?
5. Complete the action.
6. Evaluate the process and the outcome.

The ability to decide which action to take may be developed by understanding the steps and discussing situations in which there are conflicting elements. Examining ethical distress, dilemmas, and locus of authority problems provides the opportunity to base professional decisions on ethical reasoning. Examining situations systematically benefits clients, professionals, and the employer.

The case application in Box 7-1 provides an example of the ethical decision-making process.

Box 7-1   Dave: A Case Application of the Ethical Decision-Making Process

Dave, a 13-year-old boy, has reached his occupational therapy goals. He was injured in an automobile accident wherein the driver had excellent insurance coverage, so the insurance is still available. Reportedly, his home situation is not good; both parents are alcoholics and have difficulty staying employed; there is concern for his welfare. Dave enjoys the attention he receives in therapy and works hard on his goals. In the time the OT practitioner has worked with him, his whole attitude has improved. He wants to keep coming to occupational therapy, but his occupational therapy goals have been reached. The OT practitioner is meeting with the team and must make a recommendation as to whether or not to continue intervention. The practitioner enjoys working with Dave and has established a meaningful and positive therapeutic relationship.

Following is a description of how to work through this case using the ethical decision-making process.

STEPS IN THE ETHICAL DECISION-MAKING PROCESS	CONSIDERATION AND ANALYSIS OF THE STEPS
1. Gather all the relevant facts about the situation. Describe the clinical, contextual, individual, and personal preferences concerning the situation.	• *Dave will be returning home to a less than optimal situation.* • *Dave's parents are both alcoholics who have difficulty keeping employment.* • *Dave has moved frequently.* • *Dave's parents are inconsistent in visiting him.* • *Dave loves the attention he gets during occupational therapy intervention.* • *Dave is well liked by his older peers in the rehabilitation setting.* • *If Dave continues to come to occupational therapy services, he may become dependent upon a support structure that is not readily available to him upon eventual discharge. The team is concerned for the welfare of the child; social workers are involved in the case.* • *Dave has a tutor, who will make home visits upon discharge. The teacher, school psychologist, and family physician are all important members of the team.*
2. Identify the type of ethical problem (e.g., distress, dilemma, locus of authority). Determine the ethical principles involved (e.g., beneficence, nonmaleficence, justice, veracity, autonomy, confidentiality, fidelity).	• *Ethical distress is illustrated as the OT practitioner examines whether Dave should continue to receive occupational therapy services after meeting his goals. The OT practitioner, experiencing ethical distress, wonders if her integrity would be compromised by providing services to a child who may not require them.* • *The ethical dilemma can be defined as discharging Dave now that he has reached his goals or continuing occupational therapy services, which may require new goals.* • *Locus of authority problem is depicted in that the child (a minor) wants to continue with therapy, yet his parents (who have substance abuse issues) may not serve his best interest. The OT practitioner must decide if she will rely on the wishes of the parents, the child, or the institution (which supports continued treatment due to financial income) to determine intervention.* • *The OT practitioner may hypothesize that occupational therapy services could still help the child and that returning home to an unsupportive environment may do more harm. Thus, the principle of beneficence (do well) is being challenged. Furthermore, the*

Box 7-1 Dave: A Case Application of the Ethical Decision-Making Process—cont'd

the professional issue of providing services to a child who has reached his goals may challenge the principle of veracity (truthfulness). The OT practitioner may have to be less than truthful in saying the child requires occupational therapy services. Fidelity is challenged by not trusting other colleagues to serve the child.

3. Clarify professional duties in this situation that may be outlined in the *Code of Ethics* (e.g., do no harm, tell the truth, keep promises, and be faithful to colleagues).

- *The OT practitioner is responsible for helping Dave return to the occupations that he desires, including school, community activities, and activities of daily living. Although the child has reached the physical and social goals, as per his intervention plan, the practitioner believes Dave may require some modifications to be successful in school. The OT practitioner also remains concerned that Dave's support system (e.g., his parents) may not adequately assist him. After careful consideration, the practitioner acknowledges that other professionals, such as the social worker and school psychologist, may be able to address these issues.*

4. Explore alternatives, including the desired outcome and consequences of actions.

- *The OT practitioner could develop new goals for occupational therapy intervention. This way Dave would stay in the current system. He may become attached to the center and have difficulty transitioning to home, school, or the community.*
- *Dave could be discharged from occupational therapy services, and attend a new program for children with learning issues (due to head injuries), which takes place close to his community. The social worker may be able to secure transportation. However, the child may still be in a chaotic home environment and benefit from outside support. The school psychologist recommends a Big Brother/Big Sister program and a parent support group for the parents (who may be willing, with encouragement from the team).*

5. Complete the action.

- *The team meets to discuss the courses of action and the consequences for each. After a thorough analysis, the OT practitioner feels informed and prepared to discuss the options that are in Dave's best interest. Although the initial reaction of the practitioner was to continue Dave's occupational therapy by reworking several goals, the practitioner realizes that the other alternatives might benefit him. In this case, the team works together to address the issues and discharges the client to a successful situation. Dave will attend a support program in his local area for teens. This program will address his emotional needs and help him transition to the school. The OT practitioner will consult with the director and staff members concerning Dave's physical and social needs. The OT practitioner agrees to attend a session with Dave so that he feels some continuity of care.*

6. Evaluate the action.

- *The OT practitioner felt supported by the team. The careful analysis of the alternative plans provided a solution that maintained the integrity of the profession and supported the child. Dave benefited from the work of all members and saw the team as advocates. The school and community support provided the child with the independence to engage in activities with his peers.*

PRACTICING LEGALLY

At both the state and federal levels, there are different types of laws that govern certain aspects of occupational therapy practice. The US Constitution and state constitutions are the primary source of legal authority. After the federal and state constitutions, statutory law is the next source of legal authority.[13] **Statutes** are laws that are enacted by the legislative branch of a government. There are federal and state statutes. The federal congress or state legislature votes to pass a law, which then is assigned to an agency. The agency itself, or a designated board, follows up with the development of regulations to implement and enforce the law. The **regulations** describe in specific terms how the intent of the law will be carried out. In this section, we discuss both statutes and regulations that affect the practice of occupational therapy. More information on state and federal laws and regulations can be found on the Internet.

FEDERAL STATUTES

Federal statutes, which are passed by Congress in Washington, DC, pertain to all 50 states. Federal statutes can be enforced through the federal court systems. Violating a federal statute may result in fines, injunctions, or prison time. Examples of some of the important federal statutes that affect the practice of occupational therapy include the following:

- The Health Insurance Portability and Accountability Act (HIPAA) established national standards for electronic health care transactions and addressed the security and privacy of health care data.[10]
- The Individuals with Disabilities Education Act (IDEA) requires public schools to make available to all eligible children with disabilities a free, appropriate public education in the least restrictive environment appropriate to their individual needs. OT practitioners working in school systems practice under this act. Thus the role of the OT practitioner is to provide intervention that will allow the child to engage in education.
- The Americans with Disabilities Act (ADA) provides protection from discrimination on the basis of disability. The ADA upholds and extends the standards for compliance set forth in Section 504 or the Rehabilitation Act of 1973 to employment practices, communication, and all policies, procedures, and practices that impact the treatment of students with disabilities.[17]
- The Social Security Amendments of 1965 established, among other provisions, the foundation for the Medicare and Medicaid programs. Medicare is a federally subsidized health insurance program for individuals 65 and older. Medicaid is a joint federal- and state-funded program that provides health care services to the poor. Occupational therapy services are covered under both of these programs.

STATE STATUTES

State statutes are passed by state legislatures. Accordingly, regulations will vary from state to state. Most state statutes are organized by subject matter and published in books referred to as codes. Typically, a state has a family or civil code, a criminal code, a welfare code, and a probate code, in addition to many other codes dealing with a wide variety of topics.

States are permitted by the federal Constitution to regulate areas such as education, insurance (private and public), and licensing. Consequently, state statutes may affect the practice of occupational therapy through regulation of the insurance industry, including health maintenance organizations, workers' compensation insurance programs, and health care services for the indigent. Child abuse and elder abuse laws are also within the state purview. All states have passed some form of law requiring **mandatory reporting** of suspected child abuse and neglect. Mandatory reporting is the requirement that certain professionals, including health care providers, report suspected child abuse. A health care provider who fails to report suspected abuse may be criminally liable.[15]

One of the most significant statutes affecting occupational therapy practice is the state occupational therapy practice act. With the recognition that laws and regulations will vary from state to state, the next section focuses on general principles of state regulation of occupational therapy.

STATE REGULATION OF OCCUPATIONAL THERAPY

State regulation of occupational therapy practice has been in place since the 1970s and includes licensure, statutory certification laws, registration, and trademark laws. Occupational therapy is regulated through one of these forms in all 50 states, the District of Columbia, Puerto Rico, and Guam.[1] Table 7-1 shows the breakdown of state regulation as of 2006. The primary purpose of regulation is to protect the consumer from practitioners who are unqualified or unscrupulous.

Under statutory certification and registration, a person may not use the title of or proclaim to be *certified* or *registered* unless he or she has met specific entry-level requirements. State trademark laws (also called *title control*) are similar to statutory certification in that they prevent non–OT practitioners from representing and charging for occupational therapy services. Neither statutory certification nor trademark laws define the scope of practice of the profession.

Licensure, the most stringent form of regulation, is "the process by which an agency of government grants permission to an individual to engage in a given occupation upon finding that the applicant has attained the minimal degree of competence required to ensure that the public health, safety, and welfare will be reasonably protected."[16] State licensure is one way to ensure the public that the person delivering services has obtained a degree of competency required by the profession and has permission to engage in that service. In the states with licensure laws, it is illegal to offer occupational therapy services without a license.

In addition to listing the qualifications needed for a person to practice, licensure laws also define the scope of practice of a profession and, therefore, are often referred to as practice acts. The scope of practice defined in the licensure law is a legal definition of occupational therapy's domain of practice. This is another step toward ensuring consumer

TABLE 7-1 State Regulation of Occupational Therapy

	Occupational Therapists	Occupational Therapy Assistants
Licensure	46 states, District of Columbia, Guam, Puerto Rico	43 states, District of Columbia, Guam, Puerto Rico
Certification	1 (Indiana)	2 (California and Indiana)
Registration	2 (Hawaii and Michigan)	1 (Michigan)
Trademark	1 (Colorado)	0
No regulation	0	4 (Virginia, New York, Hawaii, and Colorado)

From American Occupational Therapy Association: State licensure requirements, July 24, 2006. Retrieved August 17, 2006, from www.aota.org/members/area4/links/links03.

protection. The scope of practice also defends occupational therapy from challenges of other professions that may question the qualifications of practitioners to provide particular services or that may infringe upon occupational therapy's scope of practice.[14] Most states use the *Definition of Occupational Therapy Practice for the AOTA Model Practice Act*[6] and the *Scope of Practice*[8] as model language for state licensure laws and regulations. These documents are not statutes and do not have the force of the law, but they are intended to support state laws and regulations that govern the practice of occupational therapy.

OTs are legally responsible for services provided by OTAs or aides under their supervision. The role and supervision of OTAs and aides are also delineated in state regulations. Two AOTA documents provide guidelines that are used by states to develop these regulations. *The Standards of Practice for Occupational Therapy*, which was last revised in 2005, describes the minimum standards of practice for professional standing and responsibility, screening, evaluation, re-evaluation, intervention, and outcomes.[5] *The Guidelines for Supervision, Roles, and Responsibilities During the Delivery of Occupational Therapy Services*[7] outlines parameters of supervision for OT personnel (see Chapter 6).

An appointed state regulatory board carries out the tasks involved in implementing the licensure law and regulations. These licensure boards vary in structure from an advisory board to an autonomous body. Licensure boards are responsible for writing the regulations that govern the license, collecting fees and issuing licenses, investigating complaints, and delineating requirements for continuing competency. Licensure boards cannot change the scope of practice enacted through state legislation. They may advise the legislature or make suggested amendments. In some states, OT practitioners are appointed to serve on the board. OT practitioners can provide input into the regulatory process through their state association or by attending hearings, which are typically announced ahead of time and open to the public.

To be licensed in a state generally requires that the practitioner provide proof that he or she has completed the academic and fieldwork requirements of an Accreditation Council for Occupational Therapy Education (ACOTE)–accredited occupational therapy or occupational therapy assistant program and has passed the National Board of Certification for Occupational Therapy (NBCOT®) certification exam. An application is completed, fingerprints are submitted for a background check, and a fee is paid. Upon satisfying all legal requirements, the practitioner is issued a license to practice in that state. Each state requires its own licensing, and it is not permissible to practice in a state requiring licensure without a license. A practitioner may become licensed in as many states as he or she wishes.

States require practitioners to renew their license at specific intervals, usually every 1 to 2 years. Many state regulations require that practitioners complete a number of continuing education (CE) hours or continuing competence requirements to renew licensure. It is the responsibility of the practitioner to keep his or her knowledge up to date with current practice. Again, requirements vary from state to state, and each practitioner needs to be aware of the particular continuing competence requirements for his or her state. Strategies for professional development and continuing competence are discussed in Chapter 6.

DISCIPLINARY PROCESSES

Law and professional ethics are often intertwined. This blending may be related to the highly legalistic nature of today's society in which "one in seven Americans may be embroiled in civil litigation at any given time." Another reason is the fact that consumers

---

Box 7-2 Case Study: Blending of Ethics and Law

An OT student is completing her Level II fieldwork in a mental health setting. Her clinical supervisor, Kent, repeatedly asks her if she would like to join him in activities outside of work hours. She makes up excuses or manages to avoid the question. After a group session, he makes a comment to her about her breasts. The student is afraid to say anything to her supervisor or the department manager for fear that it will affect how she is evaluated on her fieldwork. The student keeps quiet about the situation until the end of her fieldwork, when she reports the situation to the academic fieldwork coordinator. Preceding her statement to the coordinator, she asks that the information she is about to divulge remain confidential.
- Is this a legal issue? An ethical issue? Or both?
- What actions should the academic fieldwork coordinator take at this time?
- Should the student pursue any further actions? If so, what?

---

of health care services have become more aware of their rights and more willing to assert those rights, which might mean using the legal system.[13] With this blending of law and professional ethics comes the potential to process violations in a number of different ways. In Box 7-2, we present a case study that exemplifies the blending of ethics and law.

The *Occupational Therapy Code of Ethics* applies to individuals who are or were members of AOTA.[4] Therefore AOTA has jurisdiction over complaints against members who are suspected of unethical conduct. The Ethics Commission (EC) of AOTA ensures compliance with the *Code of Ethics,* and it establishes and maintains enforcement procedures. Any individual, group, or entity within or outside of AOTA may file a formal, written complaint against a member of AOTA for unethical conduct.[3] The EC conducts a preliminary assessment and determines if there is sufficient ground to carry the complaint forward to a full investigation. If the member is found to have committed an ethical violation, one of the following disciplinary sanctions is imposed: reprimand, censure, probation of membership subject to terms, membership suspension, or revocation of membership in AOTA (see Box 7-3).[3] It is the policy of AOTA to communicate with NBCOT® and state regulatory boards when disciplinary actions have been taken against an OT practitioner.

It is the responsibility of the licensure board to protect the public from direct or potential harm that may be caused by unqualified or incompetent practitioners. The regulatory board follows established disciplinary processes and guidelines that are clearly spelled out in each state's regulations. In cases in which there is not direct or potential harm to the public (e.g., practicing without a current and active license, failing to disclose a conviction

---

Box 7-3 Possible Sanctions Imposed by American Occupational Therapy Association

Reprimand: A formal expression of disapproval of conduct communicated privately by letter from the Chairperson of the Ethics Committee that is nondisclosable and noncommunicative to other bodies
Censure: A formal expression of disapproval that is public
Probation: Failure to meet terms will subject a member to any of the disciplinary actions or sanctions
Suspension: Removal of membership for a specified period of time
Revocation: Permanent denial of membership

From American Occupational Therapy Association: Enforcement procedures for occupational therapy code of ethics, *Am J Occup Ther* 59:643-652, 2005.

or convictions in the application process), the licensure board may assess a fine, which would vary depending upon the gravity of the situation. An abatement, or order of correction, is also usually given to the practitioner and must be completed in a designated amount of time. In situations in which there is clear evidence of direct or potential harm to the public, the consequences for the practitioner are more severe. Disciplinary actions that could be taken against the practitioner include public censure, suspension, or revocation of licensure or practice privileges. Each state has jurisdiction only over practitioners licensed in the state.

SUMMARY

The *Occupational Therapy Code of Ethics* provides standards of conduct for OT practitioners. This *Occupational Therapy Code of Ethics* identifies seven principles that apply to all OT personnel in all types of roles. The Ethics Commission enforces the principles of the *Code of Ethics*. The seven principles include beneficence, nonmaleficence, autonomy and confidentiality, duty, procedural justice, veracity, and fidelity. Using ethical decision-making guidelines helps practitioners make professionally sound decisions.

Standards of practice provide guidelines for the delivery of quality occupational therapy services to the consumer. State licensure is the legal means of regulating occupational therapy practice. Both the *Code of Ethics* and state licensure laws have procedures for processing disciplinary actions. OT practitioners are responsible for understanding and following the ethical and legal standards of practice.

Ethics, laws, and regulations serve primarily to protect the public from unqualified or unscrupulous practitioners. Laws and regulations in particular establish a legal scope of practice for the profession and differentiate it from other professions. OT practitioners obtain rights and protection as a result of these laws and regulations, but they must also assume the responsibilities and limits imposed by regulation.

Learning Activities

1. Obtain a series of ethical situations, including suggested solutions, from faculty members or practicing therapists. In small groups, discuss the scenarios; and, using the ethical decision-making guidelines, develop a solution. Discuss each scenario, and use the suggested solutions to provide alternatives.
2. Compare and contrast the *Occupational Therapy Code of Ethics* to those of two other allied health professions.
3. View a film such as *The Kevorkian Files*, *The Tuskegee Study*, or the *Life of David Gale* to promote discussion on ethical decision-making. Ask students to identify one or two ethical issues from the film, define them, and discuss the stakeholders and alternatives.
4. Ask students to bring in an ethical issue from current news. Using the ethical decision-making process, discuss this issue and possible solutions.
5. Research the licensure laws from three states. Compare and contrast the occupational therapy practice guidelines for each of these states.

Review Questions

1. What is a code of ethics?
2. Provide an example of ethical distress, ethical dilemma, and locus of authority problems.
3. List and describe the seven principles in the *Occupational Therapy Code of Ethics*.
4. List the six steps to ethical decision-making.

REFERENCES

1. American Occupational Therapy Association: State licensure requirements. Retrieved August 17, 2006, from www.aota.org/members/area4/links/links03.
2. American Occupational Therapy Association: Guidelines to the occupational therapy code of ethics. Retrieved July 17, 2006, from www.aota.org/members/area2/docs/codeguidelines.
3. American Occupational Therapy Association: Enforcement procedures for occupational therapy code of ethics, *Am J Occup Ther* 59:643-652, 2005.
4. American Occupational Therapy Association: Occupational therapy code of ethics, *Am J Occup Ther* 59:639-642, 2005.
5. American Occupational Therapy Association: Standards of practice for occupational therapy, *Am J Occup Ther* 59(6):663-665, 2005.
6. American Occupational Therapy Association: *Definition of Occupational Therapy Practice for the AOTA Model Practice Act,* Bethesda, MD, 2004, American Occupational Therapy Association. Retrieved August 23, 2006, from http://www.aota.org/members/area4/docs/defotpractice.pdf.
7. American Occupational Therapy Association: Guidelines for supervision, roles, and responsibilities, *Am J Occup Ther* 58(6):663-667, 2004.
8. American Occupational Therapy Association: Scope of practice, *Am J Occup Ther* 58:673-77, 2004.
9. American Occupational Therapy Association: Core values and attitudes of occupational therapy practice, *Am J Occup Ther* 47:1085-1086, 1993.
10. Centers for Medicare and Medicaid Services: HIPPA—General information, 2005. Retrieved August 18, 2006, from http://www.cms.hhs.gov/HIPPAAGenInfo/.
11. Davis CM: *Patient Practitioner Interaction: An Experiential Manual for Developing the Art of Health Care,* ed 4, Thorofare, NJ, 2006, Slack.
12. Purtilo R: *Ethical Dimensions in the Health Professions,* ed 4, Philadelphia, 2005, WB Saunders.
13. Scott R: *Professional Ethics: A Guide for Rehabilitation Professionals,* St. Louis, 1998, Mosby.
14. Slater DY, Willmarth C: Understanding and asserting the occupational therapy scope of practice, *OT Practice* 10(October 17), 2005.
15. Smith SK: *Mandatory Reporting of Child Abuse and Neglect,* Hartford & Avon, CT, June 3, 2006. Retrieved August 23, 2006, from http://www.smith-lasfirm.com/mandatoryreporting.htm.
16. United States Department of Health, Education, and Welfare, Public Health Service: *Credentialing Health Manpower [Publication No. (OS) 77-50057],* Bethesda, MD, 1977, United States Department of Health, Education, and Welfare, Public Health Service.
17. United States Department of Justice: *Civil Rights Division, Disability Rights Section: A Guide to Disability Rights Laws,* September 2005. Retrieved July 5, 2006, from http://www.ada.gov/.

I stumbled upon the profession of occupational therapy quite serendipitously. I had originally intended to pursue a law degree in college but found myself drawn to courses in the sciences and arts. A university counselor recommended that I take a series of career tests, and the profession of occupational therapy appeared. Because I had never heard of this profession, the counselor provided me with information and names of individuals to contact regarding occupational therapy. I was amazed at the range of the profession and the creativity of the occupational therapists I encountered. This profession offered such variety!

As I reflect on over 25 years as an occupational therapist (I stopped counting after the quarter century mark!), I am so grateful to that counselor who opened my eyes to a profession that has provided me with such a tremendous opportunity for growth. This profession has allowed me to be a clinician, supervisor, educator, and researcher. Throughout the years, I have been so fortunate to learn from my clients, students, and colleagues in occupational therapy and other professions. They have taught me the true importance of occupation, whether playing a card game with friends, jumping rope on a playground, studying for an exam, or discussing the efficacy of various intervention methods. I have never ceased to be thankful that I found a profession as rewarding and fulfilling as occupational therapy.

Winifred Schultz-Krohn, PhD, OTR/L, SWC, BCP, FAOTA
Associate Professor of Occupational Therapy
San Jose State University

Chapter 8

Professional Organizations

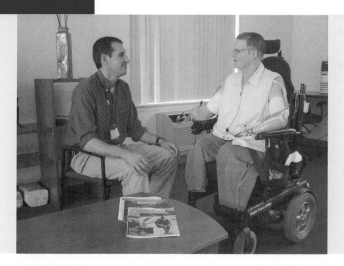

It is customary for professions to establish a professional association. The stronger and better supported the association is, the greater the benefits for the individual members. A **professional association** is organized and operated by its members for its members. It exists to protect and promote the profession it represents by (1) providing a communication network and channel for information, (2) regulating itself through the development and enforcement of standards of conduct and performance, and (3) guarding the interests of those within the profession.[1]

The professional organization for OT practitioners in the United States is the **American Occupational Therapy Association (AOTA).** Originally incorporated in 1917 as the National Society for the Promotion of Occupational Therapy, the association's name was changed to its present version in 1923. The **World Federation of Occupational Therapists (WFOT)** was established in 1952 to help OT practitioners access international information, engage in international exchange, and promote organizations of occupational therapy in schools in countries where none exists.[3,5] Each state also has a professional organization for OT practitioners living in the state. Although there is frequent collaboration between AOTA and the individual state associations, the state associations are funded and operated independently from the national association. It is beneficial for OT practitioners to have a good understanding of the professional organizations and the services they provide. Because it would be impossible to discuss each state association in this text, this chapter describes the world and national association. Readers are encouraged to join and support their professional associations at the world, national, state, and local levels. See Appendix D for the contact information for selected organizations.

AMERICAN OCCUPATIONAL THERAPY ASSOCIATION

MISSION

The mission of AOTA is "to advance the quality, availability, use and support of occupational therapy through standard-setting, advocacy, education, and research on behalf of its members and the public." In keeping with this mission statement, AOTA directs its efforts to (1) assure the quality of occupational therapy services, (2) improve consumer access to health care services, and (3) promote the professional development of its members.[1]

MEMBERSHIP

Three professional membership categories exist in AOTA: occupational therapist (OT), occupational therapy assistant (OTA), and occupational therapy student (OTS). Persons interested in the profession who are not OT professionals may join the organization as organizational or associate members. Membership categories determine the fees paid for membership and conferences and who can attend special meetings, hold office, and vote. For example, organizational and associate members do not have voting privileges. Membership fees are higher for OTs. Membership fees for the OT student are lowest to encourage them to become involved in the organization and familiarize themselves with membership benefits.

Members at all levels are encouraged to become actively involved in AOTA by serving on committees, attending the annual conference, reviewing journal articles, presenting at conferences, and holding elected and volunteer positions. Active membership helps OT practitioners become informed.[1]

ORGANIZATIONAL STRUCTURE

AOTA is made up of a volunteer sector and paid national office staff. See Figure 8-1 for a description of the organizational structure of AOTA. The paid office staff is employed at the headquarters in Bethesda, Maryland, and performs the day-to-day operations under the management of the executive director. The national office staff is organized around four divisions: Business Operations Division (membership, marketing, corporate relations, and exhibits and advertising); Division of Public Affairs (federal affairs, reimbursement and regulatory policy, state affairs, and public/media relations); Professional Affairs Division (accreditation, education, practice, and professional development); and Finance, Information Technology, and Administration Division.

The volunteer sector consists of all the members of the association and is represented by the executive board and the representative assembly. The executive board is charged with the administration and management of the association and includes elected officers. There are several standing committees of the executive board including, the representative assembly (RA), which is the legislative and policy-making body of the AOTA. The RA is composed of elected representatives from each recognized state, elected officers of the assembly and the association, a representative from the student committee, an occupational therapy assistant representative, the first delegate of the WFOT, and the chairpersons of the commissions. The standing commissions of the RA include the Commission on Education, the Commission on Practice, and the Commission on Standards and Ethics.[1]

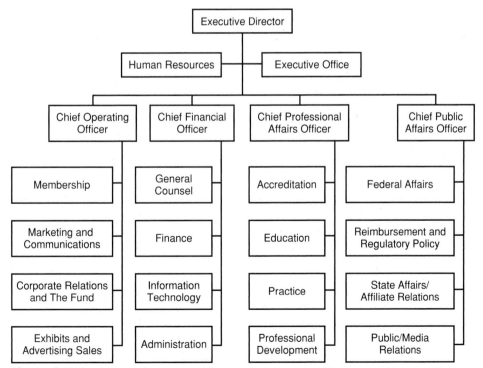

Figure 8-1 Organizational structure of the American Occupational Therapy Association. *(Courtesy of the American Occupational Therapy Association, Bethesda, MD.)*

Many occupational therapy educational programs have a club or organization for students. Student groups may participate in the **American Student Committee of the Occupational Therapy Association (ASCOTA),** a standing committee of the executive board of AOTA.

ASSURING QUALITY OF OCCUPATIONAL THERAPY SERVICES

The AOTA is responsible for ensuring the delivery of quality occupational therapy services. To this end, the association develops standards, produces official documents that identify the standards, and reviews the standards on a regular basis. Standards ensure that educational programs prepare students properly, that guidelines are in place articulating occupational therapy practice, and that a code of conduct is provided to clarify ethical issues. AOTA has developed standards of education, standards of practice, and ethical standards.

Standards for OT and OTA educational programs are developed and reviewed on a regular basis by the association's Accreditation Council for Occupational Therapy Education (ACOTE). Educational programs are accredited based on their compliance with these standards (see Chapter 5). These standards help ensure the delivery of quality educational programs in occupational therapy.

AOTA lends its support to states for the regulation of practice through licensure and other state laws. The *Occupational Therapy Scope of Practice,* developed by AOTA, is used by states as a model for their licensure laws. As discussed in Chapter 7, state regulatory laws help ensure that practitioners meet specific competencies.

PROFESSIONAL DEVELOPMENT OF MEMBERS

AOTA promotes the professional development of its members through a number of activities, including publications, continuing education, and practice information. The Commission on Continuing Competence and Professional Development (CCCPD) is the designated body of the RA that is responsible for developing standards for continuing competency and for communicating to the various stakeholders' issues surrounding competency and occupational therapy. The CCCPD was also responsible for the development of the Professional Development Tool (PDT) discussed in Chapter 6.

PUBLICATIONS

The association contributes to the professional development of OT practitioners through a variety of publications. The organization's official publication, *American Journal of Occupational Therapy (AJOT),* has traditionally served as the main source of research information for the profession. *AJOT* is distributed monthly (except for bimonthly publications in July/August and November/December) to all AOTA members, and it is also available through subscription to nonmembers and libraries. Subjects may include approaches to practice, programs and techniques, research, educational and professional trends, and areas of controversy in the occupational therapy field. Articles are written by professionals in occupational therapy or related fields and must meet the rigid standards set by its editors.

As a part of AOTA membership, each member has online access to 11 Special Interest Sections (SISs); voting privileges to 3 SIS, and 1 printed SIS quarterly that they receive by mail. The SISs are: Administration and Management, Developmental Disabilities, Education, Gerontology, Home and Community Health, Mental Health, Physical Disabilities, School System, Sensory Integration, Technology, and Work Programs. Members are eligible to participate in activities (such as meetings) held by three SISs.[1]

OT Practice is a biweekly publication designed to keep members informed about the profession in general. *OT Practice* publishes useful clinical information to members.

An extensive product catalog lists books, videotapes, audiotapes, brochures, official documents, and other materials that are available on a broad range of topics related to occupational therapy. Materials are available for purchase, rent, or loan; some are distributed free of charge.

CONTINUING EDUCATION

AOTA sponsors numerous continuing education activities, including workshops, continuing education articles (in *OT Practice*), self-paced clinical courses, and online courses. The annual meeting, held in a different city each year and hosted by the area's local or state association, provides a variety of continuing education opportunities. All members are encouraged to attend. The conference hosts presentations ranging from poster sessions, panel discussions, and workshops, to formal presentations. The national conference conducts business meetings and also includes an awards ceremony to recognize contributions to the field. The latest materials, equipment, and books are displayed. The national conference provides members with current information and a chance to network with OT practitioners around the country.

PRACTICE INFORMATION

In addition to all the publications mentioned, AOTA has developed resources for information on all the practice areas, including published practice materials, staff experts, and volunteers who provide consultation. These resources include standards for practice, handouts for parents and consumers, and fact sheets concerning occupational therapy. AOTA's official website at www.aota.org provides a wealth of information. Although some information is available to the general public, much of the information is restricted to use by AOTA members.

IMPROVING CONSUMER ACCESS TO HEALTH CARE SERVICES

The national association ensures that services are accessible to consumers through an ongoing process of communication with state and federal lawmakers, regulatory bodies, third-party payers, health care professionals, the media, and the public. For example, the AOTA keeps abreast of proposed legislation and special committees within the government, ensuring that new laws affecting practice are not passed without hearing the voice of the profession. The association is in communication with its political action committee (PAC), the legally sanctioned vehicle through which organizations can engage in political action. The **American Occupational Therapy Political Action Committee (AOTPAC)** furthers the legislative aims of the profession by attempting to influence the selection, nomination, election, or appointment of persons to public office.[2]

For example, when the federal government developed legislation outlining what services schools must provide for the Handicapped Children Act, AOTA provided information on occupational therapy services and successfully lobbied for the inclusion of occupational therapy. This professional vigilance applies not only to the government but also to the private sector. When major insurance companies write or rewrite policies regarding the health services they will cover, AOTA works to ensure that occupational therapy is included. AOTA also has a toll-free hotline for consumers to access information regarding occupational therapy.

AMERICAN OCCUPATIONAL THERAPY FOUNDATION

The **American Occupational Therapy Foundation (AOTF)** is a national organization designed to advance the science of occupational therapy and increase public understanding of the value of occupational therapy. AOTF was incorporated as a separate not-for-profit organization in 1965.[4] It is a vehicle for providing resources to programs and individuals for the purpose of carrying out occupational therapy education and research. AOTF also operates a library that contains books and journals related to occupational therapy. AOTF provides grant opportunities, scholarships, and research support.[4] Donations and bequests from AOTA members, corporations, and private foundations are collected and managed by AOTF to support these programs.

Since 1980, AOTF has published the *Occupational Therapy Journal of Research (OTJR)*, now named *OTJR: Occupation, Participation and Health,* to address the need for more publication opportunities. This journal is published quarterly and is available for a subscription fee.

WORLD FEDERATION OF OCCUPATIONAL THERAPISTS

The World Federation of Occupation Therapists was developed in 1952 with the objectives to promote and advocate for occupational therapy and establish minimum educational standards for member countries.[5] WFOT also serves as a vehicle for international information exchange among occupational therapy associations, practitioners, and other allied health personnel. The organization is responsible for many publications, including the WFOT journal. WFOT is organized into five program areas, which include standards and quality, education and research, promotion and development, international cooperation, and executive programs.[5] An international conference is sponsored by WFOT every 4 years. As the worldwide practice of occupational therapy continues to grow and develop, WFOT is a valuable mechanism for exchange of information with OT practitioners in other countries.

SUMMARY

The AOTA is the national organization representing OT practitioners. Its major activities include assuring the delivery of quality occupational therapy services, improving consumer access to health care, and promoting the professional development of its members.

AOTA ensures the delivery of quality services through the development and enforcement of standards, accreditation of educational programs, research, and support for regulation. To encourage the professional development of its members, AOTA conducts continuing education programs, publishes materials, and provides practice information. AOTA distributes information to federal and state lawmakers, insurance providers, media, public, and other health care providers.

At the international level, WFOT provides an information exchange and advances the practice and standards of occupational therapy around the world. OT practitioners are encouraged to participate in professional organizations at the international, national, state, and local levels.

Learning Activities

1. Go to AOTA's website (www.aota.org), and retrieve information on an aspect of AOTA that is of special interest to you; write a brief paper on your findings.
2. Gather information on the next AOTA conference (e.g., when, where, cost, theme), and prepare a bulletin board display or poster.
3. Hold a class brainstorming session to compile a list of topics appropriate for a 15-minute conference short paper.
4. Gather information on your state occupational therapy association; prepare an informational handout for your class.
5. Prepare an overview of a topic from the WFOT conference. Discuss the current issues and topics with classmates.
6. The following is a recommended series of exploratory *American Journal of Occupational Therapy* investigations. Each stage is a bit more demanding and thus builds an increasing familiarity with both the publication and research techniques. These can become a series of projects over a period of time. Each class member is to do the following:
   - Locate the place and manner in which *American Journal of Occupational Therapy* is housed (current and past volumes).
   - Read an article of interest from *American Journal of Occupational Therapy*; give a 5-minute oral report on the topic, the source information, and the point of interest.
   - Research an article on an assigned topic; give a 5-minute oral report. (Further research may be required to gain information on the topic before the article search.)
   - Read an article from any occupational therapy source; write a half-page summary of the topic.
   - Gather information on an intervention technique by summarizing and critiquing at least three research articles.

Review Questions

1. What are the purposes of a professional organization?
2. List five benefits to membership in AOTA, WFOT, and state organizations.
3. How can members participate in professional organizations?
4. What resources are available to OT practitioners through the professional organizations?
5. What is your local occupational therapy association? Describe the activities of this association.

REFERENCES

1. American Occupational Therapy Association: About AOTA. Retrieved July 20, 2006, from www.aota.org.
2. American Occupational Therapy Association: AOTPAC fact sheet. Retrieved July 20, 2006, from www. aota.org.
3. American Occupational Therapy Association: Frequently asked questions about the World Federation of Occupational Therapists (WFOT). Retrieved July 20, 2006, from www.aota.org.
4. American Occupational Therapy Foundation: Did you know? Facts about the American Occupational Therapy Foundation. Retrieved July 20, 2006, from www.aotf.org/html/facts.shtml.
5. World Federation of Occupational Therapy: WFOT information. Retrieved July 20, 2006, from www. wfot.org.au/inside.asp.

Section **3** | # The Practice of Occupational Therapy

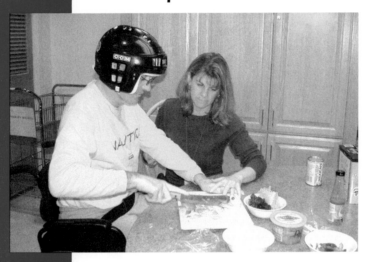

My entrance into the profession was influenced and sustained by the efforts and examples of some very remarkable mentors. My mother, a registered nurse, regaled my sisters and me with tales of her nursing experiences in the Army Nurse Corps during World War II. I read every Cherry Ames book (nurse/detective *à la* Nancy Drew), and I loved my stint as a candy striper at the local hospital, but somehow I knew that nursing wasn't quite what I was looking for in my career future. I remember first hearing about Occupational Therapy from Dr. Marian Diamond, the esteemed professor of anatomy and physiology at the University of California at Berkeley and my instructor. Based upon my high regard for her and her suggestion that I would be a perfect OT (whatever that was), I followed suit and met with Doris Cutting, the chair of the OT department at San Jose State University, who made me want to be a part of whatever it was she was. Armed with my bachelor's in humanities from Berkeley, I smiled as I picked up my OT class schedule and saw neuroanatomy, psychology, and weaving on my list—now this was a program that was meant for me!

OT school was a dream—each of the assignments a step closer to my newly chosen profession. Professors Amy Killingsworth, Lorraine Pedretti, and many others further nourished my enthusiasm for OT through their obvious passion for the profession, conveyed through stories of their caring and creative interactions with clients. I was privileged to begin my career at Rancho Los Amigos Medical Center with incomparable role models of superb OT practice, including Dottie Wilson, Lois Barber, Doris Heredia, Sarah Kelly, and numerous others who mentored their colleagues, facilitating and celebrating each other's successes. I remember driving to work with a smile on my face and eagerly looking forward to each day and the new stories I would be developing with my clients—a wish I have for every budding OT.

All of these mentors, through their example, inspired pursuit of further learning and scholarship as a commitment to furthering excellence in client care as well as advancing the knowledge base of the profession. In response, I chose to study at the graduate level and subsequently seek an academic position—both environments where I was again treated to the supportive mentoring climate I have come to know throughout my occupational therapy experience. Elizabeth Yerxa, Florence Clark, Lela Llorens, Ruth Zemke—among many others in academia—exemplified for me the importance of nurturing and celebrating the accomplishments of others to strengthen and enrich the profession we love so well. In tribute to these generous and amazing mentors, I encourage my OT colleagues and strive myself to reach out, encourage, and support developing occupational therapists.

Heidi McHugh Pendleton, PhD, OTR/L, FAOTA
Professor
Department of Occupational Therapy
San Jose State University
San Jose, California

Occupational Therapy Practice Framework: Domain and Process

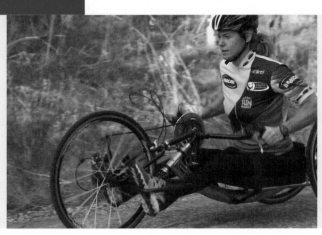

OBJECTIVES

After reading this chapter, the reader will be able to do the following:

- Define the domains of occupational therapy (OT) practice
- Outline the occupational therapy process
- Analyze activities in terms of areas of performance, performance skills, performance patterns, and client factors
- Provide examples of how contexts impact occupations
- Describe intervention approaches

KEY TERMS

Activities of daily living
Activity demands
Client-centered approach
Client factors
Client satisfaction
Consultation
Context
Education

Evaluation
Health
Instrumental activities of daily living
Occupational performance
Occupation-based activity
Performance patterns
Performance skills

Preparatory methods
Purposeful activity
Quality of life
Role competence
Therapeutic use of occupations and activities
Wellness

The *Occupational Therapy Practice Framework (OTPF)*[1] was developed as a revision to the *Uniform Terminology for Occupational Therapy.*[3] *Uniform Terminology* was developed by the American Occupational Therapy Association (AOTA) to answer OT practitioners' requests for a unified language for the profession. Although *Uniform Terminology*[3] helped practitioners "speak the same language," this document did not provide information on the process of providing occupation-based intervention. Thus the *OTPF* was developed to help practitioners use the language and constructs of occupation to serve clients and educate consumers.[1]

The *OTPF* attempts to clearly and concisely describe the occupational therapy profession, including the process and terminology, for students, clinicians, and consumers. Therefore, the emphasis is on occupation, client-centered care, and the dynamic nature of the therapy process. This chapter will provide readers with an overview of the *OTPF*. See Appendix C for a description of the terms and concepts in the *OTPF*.

PERFORMANCE AREAS

The goal of occupational therapy is to help clients engage in occupation.[1,7,9,10] Occupations are the everyday things that people do and that are essential to one's identity.[1,6,10] The performance areas of occupation include activities of daily living (ADL), instrumental activities of daily living (IADL), education, work, play, leisure, and social participation.[1] The following paragraphs provide descriptions of the areas of performance along with clinical examples.

ACTIVITIES OF DAILY LIVING

Activities of daily living refer to activities involved in taking care of one's own body and include such things as dressing, bathing, grooming, eating, feeding, personal device care, toileting, sexual activity, and sleep/rest.[1]

> Craig is a 2-year-old boy, small for his age, whose mother is concerned that he does not like many foods. Upon evaluation, the occupational therapist (OT) determines that Craig exhibits oral motor control issues (e.g., tongue thrusting) and oral hypersensitivity that interfere with his eating. The OT develops an intervention plan to address this ADL.

INSTRUMENTAL ACTIVITIES OF DAILY LIVING

Instrumental activities of daily living refer to activities that may be considered optional and involve the environment. IADLs include care of others, care of pets, child rearing, communication device use, community mobility, health management, financial management, home establishment and management, meal preparation and clean up, safety, and shopping.[1]

> Raiser is a 19-year-old man with mild intellectual deficits. He has recently graduated from a group home and will be living alone in the next few months. The OT practitioner works with Raiser on living independently by practicing how to purchase, use, and maintain household equipment (e.g., toaster, microwave). In another session, the practitioner works with Raiser on using the telephone to call the landlord for assistance with the household. These skills are part of home management.

EDUCATION

Education is an area of occupation that includes formal (e.g., school, university, course-work) and informal (e.g., obtaining topic-related information or skills, instruction/training in areas of interest) learning.

David is a 7-year-old second grader who is experiencing difficulty with handwriting. His teacher is concerned that David is falling behind others in his class and makes a referral to occupational therapy. The OT evaluates David's handwriting skills and begins intervention to improve strength and coordination for handwriting. Because children spend approximately 30% of the school day writing,[12] this is a necessary ability for his education.

WORK

Work refers to paid or volunteer activities and includes the entire range of employment activities such as interests, pursuits, job seeking, and job performance, to retirement preparation and adjustment, as well as volunteer exploration and participation.[1]

Kylie is experiencing difficulty returning to her job as a legal secretary because of her motor vehicle accident, which resulted in a traumatic brain injury. The OT practitioner emphasizes work habits such as getting to work on time, organizing her work space, limiting conversation with others, and completing her work. The OT practitioner arranges a meeting with Kylie and her supervisor to review the firm's standards and the necessary job skills. The supervisor agrees to provide the OT practitioner with a description of Kylie's "typical day" so the OT practitioner may prepare her more adequately.

PLAY

Play refers to "any spontaneous or organized activity that provides enjoyment, entertainment, amusement, or diversion."[1,14] OT practitioners work with clients on play exploration and participation.

Karl is a 12-year-old boy who does not engage in play activities with his peers at school or at home. His teachers and parents are concerned that Karl does not find any enjoyment in his childhood. The OT practitioner works with Karl to identify play activities and invites two friends to a session in which they engage in a variety of outdoor games as a means of exploring the types of play that Karl may enjoy.

LEISURE

Leisure refers to nonobligatory activity. This area of occupation includes planning as well as participating in the activity. Exploring areas of interest is considered part of leisure occupations.

Jana is a 66-year-old woman who is dealing with the loss of her husband. She and her husband retired to a new state just prior to his death, and Jana therefore has few friends. Upon evaluation, the OT discovers that Jana participates in few enjoyable activities. In fact, Jana cannot articulate any leisure interests. The OT invites Jana to several community outings that she thinks Jana may enjoy. The practitioner watches for any nonverbal or verbal indication of enjoyment so that she may elaborate or expand on areas of interest for Jana. Exploring one's options is often the first step in developing leisure occupations.

SOCIAL PARTICIPATION

Social participation refers to activities involving interactions with others, including family, community, and peers/friends.[1] OT practitioners examining social participation analyze the behaviors and standards for given social situations.

Gloria is a 52-year-old woman with a diagnosis of schizophrenia. She has difficulty in many social settings. The OT practitioner begins intervention by helping Gloria succeed in community settings by reviewing basic social manners, including dress, language, and how close she stands to others. As part of the intervention, Gloria attends several outings in the community, including the art museum, library, and a coffee shop. Standards of behavior vary with the type of social participation activity.

As shown in the above examples, performance in areas of occupation varies greatly, depending upon the client's age, motivation, interests, culture, and abilities. Thus further analysis of occupations is necessary to fully understand how to provide meaningful intervention.

ANALYSIS OF OCCUPATIONAL PERFORMANCE

The *OTPF* supports a top-down approach in that the OT practitioner evaluates the areas of performance and occupations in which the client hopes to engage first, followed by an analysis of the performance skills or client factors interfering with performance. This approach differs from reductionistic approaches that analyze components first and subsequently design intervention based upon deficits. The *OTPF* encourages practitioners to keep occupation central to practice. See Figure 9-1 for an overview of the domain of occupational therapy.

Once the practitioner has identified the occupations in which the client would like to engage, the practitioner analyzes **performance skills**—including motor, process, and communication/interaction skills—required to complete the occupation. Performance skills are small units of performance. When an OT practitioner examines performance, he or she identifies performance skills that are effective or ineffective.[1] For example, the practitioner may decide that the client's poor fine-motor skills are interfering with the ability to get dressed in the morning. The client may have difficulty problem-solving how to make breakfast or be unable to make eye contact with peers. These types of performance skills may need to be addressed before the client can engage in desired occupations. Performance skills are dependent upon client factors, activity demands, and context.[1]

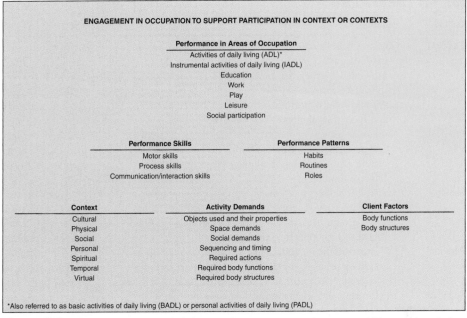

Figure 9-1 Domain of occupational therapy. *(From American Occupational Therapy Association: Occupational therapy practice framework: domain and process,* Am J Occup Ther *56(6):611, 2002.)*

Client factors are even more specific components of performance that may need to be addressed for clients to be successful. Client factors include body functions and body structures. Many of the terms from the *Uniform Terminology for Occupational Therapy*[3] are included under client factors, including range of motion, strength, endurance, posture, visual acuity, and tactile functions. OT practitioners are skilled at analyzing occupational performance at the basic level so that they can help clients fine-tune their skills and obtain the standards they wish.

Patterns of performance are another component of occupational performance analyzed by the OT practitioner. **Performance patterns** refer to the clients' habits, routines, and roles.[1] Three types of habits are described in the *OTPF:* useful habits support occupations; impoverished habits do not support occupations, and dominating habits interfere with occupations. Examining performance patterns helps the OT practitioner understand how the occupation is actually accomplished for the individual client. An example of a client with an impoverished habit is one who has difficulty consistently getting up on time and performing morning self-care in a timely manner. As a result of this, the client will have a poorly established or ineffective routine and experience difficulty carrying out his or her desired roles.

When choosing an activity to help a client reach his or her goals, OT practitioners also examine the **activity demands,** which include the objects used and their properties, space demands, social demands, sequencing and timing, required actions, required body functions, and required body structures.[1] For example, Mrs. Salazar is a client in occupational therapy who finds the occupation of baking for her family very meaningful. Due to her recent stroke, she has difficulty sequencing the steps for baking a cake. The OT practitioner modifies the demands of the activity by writing each step out very clearly on a sign that is placed in front of Mrs. Salazar while she bakes a cake. Evaluating activity demands allows

TABLE 9-1 Context or Contexts

Context	Definition	Example
Cultural	Customs, beliefs, activity patterns, behavior standards, and expectations accepted by the society of which the individual is a member. Includes political, such as laws that affect access to resources and affirm personal rights. Also includes opportunities for education, employment, and economic support.	Ethnicity, family, attitude, beliefs, values
Physical	Nonhuman aspects of contexts. Includes the accessibility to and performance within environments having natural terrain, plants, animals, buildings, furniture, objects, tools, or devices.	Objects, built environment, natural environment, geographic terrain, sensory qualities of environment
Social	Availability and expectations of significant individuals, such as spouse, friends, and caregivers. Also includes larger social groups that are influential in establishing norms, role expectations, and social routines.	Relationships with individuals, groups, or organizations; relationships with systems (political, economic, institutional)
Personal	"[F]eatures of the individual that are not part of a health condition or health status."[16] Personal context includes age, gender, socioeconomic status, and educational status.	25-year-old unemployed man with a high school diploma
Spiritual	The fundamental orientation of a person's life; that which inspires and motivates that individual.	Essence of the person, greater or higher purpose, meaning, substance
Temporal	"Location of occupational performance in time."[13]	Stages of life, time of day, time of year, duration
Virtual	Environment in which communication occurs by means of airways or computers and an absence of physical contact.	Realistic simulation of an environment, chat rooms, radio transmissions

From American Occupational Therapy Association: Occupational therapy practice framework: domain and process, *Am J Occup Ther* 56(6):623, 2002.

the OT practitioner to match appropriate activities to the client's needs and to determine how to modify, adapt, or delete aspects of the activity so the client can be successful.

The activity demands change as a result of the **context** or setting in which the occupation occurs. Context changes the requirements and performance skills, patterns, and demands of the activity. For example, cooking a meal at home for one is much different than having five friends over for a holiday dinner. According to the *OTPF*, contexts include aspects related to the cultural, physical, social, personal, spiritual, temporal, and virtual areas.[1] See Table 9-1 for definitions of each. Each context must be examined in terms of the various demands placed on the occupation.

CASE APPLICATION

The following case provides an overall view of how the *OTPF* is used in clinical practice.

An OT working at a home health agency evaluates 2-year-old David, who has developmental delays, and finds out the following:
- The parents are concerned because David does not "play like other children."
- David does not sleep through the night, does not eat a variety of foods, and is small for his age.

- David drools and is difficult to understand. He talks using one-word sentences. He still sucks his thumb.
- David reaches with and uses a palmar grasp to hold objects. He walks with a wide-based gait.
- David smiles on approach and makes brief eye contact.
- David lives at home with three siblings (ages 7, 5, and newborn).

Using the *OTPF* as a guide, the OT decides to focus intervention on play and feeding issues. Play and activities of daily living are performance areas of occupation within the domain of occupational therapy. After considering areas of performance and patterns of performance, the OT practitioner examines David's motor, processing, and communication/interaction skills (performance skills). The practitioner explores the contexts in which the activities will occur. Specifically, the clinician finds out that David will play with his 7- and 5-year-old sisters, who enjoy playing musical games and pretend. The family has a safe and well-stocked playroom. David will get plenty of practice if the sisters participate in the sessions.

Contextually, the practitioner identifies that meal times may be very stressful, as Dad has an inconsistent work schedule, leaving meal times to Mom (with four small children). Thus the practitioner decides to focus feeding intervention strategies to snack times and subsequently provides adaptations (e.g., finger foods) to compensate for poor skills to ensure successful independent meal times. The activity demands of the feeding intervention are changed by modifying the types of food served to David, for example, by having him eat finger foods instead of foods that require a utensil. Furthermore, David is gaining weight and not experiencing any malnutrition. The OT practitioner examined body functions and structures to determine how they may be impacting David's performance.

This example provides an overall look at how to use the *OTPF* to guide intervention. Much more detail can be uncovered by examining each aspect of the framework. Furthermore, many occupational therapy models of practice also provide comprehensive guidelines that are congruent with the framework (see Chapter 14).

OCCUPATIONAL THERAPY PROCESS

The *OTPF* provides a description of the process involved in occupational therapy. Specifically, OT practitioners are involved in evaluation, intervention, and outcome of services.[1] The OT is primarily responsible for the evaluation and interpretation of assessments. However, the occupational therapy assistant (OTA) may assist the OT, and he or she contributes to the evaluation by providing data, after service competency has been determined. Service competency refers to verifying that the OTA is able to produce similar consistent results as the OT. The OTA is not responsible for the interpretation of the results. The OT is responsible for developing the intervention plan.[2,4] The key points of the occupational therapy process emphasized by the *OTPF* are listed in Box 9-1.

The **evaluation** includes an occupational profile and analysis of occupational performance. An occupational profile provides background information on the client's goals, habits, occupations, and history.[1] Generally, the occupational profile is obtained through an interview. However, the OT practitioner may also administer assessments to

---

Box 9-1 Key Points of the Occupational Therapy Process

1. The process outlined is dynamic and interactive in nature.
2. Context is an overarching, underlying, and embedded influence on the process of service delivery.
3. The term "client" is used to name the entity who receives occupational therapy services.
4. A client-centered approach is used throughout the Framework
5. "Engagement in occupation" is viewed as the overarching outcome of the occupational therapy process.

From American Occupational Therapy Association: Occupational therapy practice framework: domain and process, *Am J Occup Ther* 56(6):614-615, 2002.

Box 9-2 Occupational Profile

1. Who is the client (individual, caregiver, group, population)?
2. Why is the client seeking service, and what are the client's current concerns relative to engaging in occupations and in daily life activities?
3. What contexts support engagement in desired occupations, and what contexts are inhibiting engagement?
4. What is the client's occupational history (i.e., life experiences, values, interests, and previous patterns of engagement in occupations and in daily life activities; the meanings associated with them)?
5. What are the client's priorities and desired targeted outcomes?
   - Occupational performance
   - Client satisfaction
   - Role competence
   - Adaptation
   - Health and wellness
   - Prevention
   - Quality of life

From American Occupational Therapy Association: Occupational therapy practice framework: domain and process, *Am J Occup Ther* 56(6):616, 2002.

---

obtain the information. Box 9-2 presents the information collected for an occupational profile.

The evaluation process involves a **client-centered approach;** the OT practitioner is interested in the client's viewpoint, narrative, and desires. Because the aim of therapy is to help the client re-engage in occupations, the practitioner determines from the client, if possible, the occupations of interest. A client-centered approach involves working collaboratively with clients and is considered a foundational component of occupational therapy practice.[1,10]

During the evaluation, the OT analyzes the client's performance skills and client factors to determine strengths and limitations for the client. The OT may choose to use formal assessments, including standardized tests or protocols, when evaluating clients. The OTA may assist in the process, once he or she has demonstrated competency in administering the assessment or protocol. However, the OT is responsible for the interpretation of the data.

INTERVENTION PLAN

An intervention plan is developed once the evaluation is completed and the OT has determined the client's strengths and weaknesses, and has analyzed the areas of performance and contexts in which the occupations are performed. The intervention plan is developed with the client to address those areas important to him or her.[1,10] See Table 9-1 for a definition of the contexts.

The intervention plan includes a description of the goals and objectives of intervention. Although the OT develops the plan, the OTA may also contribute to its development (upon establishment of service competency). Goals are designed to be meaningful, relevant to the client, measurable, and occupation based.

Once the goals and objectives have been established, the intervention approach is developed. The *OTPF* identifies five general approaches to intervention: create, establish, maintain, modify, and prevent. The following paragraphs describe each approach and provide a clinical example.

CREATE/PROMOTE (HEALTH PROMOTION)

This approach provides opportunities for people with and without disabilities. The OT practitioner sets up a program or activity in the hope that all those who participate will benefit by enhanced performance.

> Mary, the OT for a local school, developed an after-school handwriting program to help third though fifth graders. The program provided fun strengthening and coordination activities, along with games to do at home. Mary created this program as a service to the children. Occupational therapy students from the local university helped run the groups.

ESTABLISH/RESTORE (REMEDIATE)

The OT practitioner uses strategies and techniques to change client factors to establish skills that have not yet developed or to restore those that have been lost.[1,8]

> Brian, the OT practitioner in a local rehabilitation hospital, worked with Jasmine, a 54-year-old woman who lost use of her right side after a cerebral vascular accident. The goal of the therapy sessions included increasing the use of her right hand and arm so she could prepare meals for her children again. Brian helped Jasmine improve client factors of right arm range of motion, strength, motor control, and eye–hand coordination. Remediation of these client factors ensures that Jasmine is able to meet her goals and cook for her family.

MAINTAIN

This intervention approach provides support to allow the client to continue to perform in the manner in which he or she is accustomed. OT practitioners using this approach help clients keep the same level of performance and, therefore, not decline in functioning.

Harry is an 89-year-old man who still lives on his own in a small first-floor apartment. Harry experienced a mild heart condition, which resulted in a brief hospitalization. The physician requested an occupational therapy evaluation to determine how to help Harry. Harry informed the OT practitioner that he wants to remain living alone; his family is close by for support. The OT practitioner conducted a home evaluation and made some changes in the environment to ensure safety (e.g., removed some scatter rugs, installed grab bars). These changes allowed Harry to maintain his current living situation, despite his decreased endurance and other natural effects of the aging process.

MODIFY (COMPENSATION, ADAPTATION)

Sometimes activities are changed so that clients may continue to perform them despite poor skill level. Compensation refers to changing the demands of the activity or the way the client performs the activity.[1] This is useful when client factors are not changeable in a practical amount of time and the client wishes to engage in the activity.

Gerard, a 10-year-old diagnosed with developmental coordination disorder (DCD),* is extremely disorganized and has difficulty writing quickly. The OT practitioner provides Gerard with a simple day planner (as opposed to a large complicated system) and requests that the teacher provide a list for the child's homework. These compensations allow Gerard to be successful in a regular classroom until his handwriting skills are adequately developed.

*Developmental coordination disorder is characterized by marked motor coordination deficits that interfere with activities of daily living that are not due to physical, sensory, or neurological impairments.[5]

PREVENT

OT practitioners are interested in keeping clients well, and as such they may help clients engage in activities to prevent or slow down disease, trauma, or poor health.

Conrad is the OT practitioner in a rural community with a high percentage of families with obesity. Conrad and his colleagues develop a program for children to engage in physical activity and to educate families about nutrition. The OT practitioner grades and adapts the physical activity as necessary and provides group activities to enhance self-esteem, self-concept, and healthy choices. This program is designed to prevent childhood obesity and the complications that arise from obesity.

The previously mentioned intervention approaches show the range of possibilities for servicing clients. OT practitioners use clinical judgment, experience, and research to determine which type of approach works for the specific client within the particular setting. The OT practitioner considers the context(s), client factors, performance skills, performance patterns, and activity demands when determining the intervention approach. Once the approach is identified, the practitioner develops the intervention plan for therapeutic use of occupations. The following section describes the types of occupational therapy interventions.

TYPES OF OCCUPATIONAL THERAPY INTERVENTIONS

The *OTPF* lists therapeutic use of self (see Chapter 16), therapeutic use of occupations and activities, consultation, and education as the types of occupational therapy intervention.[1] The evaluation process helps OT practitioners determine what type of intervention strategy they will use. Furthermore, the OT practitioner bases these decisions on models of practice (ways to organize one's thoughts[11,15]) and frames of reference (ways to implement therapy). Upon determining the client's goal for therapy, the OT practitioner decides the best strategy for meeting the goals.

Therapeutic use of occupations and activities refers to selecting activities and occupations that will meet the therapeutic goals.[1] OT practitioners may use **preparatory methods** or activities designed to get the client ready to engage in occupations.[1,9] Preparatory activities may include such methods as stretching, range of motion, exercise, and applying heat or ice; and they are designed to get the client ready for purposeful or occupation-based activity. Preparatory activities should be conducted as one part of the intervention session rather than making up the entire session.[9]

Purposeful activities involve choice, are goal-oriented, and do not assume meaning for the person. **Purposeful activity** leads to occupation and may be a part of the occupation. For example, practicing folding towels is considered purposeful activity for the occupation of household maintenance.

The goal of occupational therapy is for clients to engage in occupations that they find meaningful. Therefore, **occupation-based activity** refers to participation in the actual occupation, which has been found to be motivating and which results in better motor responses and improved generalization. Occupation-based activity requires that the activity be completed in the actual context in which it occurs.

Consultation involves "a type of intervention in which practitioners use their knowledge and expertise to collaborate with the client. The collaborative process involves identifying the problem, creating possible solutions, and altering them as necessary for greater effectiveness. When providing consultation, the practitioner is not responsible for the outcome of the intervention."[1,7] **Education** involves imparting knowledge to the client.[1] This intervention type involves providing clients information about the occupation, but it may not result in actual performance of the occupation. For example, an OT practitioner who is treating a young child for a feeding problem may be at the house on one visit when it would be inappropriate to have the child eat. The practitioner can educate the mother by using pictures of the proper way to position the child during feeding.

OUTCOMES

Occupational therapy intervention is designed to help clients engage in occupations. It is important for OT practitioners to measure the outcome of their intervention and to determine whether the overarching goal of engagement in occupations has been met. This is a very broad end result, and OT practitioners use the following more specific outcomes to measure the results of intervention.

The OT practitioner can measure improvement or enhancement of the client's ability to carry out activities of daily living, or what is called **occupational performance.** For example, a client at admission to a skilled nursing facility following hip replacement may not have been able to dress himself due to decreased endurance and prescribed precautions because of the surgery. The client receives occupational therapy intervention to improve his activities of daily living and upon discharge is independent in dressing with the use of assistive devices. The outcome in this case is his ability to independently function in the activity of dressing. Occupational performance outcomes are the most commonly used outcomes in occupational therapy.

As clients improve skills and perform occupations, they show improved **role competence,** that is, the ability to meet the demand of roles.[1] Furthermore, clients become more able to adapt or change to varying situations. Another outcome that can be measured following occupational therapy intervention is **client satisfaction.** This is a measure of the client's perception of the process and the benefits received from occupational therapy services. Because occupational therapy is a client-centered approach, one hopes that the clients are pleased with the outcomes and the process.

Engagement in occupations and activities impacts a client's **health** and **wellness.** Health refers to the state of physical, mental, and social well-being, whereas wellness refers to the condition of being in good health.[1]

Because clients often become active in their lives again after occupational therapy intervention, **quality of life** may improve and thus is considered a desired outcome of intervention. Quality of life measures determine the client's appraisal of his or her satisfaction with life at that given time. Finally, another goal of occupational therapy intervention is prevention of further disease and the promotion of a healthy lifestyle. Whether or not further disease has been prevented and the person is following a healthier lifestyle are also outcomes of occupational therapy that can be measured. The type of outcomes used will depend upon the practice setting.

Outcomes are identified from the very beginning of the occupational therapy process, during the evaluation. At this point in the process, the types of outcomes and measures are selected. The focus on outcomes remains throughout the intervention, and re-evaluation as the client's progress towards the desired goal(s) is measured. Modifications to intervention and decisions (i.e., continue intervention, discontinue intervention) about further intervention are based on the client's needs and performance.

SUMMARY

The *OTPF* provides a description of the occupational therapy domain and process for OT practitioners, students, and consumers. The framework is comprehensive and emphasizes occupation-based intervention. This framework may be used with a variety of models of practice and frames of reference. Together, the OT and OTA (upon reaching service competency) develop intervention goals by collaborating with the client. Once an intervention plan has been developed, the OT and OTA provide intervention that may include therapeutic use of self, therapeutic use of occupation or activity, preparatory methods, consultation, or education. The outcomes of occupational therapy include improving occupational performance, role competence, and quality of life. Occupational therapy intervention may promote client satisfaction, health and wellness, adaptation, and prevention.

Learning Activities

1. Match a list of activities with the area of performance under which they fall.
2. Select an occupation that is important to you. Analyze the performance skills, client factors, and performance patterns required to engage in the occupation. Describe the context(s) in which you most frequently engage in this occupation.

3. Provide a clinical example for each of the five general approaches to intervention. Present these to your classmates.
4. Review research articles exploring occupational therapy intervention. Present to the class a review of how the current literature describes therapeutic use of occupation and activities. Write a three-page paper describing therapeutic use of occupations. Include a short PowerPoint slide show presentation.

Review Questions

1. What are the differences between areas of performance, performance skills, and client factors?
2. How is the occupational therapy process described according to the *OTPF*?
3. What are the types of occupational therapy intervention?
4. What are the five general approaches to intervention?

REFERENCES

1. American Occupational Therapy Association: Occupational therapy practice framework: domain and process, *Am J Occup Ther* 56(6):609-639, 2002.
2. American Occupational Therapy Association: Guide for supervision of occupational therapy personnel, *Am J Occup Ther* 48:1045, 1994.
3. American Occupational Therapy Association: Uniform terminology for occupational therapy, ed. 3, *Am J Occup Ther* 48:1047, 1994.
4. American Occupational Therapy Association: Entry-level role delineation for registered occupational therapists (OTRs) and certified occupational therapy assistants (COTAs), *Am J Occup Ther* 44:1091, 1990.
5. American Psychiatric Association: *Diagnostic and Statistical Manual of Mental Disorders,* ed 4, Washington, DC, 1994, American Psychiatric Association.
6. Christiansen CH, Baum CM (eds): *Occupational Therapy: Enabling Function and Well-being,* Thorofare, NJ, 1996, Slack.
7. Dunn W: *Best Practice in Occupational Therapy in Community Service with Children and Families,* Thorofare, NJ, 2000, Slack.
8. Dunn W, McClain LH, Brown C, et al: The ecology of human performance. In Neidstadt ME, Crepeau EB (eds): *Willard and Spackman's Occupational Therapy,* ed 9, pp. 525-535, Philadelphia, 1998, Lippincott Williams & Wilkins.
9. Fisher AG: Uniting practice and theory in an occupational framework, *Am J Occup Ther* 52(7):509-519, 1998.
10. Law M, Cooper B, Stewart D, et al: The person-environment-occupation model: a transactive approach to occupational performance, *Canad J Occup Ther* 63(1):9-23, 1996.
11. MacRae N: Unpublished lecture notes: OT 301 foundations of occupational therapy, University of New England, 2001.
12. McHale K, Cermak SA: Fine motor activities in elementary school: preliminary findings and provisional implications for children with fine motor problems, *Am J Occup Ther* 46:898-903, 1992.
13. Neidstadt ME, Crepeau EB (eds): *Willard and Spackman's Occupational Therapy,* ed 9, Philadelphia, 1998, Lippincott Williams & Wilkins.
14. Parham LD, Fazio LS (eds): *Play in Occupational Therapy for Children,* St. Louis, 1997, Mosby.
15. Solomon J, O'Brien J: Scope of practice. In Solomon J, O'Brien J (eds): *Pediatric Skills for Occupational Therapy Assistants,* St. Louis, 2006, Mosby.
16. World Health Organization: International Classification of Functioning, Disability and Health (ICF), Geneva, Switzerland, 2001, World Health Organization.

I remember my first months in practice as an occupational therapist. I simply could not believe that anyone would pay me for doing what was pure fun and enjoyment. Today, some 23 years later, I no longer mind being paid for my services as a pediatric therapist. However, I continue to love the practice of occupational therapy with children and marvel that something as fun as therapy is considered to be a "job." Perhaps we should keep it a secret!

Why does occupational therapy with children continue to be personally exciting and stimulating? First, it forces me to critically analyze and solve problems. Simultaneously, I must be concerned about (1) the child's behavior and performance; (2) the parents' perceptions, desires, and concerns; (3) the conditions in the environment that seem to relate to my first two concerns; and (4) the interests and concerns of other adults invested in the child (e.g., physical therapist, teacher, speech therapist). While analyzing all of the variables that influence the child's functional performance and behavior, I must select interaction styles, therapeutic activities, and recommendations that will optimally benefit the child and promote development. What a challenge! Understanding the child–family–environment interaction, solving problems related to the child's function and behavior, and implementing the steps that will lead to a mutually agreed-upon vision for the child is just the right challenge for me.

Jane Case-Smith, EdD, OTR/L, FAOTA
Professor
Division of Occupational Therapy
Ohio State University
Columbus, Ohio

Occupational Therapy Across the Lifespan

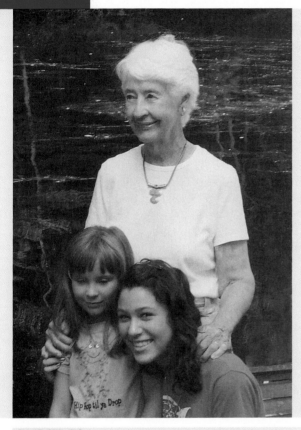

OBJECTIVES

After reading this chapter, the reader will be able to do the following:

- Understand the changes in occupation across the lifespan
- Understand the developmental tasks throughout the lifespan
- Understand client factors across the lifespan
- Describe the types of clients for each developmental stage whom occupational therapy (OT) practitioners work
- Understand the unique services provided by occupational therapy at each developmental stage

KEY TERMS

Adolescence	Developmental delays	Infancy
Adulthood	Developmental frame of	Later adulthood
Aging	reference	Learned helplessness
Cerebral palsy	Family-centered care	Least restrictive environment
Childhood	Hospice	Play

Evan is a premature infant weighing 4 pounds 5 ounces at birth. The OT practitioner works with him in the neonatal intensive care unit (NICU) to help facilitate feeding, sleep/wake cycles, and regulation. The practitioner considers the medical context of Evan's intervention sessions along with the parent and family needs. Evan's family travels far to see him each day, and the toll of the long drive to the hospital begins to show on his parents' faces. The OT practitioner carefully negotiates suggestions so as to support the family and help the client.

Meanwhile, an OT practitioner works with Grace, a 98-year-old woman who hopes to remain at home despite a recent fall. Grace has lived alone since her husband died 25 years ago. She maintains a small house and entertains family on occasion. Grace walks to the post office for her mail daily. She has lived in the small rural town all her life. The occupational therapist (OT) evaluates the safety of her home and makes simple suggestions to Grace and the family so that Grace may remain at home.

These examples illustrate the varied approaches an OT practitioner may take with clients who range in age and ability. Because OT practitioners work with clients of all ages, practitioners need to understand the developmental tasks throughout the lifespan. The following paragraphs provide descriptions of the developmental tasks expected of typical age groupings. Not all persons fit exactly into these groupings. Thus practitioners must view each person individually while being aware of developmental progressions.

INFANCY

Were you a "good" baby? How big were you at birth? At what age did you roll, sit, crawl, walk, talk, or feed yourself? When did you sleep through the night? What were your favorite play things? With whom did you like to play? Were you a picky eater? How was your temperament? OT practitioners ask these questions to learn about infants. Frequently, parents of infants wonder if their child is developing "typically." Because a wide range of "typical" behavior exists, OT practitioners must understand the normal range of development to provide parents with answers for promoting infant development and to provide effective intervention.

DEVELOPMENTAL TASKS OF INFANCY

Infancy represents the period of birth through 1 year. During this period, infants grow rapidly and achieve motor, social, and cognitive skills (Box 10-1). Gross and fine motor skills develop as infants begin to voluntarily reach, grasp objects, roll, sit, crawl, and eventually walk. Notably, infants grow in size, height, and weight. Frequently, pediatricians chart the infant's growth pattern as a sign of early development. Pediatricians also test an infant's reflexes. Primitive reflexes are present at birth or soon after, which is an indication of the infant's neurological development.[1] Reflexes are motor responses to sensory stimuli, such as moving one's foot when the sole of the foot is stroked or quickly putting one's hands in front to avoid falling. Infants possess a variety of reflexes. For example, the sucking reflex, which promotes nutrition, is present.[1] Over the course of the first year, the primitive reflexes typically disappear. Thus the practitioner evaluates for the presence or absence of reflexes as an indicator of development. An infant who continues to have reflexes past the "typical" age may have sustained neurological trauma.[1]

Box 10-1   Developmental Tasks of Infancy (0-1 Years of Age)
Exploration phase: child explores self and environment Motor milestones: integration of primitive reflexes, rolling, prone-on-elbows, sitting, crawling, walking Oral motor control: learning to eat different textures and types of food Social trust develops, including smiling and interactions with others Regulates sleep/wake cycle Fine motor development: holding and releasing objects, picking up objects Engages in solitary play and sensory movements

Adapted from Llorens L: *Application of a Developmental Theory for Health and Rehabilitation,* Rockville, MD, 1982, American Occupational Therapy Association.

Typically, developing infants establish a sleep/wake cycle, and they experience periods of playfulness and express discomfort through crying.[2] However, typical infants can be consoled and stop crying once their needs are met. Infants who are not consolable may have sensory regulation disorder. These children may benefit from occupational therapy to help regulate their behaviors.

Socially, infants interact by smiling and expressing emotions to family members. Infants play pat-a-cake, make eye contact, and smile. Between 8 and 10 months, infants develop stranger anxiety and may cry when approached or held by strangers. Social language begins in infancy with sounds, vocalizations such as cooing, listening, speaking words, and learning to respond to simple verbal directions.[5] Infants begin to reciprocate by taking turns vocalizing or smiling, which is observed when they play "peek-a-boo."

Activities of daily living develop as infants learn to recognize food sources and begin to hold utensils. They may allow caregivers to dress them, and they may enjoy bath time. Infants may begin to pick up food and put it in their mouth. However, infants are dependent on adults to maintain their self-care tasks.

Cognitively, infants develop awareness of objects, and they recognize familiar people. They begin to use toys and bring their hands to their mouths. The infant responds to his or her parent or caregiver. As infants begin to reach for and grasp objects, they learn cause and effect, an important concept for future learning. Infants learn by observing their surroundings and acquire the cognitive skills of object permanence (e.g., the object may be there even if it is out of sight). At this stage, infants begin to look for hidden objects.

DIAGNOSES AND SETTINGS

OT practitioners working with this age group work in neonatal intensive care units (NICU), hospitals, early intervention programs, and home health agencies. The NICU is a specialized environment with the main concern being the medical condition of the client. OT practitioners working in the NICU must receive advanced, specialized training. Pediatric hospitals serve children with numerous medical conditions for brief or extended times. Many pediatric hospitals offer outpatient care for children. This care is intended to maximize the child's development or monitor his or her progress. Some infants discharged from the hospital may receive periodic check-ups at outpatient clinics to monitor their development and growth. Early intervention programs provide services for children 0-3 years of age and may provide services at home or in specialized day care settings. Children may receive early intervention services from a team of professionals. The focus of early intervention is on family-centered care; therefore, empowering parents to advocate for their children is an emphasis of these programs. Infants may be seen in the home by OT practitioners who work for home health agencies.

Because infants are developing, many OT practitioners work in diagnostic clinics to evaluate and provide input into the diagnoses of children. Diagnosing children early may help with payment, care, course of intervention, and support for parents. Diagnosing is meant to help parents and caregivers understand and consequently intervene on behalf of children. However, children will function at different levels despite being given particular diagnoses.

OT practitioners work with infants who may have experienced birth trauma, disease, or genetic conditions that affect their development. Infants with **cerebral palsy** continue to be the largest referral to OT practitioners working in pediatrics. These children experience motor abnormalities caused by an insult to the brain before, during, or soon after birth. Infants with cerebral palsy do not reach milestones as expected for their age. Their motor deficits may result in slow, awkward, or asymmetrical movements. Although the progression of the disorder does not worsen, the child may appear to be getting worse as he or she ages because more is expected as children age. Other diagnoses requiring occupational therapy services include Down syndrome, spina bifida, Erb's palsy, and a host of genetic disorders.

Infants may experience **developmental delays,** which refers to a general slowing of skills. Children with syndromes may be treated by OT practitioners and frequently exhibit developmental delays, cardiac difficulties, and intellectual delays (previously referred to as mental retardation). OT practitioners also work with infants who have failure to thrive, head injury, HIV, or congenital anomalies, such as cleft palate.

The OT practitioner does not treat the diagnosis but rather works with infants and families to help the child function at the highest possible level and actively participate in infant occupations.

INTERVENTION

The OT practitioner works with the infant and the family to facilitate development or, as Llorens suggests, "close the gap."[5] OT practitioners frequently use the developmental frame of reference to evaluate infants.[4,5] The **developmental frame of reference** postulates that practice in a skill set will enhance brain development and help the child progress through the stages. The OT practitioner using a developmental frame of reference begins by evaluating the current level of motor skill development. Once the practitioner has determined the skill level, the underlying client factors that may influence development are examined.[5] Such things as muscle tone, coordination, symmetrical movements, and posture may influence development. Intervention is aimed at improving the underlying factors so the infant may perform the desired skill.[3] Occupational therapy intervention with children is generally playful in nature, but it can include medically based intervention such as splinting, positioning, or cardiac rehabilitation.

OT practitioners working with infants provide **family-centered care,** entailing that they collaborate closely with the family. Family-centered care involves working with family members on goals that are considered important to them. This collaboration works best when members of the team respect and listen to each other. This philosophy of care supports parents as being the "expert" on their child and urges practitioners to listen and respond to family requests.

Although direct intervention using therapeutic use of self and therapeutic use of occupations and activity with infants frequently targets play, behavior regulation, feeding, motor skill development, and sensory regulation, practitioners also intervene through consulting and educating parents. Consulting with parents to address questions and concerns with the infant's development requires the expertise of an experienced OT practitioner. Consulting involves providing suggestions that the OT practitioner is not directly responsible for, such as suggesting an infant attend an infant massage program. The OT practitioner does not provide the infant massage, but he or she may discuss strategies to enhance the infant's success in the activity. The OT practitioners may consult with other programs to collaborate on strategies that will benefit the infant.

Parents may need education about caring for their infant and addressing the special needs of the infant. OT practitioners frequently teach parents how to hold, handle, and calm their infant. Education on feeding techniques and developmentally appropriate activities is common practice. Education may include providing parents with information on the infant's diagnosis, prognosis, and intervention strategies. OT practitioners are skillful at providing this information in a language and format that is understandable to the parents and sensitive to their emotional needs. OT practitioners may also have to educate parents on the data supporting a given intervention. This may involve teaching parents what to look for in terms of outcomes or service from providers. Not only do OT practitioners consult and educate others, they also provide parents with resources. For example, OT practitioners may provide specialized equipment to help infants with positioning, feeding, bathing, and mobility. Infants may require adapted toys that make it possible for them to grasp or manipulate. Practitioners may help support parents by recommending support groups, respite care, and assistance in making things easy at home. OT practitioners must consider the demands of parents when providing home programs. Box 10-2 provides a list of suggestions for home programs.

Box 10-2   Suggestions When Providing Home Programs

Keep it simple; parents are busy and may be overwhelmed.
Provide playful, fun, and easy suggestions that can easily be incorporated into the day.
Provide suggestions that will make things easier for the parent.
Provide suggestions when asked.
Limit suggestions.
Write down home program suggestions.
Be sure the parent will be successful when implementing the suggestion (grade the activity so that it is easy to accomplish).
Ask the parent to demonstrate the activity to you before suggesting it as a home program.
Request that the parent demonstrate it to you when the family returns for the next session, and make sure you ask how it went. Let the parent show you how well the infant is doing. Praise the parent for being successful, and thank him or her for following through.
If the parent did not follow through with the program, be sure to empathize and ask what interfered with the ability to do this. See if you can adapt the activity or provide a suggestion that will be more easily implemented.
Try to provide the parent with activities for carry through, not activities that are really therapy. If the child does not like doing something with you, do not give that as a home suggestion. However, you may give a portion of the activity (in which the child is successful) so that the child is more ready for the next session.

CHILDHOOD

Childhood includes early childhood (1-6 years) and later childhood or school-aged children (6-12 years). Childhood represents a time of growth and refining of skills.[5] Children develop more coordination and strength and are therefore able to perform such skills as running, jumping, and more coordinated games. **Play** is the occupation of childhood; it is characterized as a spontaneous, enjoyable, rules-free, internally motivated activity in which there is no goal or purpose.[2] For example, children may spontaneously engage in playing and singing joyfully in the rain or at the beach (Figure 10-1, *A* and *B*). Furthermore, children progress from playing independently (solitary play), to playing alongside peers (parallel play) in early childhood. After parallel play, children gain more abilities and engage in cooperative play (play towards an end goal), and in later childhood, games with rules become important. The stages of childhood development are continuous and influenced by culture, family, and environmental variables (Box 10-3).

DEVELOPMENTAL TASKS OF CHILDHOOD

Motor skills develop during early childhood as children learn to sit, walk, run, climb, and jump. School-aged children refine motor coordination and develop strength and endurance for activities.

Play is the occupation of childhood and the manner in which they learn and practice social, cognitive, and motor abilities.[4,5] Early childhood is a time of intense play, and children move from parallel play to cooperative play activities. The nature of play changes as the child develops expertise. This is easily observed when comparing the difference between 2-year-olds trying to share toys (something that may not be easily accomplished) and the behavior of 4-year-olds (who are able to skillfully negotiate sharing). As children enter school, they begin to participate in cooperative play. For example, school-aged children spend large amounts of time working out the "rules" to games and developing elaborate themes and scenarios for their play.[2] Sports and competitive games become important as children begin to test their new skills.

Imaginative play develops around 3-5 years of age. This type of play involves "pretending" or make-believe scenarios, which requires cognitive problem-solving and sequencing. As children develop storylines, they may actually role-play concerns and consequently deal with stressful situations through play. Thus, imaginative play helps the child work through daily issues. Interestingly, children with special needs often do not exhibit imaginary play. Thus the OT practitioner may want to promote the creativity and problem-solving skills that come with imaginative play.

As children go to school, they engage in the occupation of education, which involves interacting with others, following rules, reading, writing, playground activities, and socialization. Children must follow the routine and communicate their needs to a new authority figure (i.e., teacher). They must pay attention to verbal directions, take turns, and transition to new activities. Remembering the rules, routines, and tasks associated with learning may challenge children. Such tasks as remembering sneakers for gym, the note from the teacher, or the homework assignment may appear straightforward to an adult, but may actually be stressful to a child and difficult to remember. However, these tasks are part of childhood and, therefore, all children must have the opportunity to show they can complete them. Education requires children to remember academic facts and to participate in the cognitive processes entailed in learning.

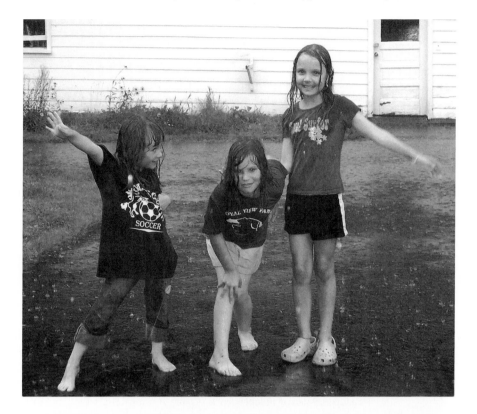

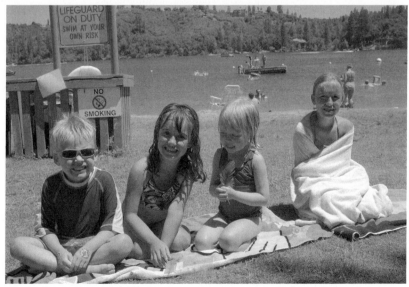

Figure 10-1 A, Molly, Alison, and Lydia enjoy playing in the rain. **B,** Cameron, Andie, Natalie, and Jamie enjoy a day playing at the beach.

Box 10-3 Developmental Tasks of Childhood

Early Childhood (1-6 Years of Age)
Competency phase: children begin to regulate their behavior
Differentiates choices based upon inner images
Fluctuations in behavior ("terrible twos") may be observed as child tries to assert him or herself
Refinement of existing motor, cognitive, and social skills
Play is symbolic, dramatic, and constructive with pre-games
Fantasy play is a precursor for occupational choice; pretend play becomes more prevalent between the ages of 4 and 6
Learns sex differences
Learn concepts of social and physical reality
Learns to relate emotionally to parents, siblings, and others
Learns to distinguish right from wrong
Develops conscience

Late Childhood (6-12 Years of Age)
Achievement stage: children enter into the student role; there is a concern for standards of performance
Learns physical skills for ordinary games
Increases speed, accuracy, and coordination
Learns to get along with peers
Learns appropriate masculine or feminine social role
Develops wholesome attitude toward self
Develops skills in reading, writing, and calculating
Develops concepts necessary for everyday living
Develops conscience, morality, and scale of values
Achieves personal independence
Separates from family environment (toward school)
Develops attitudes toward social groups and institutions

Adapted from Llorens L: *Application of a Developmental Theory for Health and Rehabilitation,* Rockville, MD, 1982, American Occupational Therapy Association.

Cognitive skills for learning require memory, attention, problem-solving, sequencing, calculation, categorizing, language, and communication. Children must be able to show their cognitive skills through verbal and written communication. In addition, sensory perception is necessary for making sense of one's environment. For example, children must not only identify the letters but be able to use visual perception to ascribe meaning to them so that they can read.

Asserting one's needs is necessary to be successful in the classroom. Children need to ask questions when they are confused or curious. Furthermore, they need to hear answers and make sense of what they hear. Children with special needs are frequently passive, and often the OT practitioner helps them indicate their wants. Advocating for oneself is an important educational and life skill.

Along with the cognitive skills required for education, children engage in motor skills such as writing, tying their shoes, and carrying a book bag. Children move around the classroom. Motor requirements of gym or singing may pose difficulties for children. Children must be able to independently use the bathroom and eat in the lunchroom. Frequently, adaptations may allow all children to participate in these activities. OT practitioners help children in schools who may have difficulty with these tasks. Childhood can be an exciting time for children. Yet children may require support and assistance in learning how to work with their strengths and weaknesses. Empowering children through play and successful experiences may lay the foundation for a strong sense of self and lead to positive self-esteem and self-concept.

Social participation is an important occupation of childhood. Children learn to get along with others through play as they express emotions, communicate, negotiate, and work out play issues. Children must learn to take turns, listen to others, and express their needs. Through play, they may begin to realize that everyone is different, with different strengths and weaknesses. In addition, children begin to figure out how the social systems work; consequently, children may be "best friends" one day and not speaking to each other the next day. These issues are important and emotional, and children may require support from the OT practitioner, parent, and teacher.

DIAGNOSES AND SETTINGS

OT practitioners working with children provide intervention to children with such diagnoses as cerebral palsy, autism, Down syndrome, intellectual disabilities, developmental coordination disorder, developmental delay, and others. Some children experience childhood illnesses, such as cancer, asthma, sickle cell anemia, or have rare medical conditions such as William's, Angelman's, or Tourette's syndrome. Still others may experience physical disabilities such as spinal cord injuries, head injuries, amputations, burns, or orthopedic deformities. Finally, children may experience a host of behavioral and psychological disorders that may impact their ability to function in a school, such as attention deficit hyperactivity disorder, conduct disorder, learning disorder, or post-traumatic stress disorder.

Children are treated primarily by OT practitioners in school systems and clinics, but they may also receive occupational therapy in hospitals, depending on the diagnosis.

INTERVENTION

OT practitioners working with children focus intervention on play development.[2] Through play, children learn motor, cognitive, social, psychological, and language skills. Children who exhibit play deficits may have difficulty interacting with others, sharing toys, maneuvering around objects, and exhibiting signs of joy.

OT practitioners may use play as the end goal of therapy or as a means to improve motor, social, or cognitive skills.[2,6] When play is the goal of the therapy session, the practitioner is trying to improve the child's play skills. When play is the means used in the session, the practitioner is trying to reach another goal through play.[2,4,6]

Consider the case of 3-year-old Donovan, whose parents are concerned that he does not play well with other children, does not share his toys, and frequently throws toys at others instead of manipulating them. The OT practitioner using *play as a means* may design a play session aimed at improving Donovan's ability to pick up objects and use them as they are intended. The practitioner begins by playing a game of catch with large balls, showing Donovan that this is fun. Next, the practitioner introduces a variety of large-sized Legos and playfully tries to get Donovan to build. Play is the means used to improve Donovan's reaching and grasping skills. The OT practitioner may use *play as the goal* of the therapy session by focusing the entire session on improving Donovan's ability to engage in play. In another scenario, the goal of the session may be for Donovan to share his toys with the practitioner. The practitioner plays ball and a variety of games involving sharing of toys. Play is the goal of this session (specifically, sharing).

School-aged children must be able to function in a school system. Therefore OT practitioners help children obtain the necessary foundational skills for sitting at a desk, reading, writing, eating in the cafeteria, playing on the playground, and participating in music, gym, and other academic learning. Occupational therapy services provided in the schools are considered related services, and the role of the OT practitioner is to help the child function within the classroom in the **least restrictive environment.** The least restrictive environment is the classroom closest to a regular classroom in which the student can be successful. Inclusive environments, in which children are in regular classrooms as much as possible, are considered ideal for children with special needs, although some children require specialized classrooms for at least part of the academic day.

Practitioners working with children are creative, playful, and able to promote structure and limits. They are sensitive to the child's and parents' needs and attentive to the family. Intervention is aimed at play; school-aged tasks; and independence in playground behavior, handwriting, skills for learning (e.g., perception), and self-care skills.

OT practitioners working in schools are skillful at consulting with teachers, providing overall suggestions that may benefit all or one of the students. For example, the OT practitioner may suggest that the teacher promote handwriting warm-up exercises in the middle of the day prior to writing. This may benefit many children, but not all. The OT practitioner provides the warm-up exercises and reviews them with the teacher, but does not directly implement the intervention. An OT practitioner may work with children in the classroom or provide direct service to prepare children to be more successful.

ADOLESCENCE

Adolescence may be considered a time of turmoil as the person tries to develop a sense of self that is independent from his or her parents. Searching for one's identity is the primary role of adolescence (Box 10-4).[5,6] This period of striving for independence is characterized by peer group pressures to conform or fit in. Subsequently, adolescents focus on the peer group. Clothing, hair, and language may imitate other members of the peer group. Adolescents may engage in competitive games and enjoy group play and team activities (Figure 10-2). The adolescent enjoys games with rules and is concerned with

---

Box 10-4 Developmental Tasks of Adolescence (12-20 Years of Age)

Learns habits for adequate performance in adult roles
Role transition, ambiguity, and experimentation
Develops more mature relationships with peers
Masculine/feminine social roles are defined
Acceptance of one's physique and using body effectively occurs
Achieves assurance of economic independence
Selects and prepares for occupation
Prepares for marriage and family life
Develops intellectual skill and concepts necessary for civic competence
Desires and achieves socially responsible behavior
Acquires a set of values and ethics

Adapted from Llorens L: *Application of a Developmental Theory for Health and Rehabilitation,* Rockville, MD, 1982, American Occupational Therapy Association.

group standards rather than adult standards. Adolescents begin to show interest in town, state, and country, rather than just focusing on the family (as in childhood).[5]

Adolescence is a period of role confusion in relationships with adults and a time of developing a sexual identity.[5,6] In general, adolescents are striving to develop their own identity apart from their parents. Therefore intense variability and insecurity occur during adolescence. Puberty occurs in early adolescence; and, with this change, adolescents demonstrate a strong desire for attention, an increased interest in the opposite sex, and frequent "crushes." They seek out support from their peers while trying to establish independence from their parents.

OT practitioners working with adolescents are aware of the challenges of this period of development when creating an intervention plan. OT practitioners work with adolescents who may have suffered disease, trauma, or a psychological event; they thus require help to face the expected challenges of adolescence in addition to those presented by the disability.

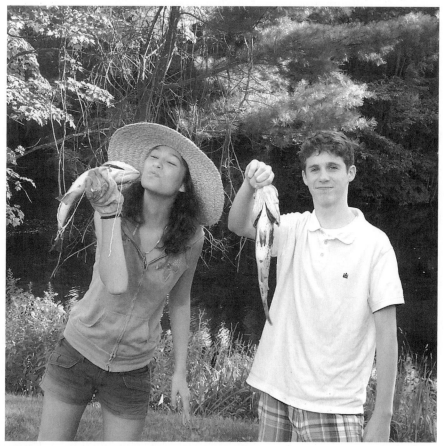

Figure 10-2 Cousins Abby and Keegan "compete" over who has the biggest fish—a typical behavior of adolescents.

DEVELOPMENTAL TASKS OF ADOLESCENCE

Physically, adolescents are growing and becoming stronger.[5,6] Children going through the awkward phase of puberty may be physically self-conscious and require assistance in understanding changes in their bodies. Postural changes, awkward motor movements, and rapid growth all make movements somewhat challenging. As the adolescent is concerned with how he or she is viewed by the peer group, the adolescent may spend more time on self-care, grooming, and hygiene issues. Girls will have to address menstruation issues. Boys will have to address the changes in their bodies as well. Furthermore, puberty is a time in which children develop a sexual identity.[4-6] Thus parents and therapists working with adolescents will need to address these issues. Adolescents can be self-conscious and egocentric. Safety issues may become important because an adolescent may make decisions that may appear impulsive and immature. Leisure activities and social participation become very important to adolescents.

Adolescence is a period of self-identity. These children start thinking about what they want to be when they grow up. Peer groups are important and influence the adolescent's dress, behavior, habits, choices, and routines.[2,6] Adolescents who experience psychological disturbances beyond those that are typical of adolescence may need intervention to develop self-concept, identity, and social skills.[2,6]

DIAGNOSES AND SETTINGS

OT practitioners working with adolescents may be working with them in hospitals, day treatment centers, school systems, or rehabilitation centers. Because adolescence is a time of transition, the OT practitioner may assist adolescents in transitioning to high school or with work readiness such as vocational rehabilitation. Adolescents with whom OT practitioners work may require firm limits, choice, understanding, and positive role models. The OT practitioner will want to relate to the adolescent without acting like a peer. Adolescents going through puberty may have questions about sexuality, which the OT practitioner may need to address.[5,6]

Mental health issues and psychological disorders such as bipolar or borderline personality disorder[4-6] may arise during puberty. Furthermore, adolescents may exhibit signs of anorexia, bulimia, or other eating disorders. They may become conflicted and show signs of suicidal depression. Finally, adolescents who experience physical disabilities may require special attention to deal with issues of sexuality, body image, and future goals and aspirations. The OT practitioner may help adolescents with all of these issues.

INTERVENTION

OT practitioners working with adolescents must set firm yet fair limits. Because adolescents typically question authority figures, the OT practitioner must be firm about expectations and consequences.[6] Generally, adolescents with whom OT practitioners work are experiencing an emotional or physical trauma. This, along with the emotions associated with adolescence, may magnify feelings. Finding opportunities for the adolescent to express himself or herself appropriately (e.g., writing, reflection, small group, individual sessions) may be beneficial.[6]

Teens may push limits and question authority. However, they must learn to trust the practitioner. Practitioners may gain trust by following through with tasks and checking in with the adolescent. It is helpful to give the adolescent control where possible.[6] In occupational therapy practice, this may be as simple as providing the adolescent a choice of activities.

OT practitioners must consider how adolescents will interact in a group situation.[6] Sometimes, involving teens in healthy group activities provides them with the support and mentoring they need. For example, Special Olympics provides teens with disabilities a feeling of competition and team membership. Adolescents with special needs may need help in all areas, such as self-care, leisure, and independence. OT practitioners may lead groups to teach teens the necessary skills for grooming, hygiene, and other self-care tasks. The practitioner may use an educational approach or may have to adapt the tasks so the teen with physical problems is able to complete them. For example, providing adaptive clothing may be a good solution when a teen is unable to button or zip. However, the OT practitioner should include the teen's clothing preferences in this intervention strategy. Perhaps the teen would prefer to struggle with regular clothing so that he or she could wear a special outfit. The clinician must be aware of the client's motivations.

Other interventions may be targeted to work-related activities to prepare the teen for the workplace.[6] Perhaps the teen is in need of social skills for work, refined work habits, or skills in filling out a job application. OT practitioners examine all aspects of gaining employment by analyzing what is required and by determining areas in which the client may need assistance.

Other teens may experience lack of leisure activities. In particular, troubled teens may engage in unhealthy leisure activities. Exploring healthy leisure opportunities may open up new experiences for teens.

YOUNG AND MIDDLE ADULTHOOD

Where do you work? What do you do? Do you have a boyfriend or girlfriend? These questions represent the challenges of young and middle adulthood. Adults assume responsibility for their own development or deterioration. **Adulthood** is generally considered a time of achievement, a time when the adult makes employment decisions. Group affiliations continue to be important (family, social, interest, civic). Adults are concerned with guiding the next generation, with creativity, and with productivity.

DEVELOPMENTAL TASKS OF YOUNG AND MIDDLE ADULTHOOD

Adulthood can be separated into young (20-40 years), middle (40-65 years), and late adulthood (over 65 years). The developmental tasks may differ slightly among these stages of adulthood. In young adulthood, the developmental tasks include finding a significant relationship, securing employment, and developing a career path (Box 10-5). Adulthood includes establishing one's home—buying a home or renting an apartment. Typically, adults have an established identity, live independently, and may choose to marry and start a family.[4,5] Families can differ in configuration (Figure 10-3). For example, a "traditional" family consists of husband, wife, and children. Today, however, families may consist of two men raising children or two women raising children. Some children are raised by grandparents or aunts and uncles. Adults make these decisions about whether and how they will raise children, and what type of family configuration they wish to have.

A major focus of adulthood is selecting and establishing a career. In young adulthood, individuals may be completing educational or other work requirements for the career. Middle adulthood is generally considered a time when the adult has met the requirements for the career or job and has an established track record. However, many adults will change careers, and seeking a new career is also considered a task of middle adulthood.

Box 10-5 Developmental Tasks of Adulthood

Young Adulthood (20-40 Years of Age)
Ability to function independently
Selecting and establishing career; work is a major source of meaning
Formation of significant relationships
Development of self-identity
Acceptance of parents' limitations
Leaving home
Personal grooming and hygiene
Managing a home
Establishing a family
Child rearing
Middle Adulthood (40-65 Years of Age)
Achieving civic and social responsibility—legacy
Midlife crisis—reformulates direction
Establishing and maintaining an economic standard of living
Assisting teenaged children to become responsible, happy adults
Developing adult leisure time activity
Accepting and adjusting to physiological changes of middle age
Adjusting to aging parents
Emotional responsibilities as parents end as children leave home
Ongoing financial responsibility becomes finite and predictable
Women lose capacity to bear children

Adapted from Llorens L: *Application of a Developmental Theory for Health and Rehabilitation,* Rockville, MD, 1982, American Occupational Therapy Association.

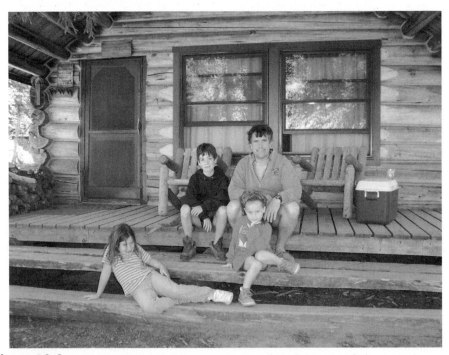

Figure 10-3 Scott, Alison, and Molly enjoy camping with Dad. (Mom took the picture.)

Middle adulthood is a time when the adult has maintained employment, established a satisfying lifestyle with loved ones, and is contributing to society. Successful adults may be financially secure and have friends and engage in leisure (Figure 10-4).

Interestingly, at some point many adults question decisions and examine their life progress. This is frequently referred to as the "midlife crisis." This may be a period when the adult changes jobs, goes back to school, or moves to another state. OT practitioners working with adults may encounter clients who have experienced a serious disruption due to illness, trauma, or a psychological event, and the practitioner may need to help the client re-evaluate his or her abilities. Furthermore, middle-aged adults must accept the physical changes of middle age. This frequently presents as decreased strength, decreased endurance, and signs of aging (e.g., wrinkles, weight gain, and hair loss).

Adults in this stage may be raising teenagers. Adults may also be adjusting to aging parents. This is sometimes referred to as the "sandwich generation" because adults may be caring for their children and their parents at the same time. Some middle adults may be experiencing the "empty nest syndrome," in which their children have all moved out of the house. One phenomenon today is that children who have left the house may return to live at home as young adults.

DIAGNOSES AND SETTINGS

Adults may experience a whole range of physical illnesses affecting functioning, including heart disease, neurological impairments, orthopedic disabilities, and psychological disturbances. Schizophrenia, bipolar disorder, borderline personality, obsessive-compulsive

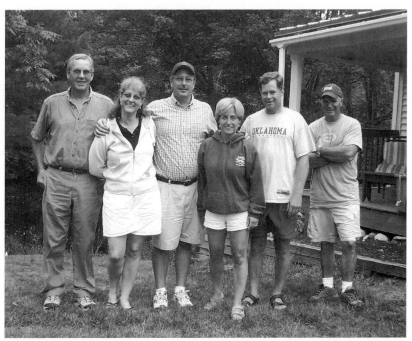

Figure 10-4 Classmates from the Yarmouth class of '77 enjoy spending time together during a recent reunion. The classmates have established their own families and careers and some have children entering college.

disorder, and a wide variety of psychiatric disorders may emerge during adulthood. Furthermore, clients may have such diagnoses as obesity, substance abuse, and other unhealthy life choices, which impact their occupational performance. Adults may have experienced physical or psychological trauma that has left them ill prepared to function in their various roles.

INTERVENTION

The goal of occupational therapy intervention with adults is to help them re-engage in occupations that they find meaningful.[3-5] This involves examining the neuromusculoskeletal, social, psychological, and cognitive aspects of occupations within the contexts of the client's environment. Thus occupational therapy intervention may focus on psychological functioning and take place in psychiatric settings, group settings, day treatment settings, or outpatient clinics. Adults may experience motor dysfunction due to illness, trauma, cerebral vascular accident, or other causes. Clients with motor dysfunction may be treated at hospitals, clinics, rehabilitation settings, and specialized programs. Adults may also be served by OT practitioners at home or at work. Many work settings have ergonomic programs that employ an OT practitioner.

LATER ADULTHOOD

Later adulthood is a time of reflection and evaluation of one's life. Many physical changes occur during this period, and the elderly must also adjust to and accept their impending death. Furthermore, older adults value group affiliations and may be concerned with what they will leave behind to the younger generation.

DEVELOPMENTAL TASKS OF LATER ADULTHOOD

Later adulthood is characterized by retirement and decrease in workload, and the emphasis shifts to community. Older adults deal with loss of spouse or peers, and this loss of others may result in depression, sadness, and prolonged grief. Some older adults have difficulty adapting to these changes; however, many healthy older adults are able to deal with loss and grief when supported by family and friends (Box 10-6).

Individuals struggle with physical declines, although this does not have to mean a loss of independence. Physical declines common with later adulthood include impaired hearing, poor balance and strength, and visual decline. Adults in later adulthood may experience tactile changes or poor circulation issues interfering with their ability to feel changes in terrain.

Box 10-6 Developmental Tasks of Late Adulthood (Over 65 Years of Age)

Adjustment to decreasing physical strength and health
Adjustment to retirement and reduced income
Adjustment to death of spouse and peers
Adjustment to one's own impending death
Establishment of affiliations with one's own age group
Meeting social obligations
Volunteerism
Independent living

Adapted from Llorens L: *Application of a Developmental Theory for Health and Rehabilitation*, Rockville, MD, 1982, American Occupational Therapy Association.

Some older adults experience cognitive changes, such as difficulty with memory and attending to multiple stimuli. Older adults are able to learn, however, and remaining active is important to staying independent and well.

Many older adults stay active in community activities and family events (Figure 10-5).[3] Those who continue to be physically and cognitively active live longer and with fewer hospitalizations.[3]

DIAGNOSES AND SETTINGS

OT practitioners working with older adults consider safety in the home and community. Wellness programs may be beneficial to older adults, such as those offered by senior citizen centers or local recreational leagues.[3-5] Clients with whom OT practitioners work may need assistance in modifying activities and help in obtaining education on the various diseases, diagnosis, and prognoses associated with them.

The **aging** process provides older adults with challenges not found in the other age levels. For example, older adults experience sensory and physical declines. Older adults may lose social supports, and they frequently lose income due to retirement. The OT practitioner may work with older adults who are experiencing difficulty transitioning into new roles, or who have lost roles and are experiencing loss and grief. The OT practitioner working with older adults helps the client remain active and engaged in his or her occupations, despite physical limitations. Such diagnoses as Alzheimer's disease, Parkinson's disease, stroke, cardiac conditions, rheumatoid arthritis, and diabetes may take a toll on the older adult.

Some clients with terminal illnesses may be served through **hospice,** which provides services to help the client be comfortable during the last stages of life. OT practitioners may help clients be comfortable while others are caring for them. It may be that the practitioner provides adaptive equipment (e.g., specialized lift) so that a client may be cared for more easily. Older adults with cancer may receive hospice care toward the end

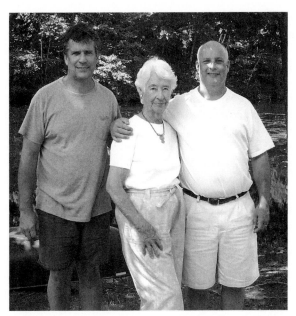

Figure 10-5 Jean enjoys spending time with her sons.

of the process. In these examples, the role of occupational therapy is to aid in the care of the client. This frequently involves prescribing adaptive equipment to make self-care easier and safer.

INTERVENTION

The OT practitioner is skilled at remediating dysfunction, compensating for lack of function, or adapting and modifying activities so that clients can be successful. Falls in the elderly and general safety issues are important concerns of occupational therapy. Practitioners may be called upon to conduct a home visit to analyze the safety of the environment. Practitioners search for unsafe walking areas, which may include stairs, scatter rugs, and uneven floors. Older persons may require changes in lighting to help with safety issues. The practitioner evaluates whether the person is able to contact someone in case of emergency and determines if extra precautions or accommodations need to be made in case of a fire or other home emergency.

Driving is important to older adults. Frequently, the physical changes of aging—such as delayed reaction time, slower movements, poor vision, and decreased hearing—make driving unsafe for older adults. Older adults who have suffered from cerebral vascular accidents (i.e., stroke) may have impaired physical abilities, such as decreased range of motion, causing them to have difficulty turning their heads to observe the road fully. They may have poor range of motion to depress the brake pedal adequately or a host of other issues. OT practitioners frequently analyze the numerous skills and client factors required for safe driving. The practitioner may help older adults regain skills for driving or address with the client how to use other means of transportation.

Because many older adults experience sensory changes, OT practitioners may help by providing instructions in large print and speaking loudly (although not infantilizing). Making visual accommodations, such as using contrasting materials, may be helpful to clients. Furthermore, limiting background noise, which may interfere with clarity of hearing, is beneficial to older adults. Older adults may experience difficulty maneuvering in crowded rooms with miscellaneous obstacles. Thus the OT practitioner should ensure that the physical space in which the activity occurs is not cluttered.

Learned helplessness is a phenomenon many elderly people manifest. This results when others do everything for the older individual and do not allow him or her to make decisions and engage in activities. Thus the senior begins to feel and act helpless and relinquishes control over things that previously held value. Some elders are put into positions that do not feel comfortable to them. For example, if one spouse becomes ill, the other spouse may need to make financial and health decisions, which they have not done before. This can cause stress on the spouse and hinder his or her health. Keeping clients active and engaged is important, and it is the foundation of occupational therapy practice. For those older adults who do not want to participate, OT practitioners may ask them to help out a peer, which is frequently motivating for others. Furthermore, exploration of volunteer opportunities may prove rewarding for many older adults (e.g., reading programs, tutoring).

SUMMARY

OT practitioners consider the stage of life of the client when conducting an evaluation and interventions. Each person enters different stages of life at different ages and for varied time periods. Clients may identify significant life events as turning points. Kielhofner suggests exploring the occupational profile of a client by examining the plots and trajectory of the person's life.[4] This provides the OT practitioner and client with a picture of a whole life to review. Understanding the developmental tasks over the lifespan provides important insight into the occupations associated with the period in a person's life.

Learning Activities

1. Divide the developmental stages among members of the class. Ask each group to present the developmental tasks for the respective developmental stage.
2. Divide the class into five groups and assign a developmental stage to each group. Ask each group to identify a variety of age-appropriate activities for their particular stage. Then have each group present their activities to the class, explaining why the activities are suited for their particular developmental stage.
3. Research some physical and psychological changes associated with a given age group. Summarize the findings in a short paper.
4. View movies such as *On Golden Pond, Father of the Bride,* and *The Breakfast Club.* Discuss the developmental issues displayed in each. Did the characters adjust to the tasks?
5. Develop a handout describing the expectations for each age group.

Review Questions

1. What are the developmental tasks associated with each age group (infancy, childhood, adolescence, adulthood, later adulthood)?
2. In what settings do OT practitioners who provide services to infants work?
3. What are some of the physical changes associated with later adulthood?
4. What are some suggestions for OT practitioners working with children or adolescents?
5. What are some of the occupational concerns of adults?

REFERENCES

1. Anderson R, Boehme R, Cupps B: *Normal Development of Functional Motor Skills,* Austin, 1993, Therapy Skill Builders.
2. Bundy A: Assessment of play and leisure: delineation of the problem, *Am J Occup Ther* 47:217, 1993.
3. Christiansen C, Baum C: *Occupational Therapy: Enabling Function and Well-being,* ed 2, Thorofare, NJ, 1997, Slack, Inc.
4. Kielhofner G (ed): *A Model of Human Occupation,* Baltimore, MD, 2002, Williams & Wilkins.
5. Lorens L: *Application of a Developmental Theory for Health and Rehabilitation,* Rockville, MD, 1982, American Occupational Therapy Association.
6. Vroman KD: Adolescent development: the journey to adulthood. In Solomon J, O'Brien J, (eds): *Pediatric Skills for Occupational Therapy Assistants,* ed 2, St. Louis, 2006, Mosby.

I have always been interested in *why* and *when* people choose occupational therapy as their career. I chose occupational therapy early on, but it took years for me to realize that it was, indeed, the career for me. My first love was art. However, when I was nearing the end of my sophomore year, I ran out of funds and could not continue as a contemporary crafts major at the University of Kansas. My aunt, an occupational therapist at the Menninger Foundation in Topeka, was supervising a fieldwork student from Texas Woman's University, and in her observation, there was money for OT students at TWU, and in that era OT was synonymous with crafts.

I graduated with my BS in Occupational Therapy from TWU 2 years later, in 1964. I set out to be an artist/craftsman, financing my studio work by working as an occupational therapist. My next venture was graduate study in anthropology with an emphasis on American Indian textiles and textile conservation, then teaching fiber constructions in continuing education but also working as a part-time occupational therapist. The next degree was in counseling. As I moved from one discipline to another, I continued to work as a clinical occupational therapist across the country, and then as an educator. It was somewhere around 1982, when I had returned to TWU as an instructor and was preparing to teach an occupational therapy history course, I realized that my own personal evolution mirrored that of the profession. I didn't *discover* occupational therapy . . . for me; it was a process—not of immediate discovery and ownership but of entering through the "back door" without much fanfare. It took some time for me to realize that *occupation* was the consistent thread that connected all of my interests: art, crafts, anthropology, and counseling. People and their occupations, their engagement in meaningful activities, these were the things that interested me; no matter what path I took along the way . . . I *was an occupational therapist*, or, as I prefer, an *occupation-centered practitioner,* and continue to be, quite happily!

Linda S. Fazio, PhD, OTR/L, FAOTA
Professor of Clinical Occupational Therapy
Assistant Chair and Coordinator of the Professional Program
Department of Occupational Science and Occupational Therapy
University of Southern California
Los Angeles, California

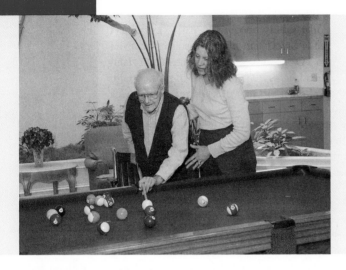

OBJECTIVES

After reading this chapter, the reader will be able to do the following:

- Describe how the holistic approach influences the ways in which occupational therapy (OT) practitioners practice
- Characterize settings in which OT practitioners are employed by types of administration, levels of care, and spheres of practice
- Identify the primary health problems addressed in different settings
- Identify various occupational therapy employment settings

KEY TERMS

Acute care
Biological sphere
Continuum of care
Diagnosis-related groups
  (DRGs)

Long-term care
Private for-profit agencies
Private not-for-profit agencies
Psychological sphere
Public agencies

Sociological sphere
Subacute care

As discussed in Chapter 3, occupational therapy subscribes to a holistic approach in that practitioners examine the biological, social, and psychological aspects of the person and how they influence the individual's ability to engage in occupations. Because of this outlook, OT practitioners work with clients of all ages, disabilities, and in many different settings. Furthermore, OT practitioners continue to develop service in nontraditional settings to better serve clients. This chapter provides an overview of the types of settings in which OT practitioners work.

CHARACTERISTIC OF SETTINGS

The different types of settings in which OT practitioners are employed can be characterized according to (1) administration of the setting, (2) levels of care, and (3) spheres of practice. Administration refers to the system's organization and management. Levels of care define the type of service and length of time a client receives services. Spheres of practice relate to the types of conditions that the setting serves. Each of these characteristics influences the occupational therapy services provided to clients.

ADMINISTRATION OF SETTING

Health care agencies can be categorized as public, private not-for-profit, or private for-profit (also called proprietary). This categorization affects the agency's mission and purpose, reimbursement mechanisms, and organizational structure.

Public agencies are operated by federal, state, or county governments. Federal level agencies include the Veteran's Administration Hospitals and Clinics, Public Health Services Hospitals and Clinics, and Indian Health Services. State-run agencies may include correctional facilities, hospitals for persons who are mentally ill or have developmental disabilities, and medical school hospitals and clinics. The county may operate county hospitals, clinics, and rehabilitation facilities that deliver services to clients in the same way as federal and state facilities. However, the administration must follow different rules and regulations, which may affect employment or method of reimbursement.

Private not-for-profit agencies receive special tax exemptions and typically charge a fee for services and maintain a balanced budget to provide services. These agencies include hospitals and clinics with religious affiliations, private teaching hospitals, and organizations such as the Easter Seal Society and United Cerebral Palsy.

Private for-profit agencies are owned and operated by individuals or a group of investors. These agencies are in business to make a profit. Large for-profit corporations may form multi-facility systems. These corporations may focus on one specific level of care (e.g., all hospitals or all nursing homes) or own multiple facilities across the continuum of care (e.g., a hospital, a skilled nursing facility, an outpatient facility). A multi-facility system is able to buy supplies and equipment in bulk at a lower volume rate. Because these systems provide a wider range of services, they have an advantage when it comes to developing contracts with third-party payers to provide health care services.

LEVELS OF CARE

Another way of characterizing health care settings is by the level of care required by the client. Health care is provided to the consumer along a continuum, as the client's needs dictate, referred to as the **continuum of care. Acute care** is the first level on the continuum. A client at this level has a sudden and short-term need for services and is typically seen in a hospital. Services provided in the hospital are expensive because of the high cost of technology and the number of services provided. The Prospective Payment System, introduced under Public Law 98-21 and passed in 1983, changed the way in which hospitals were paid through Medicare. Under this system, a nationwide schedule defines how much Medicare reimburses hospitals. Depending on the client's diagnosis, hospitals are paid a predetermined, fixed fee, based on **diagnosis-related groups (DRGs),** regardless of the services provided. The system provides an incentive for hospitals and physicians to reduce costs and to discharge clients from the hospital as soon as possible. As a result, the average length of a hospital stay has decreased since 1983.[6] The move to short hospital stays and the implementation of cost-cutting measures have resulted in a decrease in the number of OT practitioners working in hospital-based settings.[5,6,7]

Shorter hospital stays also created a need for an interim level of care, referred to as **subacute care.** At this level, the client still needs care but does not require an intensive level or specialized service, thereby reducing hospital costs. Persons receiving subacute care are "medically complex cases requiring a longer period of rehabilitation and recovery, usually from 1 to 4 weeks." Hospitals with excess acute care beds have converted beds to less expensive subacute care beds, whereas skilled nursing facilities have upgraded some beds to the subacute level.[4] Freestanding subacute care facilities have been established to address client needs. The client typically served by a subacute care facility may be a person who has sustained a stroke or hip fracture, or one who has a cardiac condition or cancer. Rehabilitation services, including occupational therapy services, are a major component of subacute care.

Long-term care includes clients who are medically stable but who have a chronic condition requiring services over time, potentially throughout life. Persons who have developmental disabilities, history of mental illness, or injury resulting in a severe disability may require this level of care. Elderly persons may also require long-term care. Services provided at this level may take place in an institution, skilled nursing or extended care facility, residential care facility, client's home, outpatient clinic, or community-based program.

SPHERES OF PRACTICE

Employment settings may be characterized according to "spheres of practice."[8] The categories are not meant to be exclusive of each other, but to help describe settings of practice. The value of this type of grouping is that it enables the OT student to categorize problems addressed in occupational therapy and to begin to interpret the nature of these problems.[8] The spheres of practice are (1) biological (medical), (2) psychological, and (3) sociological (social). As the concept is illustrated (Figure 11-1), the center of these three overlapping spheres represents *occupational performance,* the profession's central concern. Health problems occurring in any of the spheres affect the person's ability to engage in occupations. OT practitioners help clients make adjustments and find new ways to function by planning and guiding improvement of function in any or all of the three spheres of practice.

The **biological sphere** refers to medical problems caused by disease, disorder, or trauma. Primary limitations addressed by the OT practitioner include such things as loss of capacity, loss of sense, limitation in development or growth, limitation in movement, pain, damage to body systems, or neuromuscular disorders.

Problems within the **psychological sphere** include emotional, cognitive, and affective or personality disorders. These problems may be caused by an inability to cope with stress,

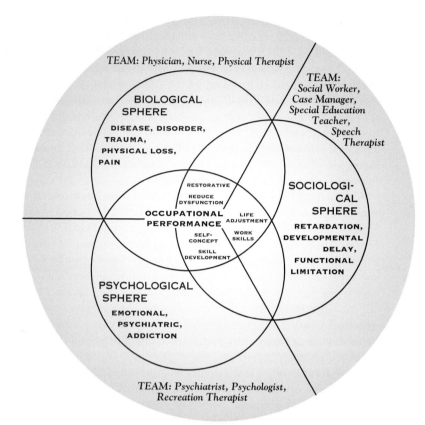

Figure 11-1 Spheres of practice diagram. *(Data from Reed K, Sanderson SR:* Concepts in Occupational Therapy, *ed 3, Baltimore, 1992, Williams & Wilkins.)*

biochemical imbalance, disease, or a combination of developmental and environmental factors. OT practitioners address problems that affect thinking, memory, attention, emotional control, judgment, and self-concept.

The **sociological sphere** refers to issues meeting the expectations of society. These social problems may result from severe physical or cognitive disability that limits functioning, developmental delays, mental retardation, long-term emotional problems, or any combination of the above. OT practitioners address such things as the absence of the ability to take care of one's own needs, lack or loss of life skills, poor interpersonal skills, failure to properly adapt to environmental changes, lack of capacity for independent functioning, and improper or detrimental behavior patterns. In general, these problems require long-term life adjustment.

To illustrate the difference between these three spheres, consider the client who is treated in occupational therapy to improve work skills with a long-term goal of employment. The OT practitioner examines whether his or her lack of work skills is due to biological (e.g., limited range of motion, loss of sensation, increased muscle tone), psychological (e.g., poor organization, intrusive thoughts, limited problem-solving, lack of motivation), or sociological problems (e.g., inability to follow directions, lack of awareness of social norms, limited life skills). The goals, objectives, and techniques of intervention differ with regard to the type of problems the client possesses.

These practice spheres are *not* mutually exclusive. For example, the OT practitioner employed in a medical setting should not ignore psychological and sociological factors when treating a client with biological limitations. To provide therapy to the whole person means including all factors in intervention planning. For example, a person who has undergone an amputation (biological) may exhibit psychological problems such as denial and anger, which must be addressed before a prosthesis (artificial limb) is accepted and a restoration program is successful.

In another example, the OT practitioner working in a group program teaching life skills to adults who have mental retardation generally addresses sociological aspects. However, while working with the client on hygiene and simple job skills, the OT practitioner discovers specific upper extremity weakness. Even though the program goal is life-skills training, the discovery of a weakness in the upper extremity requires further evaluation of and work on a goal that is considered biological—strengthening. Because decreased upper extremity functioning will interfere with the client's ability to complete life tasks, the clinician must address this through strengthening.

Many settings that employ OT practitioners may be grouped according to biological, sociological, or psychological treatment emphasis (Table 11-1). Although intervention concerns all three spheres, some distinctions in emphasis may be useful.

TABLE 11-1   Employment Settings

Sphere of Practice	Settings
Biological (medical)	Hospitals (general, state and federal, specialty)
	Clinics
	Work sites (industry)
	Home health
	Skilled nursing facilities
Sociological (social)	Schools (public, special—visual impairment, hearing impairment, cerebral palsy)
	Day treatment
	Hippotherapy centers
	Workshops
	Special Olympics
	Special camps (e.g., summer camps)
Psychological	Institutions (psychiatric, mental retardation)
	Community mental health
	Teen centers
	Supervised living
	After-school programs
All-inclusive	Long-term care
Private practice	Self-defined
Nontraditional	Correctional facilities
	Hospice
	National societies

Note: The categories do not indicate specialization. There are overlapping services in all spheres; the classification highlights the setting's primary concern.

Settings with a Biological Emphasis

The first employment setting that comes to mind is a medical facility, where rapid client turnover is expected. Medical facilities address biological or medical issues of clients. Intervention follows a medical model of identifying and addressing the problem. Medical concerns include examination of neurological, musculoskeletal, immunological, hematological, pulmonary, or cardiac systems.

Hospitals

Clients in hospitals receive care for acute illnesses. Thus occupational therapy evaluation and intervention in hospitals are generally focused on medical and functional concerns. For example, the OT practitioner in this setting evaluates such things as independence in self-care, range of motion, and muscle and perceptual functioning. The practitioner may provide activities to increase strength, coordination, or independent self-care. With shortened hospital stays, the OT practitioner immediately addresses concerns regarding the client's ability to return home (e.g., home equipment needs, family training). Acute-care hospital stays may include clients who have had hip replacements or who have heart or neurological conditions. The skilled practitioner who is alert to a holistic perspective will also address health-promoting concerns.

In addition to inpatient acute care, some hospitals provide rehabilitation services over a longer period of time; these are designed to help clients gain functioning or rehabilitate. Occupational therapy services in these specialty units occur within the general hospital. A typical rehabilitation unit provides services to clients who have sustained a disabling condition, such as stroke, head trauma, burns, or spinal cord injury. Rehabilitation services are also provided in the neonatal intensive care unit (NICU) for premature infants. The OT practitioner working in a NICU provides sensory stimulation, positioning, and feeding intervention. Training parents is also part of the intervention.

OT practitioners are also employed at specialty hospitals designed to provide services to a particular group of clients, such as those with spinal cord injuries, head traumas, burns, or childhood disorders. OT practitioners acquire the special skills needed to practice in such settings through education, workshops, reflection, experience, and on-the-job training.

Clinics

Clinics generally serve clients with disabling conditions on an outpatient basis and may focus on medical issues. Oftentimes, clients seen in outpatient clinics have been recently discharged from a hospital setting. They are still in need of therapy services, which can be provided at a lower level of care in an outpatient clinic. Outpatient clinics may be affiliated with a hospital, or they may be a separate entity. In a clinic, long-term functioning is an important consideration. The OT practitioner may be expected to teach adaptive behavior and may need to develop mechanical adaptations, in addition to the usual tasks performed for inpatient clients.

Rehabilitation clinics focusing on improving abilities include the Easter Seal Society Clinics, hand clinics, orthopedic clinics, and children's developmental clinics.

Home Health Agencies

Home health agencies serve clients who must receive therapy in the home. OT practitioners working for home health agencies provide therapy in the client's natural home environment, which is especially important when the practitioner works on problems related to performance in self-care, work and school, or play and leisure. Because clinicians working for home health agencies travel to clients, it may be difficult to communicate with team members as often as in other settings. It is the practitioner's responsibility to maintain close communication with team members. The practitioner working in a client's home also needs to plan ahead to ensure that he or she has the necessary equipment and supplies for the intervention. The OT practitioner may also work in the home of a person who receives hospice care. In this case, the emphasis of occupational therapy services is to maintain the person's abilities while making him or her comfortable. Thus the OT practitioner may provide modifications and compensations for decreased ability instead of trying to gain skills and improve functioning.

Settings with a Social Emphasis

Some clients experience functional limitations that impede their ability to satisfactorily interact with others. Frequently, these clients have long-term needs requiring that the OT practitioner help them with life adjustments to increase their daily functioning despite limitations. Thus the main concern for intervention is a social focus rather than a medical one, and therapy is directed toward a way of "being in the world."

Schools and Special Education

In 1975, the Education for All Handicapped Children Act, known as Public Law (PL) 94-142, passed, making public school education available to all children, regardless of handicap or disability. Related services, such as occupational therapy, physical therapy, and speech and language pathology, are included in this law, which mandates that children have the services they need to be successful in the classroom. Thus OT practitioners work in school systems to help children engage in education. OT practitioners may work in standard schools with children who are mainstreamed or in specialty schools for children with autism, visual impairment (blind or low vision), hearing impairment (deaf), and cerebral palsy (CP).

How a school provides these services is determined by state and local policies, but to receive federal funding, every county in every state must provide therapy services to children with disabilities. OT practitioners are either hired as an employee of the school district or contracted independently to provide services.

Day Treatment

Day treatment facilities serve people who need daytime supervision or are able to live in the community (rather than in an institution or full-care facility) but who require some assistance. Some individuals may live at home with families whose members work, whereas others live in board and care homes but cannot plan their own activities. OT practitioners are employed in day treatment settings to develop and provide structured programs of activities for the clients. Day treatment programs may specialize in intervention activities for children with behavioral disorders, persons who have mental illness, persons with Alzheimer's disease, and the elderly.

Workshops

Some communities provide special workshops for people who are not able to seek employment in the competitive job market. These may be sheltered workshops, training centers, or retirement workshops. Many clients in sheltered workshops have some type of developmental disability. Here, OT practitioners may be employed for work-skill development, work hardening, adapting to the environment, task modification, or a variety of other functions.

Settings with a Psychological Emphasis

In the next cluster of settings, the focus is on improving psychological functioning for occupational performance. These settings are regarded primarily as psychiatric or mental health settings but also address social difficulties.

Institutions

Deinstitutionalization was implemented in the 1970s. However, some state hospitals continue to provide services for those with severe developmental or emotional disabilities. These institutions (or state hospitals) may offer traditional psychiatric occupational therapy programs wherein the practitioner plans activities (e.g., crafts, recreation, outings) for the purposes of skill development, self-awareness, leisure exploration, and social participation.

Community Mental Health Centers

Community mental health centers emerged with the closing of institutions and are organized differently in regions and towns. Community mental health centers may offer medication clinics and counseling, crisis units, or day treatment programs. In community mental health settings, OT practitioners work with a client or group to develop life skills, to encourage social participation, to explore leisure opportunities, and to develop abilities to engage in areas of performance.

Supervised Living

Supervised living refers to partially or fully supervised housing for people whose problems do not warrant institutional care but who are not ready or able to manage on their own. Programming may vary from limited guidance to fully structured programs. Supervised living may include substance-abuse programs (often with a specific time limit) for alcoholics or drug addicts; half-way houses, which are usually a temporary living arrangement for someone leaving an institution but before going on to independent living; or group homes, which are expected to be more or less permanent for the client. In these settings, the OT practitioner may work with the client on general planning, such as organizing household chores, outings, and recreational activities, and on engaging the residents in life-skills training.

Elderly persons may live in assisted living facilities and may require occupational therapy services for physical, social, or psychological difficulties. OT practitioners may design activities for groups or individuals.

All-Inclusive Settings

All-inclusive settings may include long-term care facilities that provide occupational therapy services that address biological, psychological, and sociological functions. An all-inclusive facility provides residence for people for long periods of time and includes extended, residential, specialty, and skilled nursing facilities. The special skills needed by the OT practitioner in these settings depend on the nature of the facility.

Nontraditional Settings

OT practitioners work in settings such as correctional facilities, industrial settings, hospice, health maintenance organizations, community transition, and as case managers in various settings. Practitioners are working with therapeutic riding, aquatherapy, in gymnasiums, and in senior citizen centers. Some practitioners have begun to work with migrant workers, in homeless shelters, and with victims of disasters. The role of the practitioner varies according to the setting, but the aim is to help the individuals function more fully in their lives.

Private Practice and Consulting

Self-employment, or private practice, addresses aspects of client functioning, which vary and may include clients of all ages and diagnoses. Private practice for occupational therapy has increased since 1988, when the federal government, through the Health Care Financing

Administration, implemented Medicare Part B coverage. This enabled OT practitioners to fully participate in Medicare programs by permitting qualified practitioners to apply for Medicare provider numbers. A provider number allows a practitioner to become an independent provider and to bill directly for services.

OT practitioners work in privately designed practice according to personal interests or desires. For example, some therapists take individual referrals and administer treatment in private homes, whereas others ask clients to come to their facilities. Other clinicians may contract with other agencies to spend a specific number of hours at a school or a number of days at a nursing home. Some private practice companies employ practitioners from many disciplines and market therapy services as a business enterprise. Consultation requires highly developed professional expertise and management skills; the consultant and agency negotiate the parameters of service and set their own limits.[3] OT practitioners also consult with organizations in areas such as ergonomics, facility design, and wellness.[1,5,9] Many OT practitioners work in private practice and consult with agencies to provide services.[9]

OCCUPATIONAL THERAPY EMPLOYMENT TRENDS

Money magazine named occupational therapy one of the 50 best jobs.[1] One third of OT practitioners work with children in school systems, pediatric hospitals, and other pediatric settings, whereas another one third of practitioners work with older adults in skilled nursing facilities, hospitals, and clinics.[1,9] Approximately 15% of entry-level occupational therapists (OTs) work in school systems; rehabilitation and skilled nursing facilities are the most popular settings of employment (Figure 11-2, *A*). Since 2003, there has been an increase in the percentage of entry-level OTs working in private practice, outpatient, long-term, and acute care facilities. Skilled nursing facilities are still the most popular setting of employment for occupational therapy assistants (OTAs) (Figure 11-2, *B*). Since 2003, there have been increases in entry-level OTAs working in rehabilitation, acute care, outpatient facilities, and private practice.[7]

Employment in occupational therapy is "expected to increase much faster than the average for all occupations through 2014."[9] Although federal legislation limiting reimbursement for therapy may affect the job market in the short run, the long-term outlook for occupational therapy is very good. Specifically, growth in the older population, the baby-boom generation's move into middle age, and medical advances continue to increase the demand for occupational therapy.[2,9] Furthermore, evidence-based practice supporting the effectiveness of occupational therapy intervention continues to support therapy.[2]

Future practice areas targeted for growth include: ergonomics, accessibility design, driver assessment and training, assisted living, technology, health and wellness, low vision, Alzheimer's, children and youth needs, and community service (see Chapter 4).[2,3,5]

SUMMARY

Settings in which OT practitioners are employed may be characterized according to (1) administration of the setting, (2) levels of care, and (3) spheres of practice. Characterizing employment settings by the sphere of practice (i.e., biological, social, or psychological) provides some indication of the type of occupational therapy services provided at that setting.

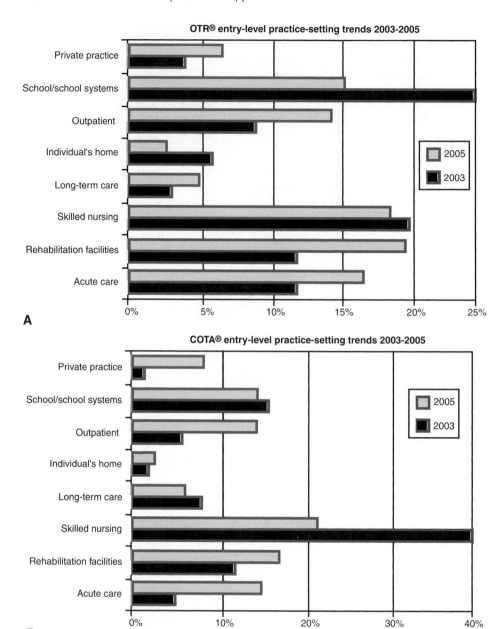

Figure 11-2 **A,** OTR® entry-level practice-setting trends, 2003-2005. **B,** COTA® entry-level practice-setting trends, 2003-2005. *(From National Board for Certification in Occupational Therapy, Inc.: Report from NBCOT® practice metrics survey, Fall 2004 Newsletter, pp. 1-3. Retrieved December 4, 2006, from www.nbcot.org.)*

OT practitioners view the biological, sociological, and psychological functioning of clients within the context of their environment. Thus OT practitioners work in a variety of intervention settings with many types of clients who have varying abilities. As such, care is tailored to the client's needs and may take place in acute, subacute, long-term, and rehabilitation settings. OT practitioners work primarily in hospital and school settings. However, many OT practitioners are expanding services into nontraditional settings, and the future of the profession looks bright.

Learning Activities

1. Research occupational therapy employment settings in your area. Describe the types of settings, types of clients the practitioners serve, and the level of care provided.
2. Make salary comparisons for entry-level practitioners (OTs and OTAs) in different kinds of employment settings. (Note: These data may not be available in some states.)
3. Review a series of case studies (many can be found in *Willard and Spackman's Occupational Therapy* and *American Journal of Occupational Therapy*). Photocopy the narrative history (minus any treatment plan); identify and group the occupational problems according to the sphere from which they arise.
4. Determine a need in your community, and define the type of services an OT practitioner could provide.
5. Review the job requirements for a particular setting that interests you. Present a brief description to the class.

Review Questions

1. What are the levels of care provided to clients?
2. What are the types of settings in which OT practitioners work?
3. What are the three spheres of practice? Provide examples of the type of factors considered within each sphere.
4. What are some nontraditional settings in which OT practitioners work?

REFERENCES

1. American Occupational Therapy Association: A consumer's guide to occupational therapy, Retrieved August 15, 2006, from www.promoteot.org/CGConsumerGuide.html.
2. Brachetesende A: The turnaround is here! *OT Practice*, January 24, 2005.
3. Jaffe EG, Epstein CF: *Occupational Therapy Consultation: Theory, Principles and Practice*, St. Louis, 1992, Mosby.
4. Joe B: Subacute care fills growing niche, OT Week, Feb 27, 1997, American Occupational Therapy Association.
5. Johansson C: Top 10 emerging practice areas to watch in the new millennium. OT Practice, January 31, 2000. Retrieved December 4, 2006, from www.aota.org.
6. Levy LL: Occupational therapy's place in the health care system. In Hopkins HL, Smith HD (eds): *Willard and Spackman's Occupational Therapy*, Philadelphia, 1993, JB Lippincott.
7. National Board for Certification in Occupational Therapy, Inc.: Report to the profession: results from NBCOT® practice metrics survey, Fall 2004 Newsletter, pp. 1-3. Retrieved December 4, 2006, from www.ncbot.org.
8. Reed K, Sanderson SR: *Concepts in Occupational Therapy*, ed 3, Baltimore, 1992, Williams & Wilkins.
9. U.S. Department of Labor, Bureau of Labor Statistics: Occupational outlook handbook, 2006-07 edition. Retrieved August 15, 2006, from www.bls.gov/print/ocos078.htm.

I was attracted to the profession when I realized the power of its medium—occupation. Life is, essentially, a chain of occupations. Occupation gives the context in which people build their skills, discover their interests, and reveal their hopes. Purposes in life are worked out through occupation. At the same time, occupation can influence and transform these purposes. The power of occupation lies in its intertwining of the person's body, mind, soul, and world. The work of the occupational therapist is to be an expert on the complexity of occupation and to use that knowledge artfully to help others achieve a life that is purposeful and meaningful. It is within this process that the therapist finds purpose and meaning; it is within this process that curiosity and wonder about how people create occupation grow.

René Padilla, PhD, OTR/L, FAOTA
Associate Professor
Department of Occupational Therapy
Creighton University
Omaha, Nebraska

Occupational Therapy Process: Evaluation, Intervention, and Outcomes

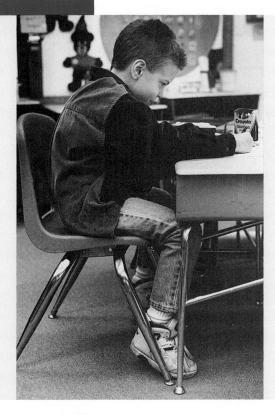

OBJECTIVES

After reading this chapter, the reader will be able to do the following:

- Identify the steps for gathering data on clients
- Recognize the type and value of the information collected for the initial evaluation
- Understand the importance of observation skills in the evaluation process
- Understand how to create a desirable atmosphere for interviewing
- Identify the steps in a generic problem-solving approach and recognize the relevance to the occupational therapy (OT) process
- Identify the five general treatment approaches used in occupational therapy
- Identify and describe the stages in the occupational therapy process
- Characterize the roles of the occupational therapist (OT) and the occupational therapy assistant (OTA) as they engage in the occupational therapy process

KEY TERMS

Assessment procedures	Normative data	Screening
Assessment instruments	Nonstandardized tests	Standardized tests
Discharge plan	Observation	Structured observation
Interrater reliability	Occupational therapy process	Test-retest reliability
Intervention	Referral	Transition services
Interview	Reliability	Validity

The **occupational therapy process** is the interaction between *two* active agents, the practitioner *and* the client, involved in a course of action. The interaction is not something *done to* the client, rather the interaction engages *with* the client. The relationship between the practitioner and the client is a collaborative one that involves problem-solving to support an enhancement in occupational performance of the client. The process is not viewed as a linear step-by-step process, but rather as a dynamic, nonlinear interaction. Throughout the occupational therapy process, the focus is on occupation and on the client as an occupational being.[2] Whether the client is an individual, a caregiver, a group, or a population, the same basic process is followed.

The occupational therapy process can be divided into three components (Figure 12-1). The first component, the evaluation process, includes referral, screening, developing an occupational profile, and analyzing occupational performance. The intervention process is the second component, and it includes intervention planning, implementation, and review. The third component is the outcomes process, which includes measurement of outcomes and decision-making related to the future direction of intervention (i.e., continue, modify, or discontinue). An overview of these stages is provided in Chapter 9. In this chapter, we describe in greater detail the components of each stage and delineate the roles of the OT and the OTA.

EVALUATION PROCESS

The purpose of the evaluation process is twofold: (1) to find out what the client wants and needs; and (2) to identify those factors that support or hinder occupational performance.[2] To determine what the client's needs are and to gain an understanding of the client's background, the OT practitioner develops an occupational profile of the client. An analysis of occupational performance provides information related to the client's skills and ability to carry out activities of daily living.

The OT bases the evaluation procedures on the client's age, diagnosis, developmental level, education, socioeconomic status, cultural background, and functional abilities. In this section, the steps to the evaluation process are reviewed, and the various methods used to gather information are described.

REFERRAL

The occupational therapy process is initiated when a **referral,** a request for service for a particular client or a change in the degree and direction of service, is made.[3] The OT is responsible for accepting and responding to the referral. Referrals may come from a physician, another professional, or the person himself or herself. Depending on the setting, referrals may range from a specific prescription for a dynamic splint to general suggestions for fine-

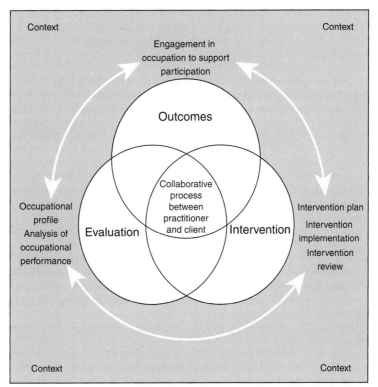

Figure 12-1 Framework collaborative process model. Illustration of the framework emphasizing the interactive nature of the client–practitioner relationship and of the service delivery process. *(From American Occupational Therapy Association: Occupational therapy practice framework: domain and process,* Am J Occup Ther *56(6):614, 2002.)*

motor problems. Federal, state, local regulations, and the policies of third-party payers determine the type of referral required (e.g., whether a physician's referral is necessary) and the role an OTA can have in the referral process.

SCREENING

Through **screening,** the OT practitioner gathers preliminary information about the client and determines whether further evaluation and occupational therapy intervention are warranted. The objective of a screening is to determine whether the person can benefit from occupational therapy in that setting.

Screening typically involves a review of the client's records, the use of a brief screening test, an interview with the client or caregiver, observation of the client, and/or a discussion of the client with the referral source. The client should also have the opportunity to ask questions. Information gathered during the screening includes the client's prior level of function in performance of occupations, his or her current level of occupational performance, and the future occupational performance needs of the client. The results of the screening are communicated to the appropriate individuals, including the party who made the referral.[1]

The OT is responsible for initiating and directing the screening process, using methods that are appropriate to the client's developmental level, gender, cultural background, and medical and functional status.[1] The OTA contributes to the screening process under the direction of an OT. Before screening tasks are performed by an OTA, he or she must achieve service competency in the particular tasks.

If screening suggests the client is in need of services, a comprehensive evaluation is arranged. The OT identifies a model of practice (see Chapter 14) from which the evaluation is based. The model of practice helps organize the practitioner's thinking. From the model of practice, the practitioner selects a frame of reference and chooses **assessment instruments** consistent with the frame of reference.

OCCUPATIONAL PROFILE

The goal of this step in the process is to gather information on the client so that an occupational profile can be developed. If a screening has not been completed, the OT practitioner obtains initial information about the client. The information includes the client's age, gender, and reason for referral; diagnosis and medical history (including date of onset); prior living situation and level of function (e.g., independent at home or in a care home); and social, educational, and vocational background. The initial review may provide information regarding precautions that need to be adhered to during the occupational therapy process. This background information is usually recorded in the client's occupational therapy chart and on the evaluation form. Figure 12-2 illustrates an example of an evaluation form used in an occupational therapy setting.

An occupational profile provides the practitioner with a history of the client's functioning and background information with which to design intervention. The following questions from the *Occupational Therapy Practice Framework (OTPF)* help the practitioner develop the occupational therapy profile[2]:

- Who is the client (individual, caregiver, group, population)?
- Why is the client seeking service, and what are the client's current concerns relative to engaging in occupations and daily life activities?
- What areas of occupation are successful, and what areas are causing problems or risks?
- What is the client's occupational history (i.e., life experiences, values, interests, previous patterns of engagement in occupations and in daily life activities, the meanings associated with them)?
- What are the client's priorities and desired targeted outcomes?

OCCUPATIONAL PERFORMANCE ANALYSIS

From the information gathered during the occupational profile (e.g. client's needs, problems, and priorities), the practitioner makes decisions regarding the analysis of occupational performance. This information provides direction to the practitioner as to the areas that need to be further examined. From this information, the practitioner can select the specific assessment instruments that will be used to collect further information.

The OT practitioner employs these assessment instruments to gather information on the individual as related to the individual's performance areas, performance skills, performance patterns, contexts, client factors, and activity demands (see Chapter 9).[2] Results of the assessment procedures are documented on a form typical to that shown in Figure 12-2. This evaluation information forms the basis for the intervention plan.

Occupational performance analysis entails analyzing all aspects of the occupation to determine the client factors, patterns, contexts, skills, and behaviors required to be successful. Once the practitioner has thoroughly analyzed the occupation, the practitioner can more easily determine what is interfering with the client's ability to engage in the occupation.

Occupational Therapy Initial Assessment

Name: _____ DOB: _____ Start of Service Date: _____

HICN: _____ Onset: _____

Medical Dx/ICD-9# _____Treatment Dx/ICD-9# _____

Past Medical History:_____

Occupational Profile:

Areas of Occupation:

ADL Status	dep	max	mod	min	sup	indep	comments:
Self-feeding							
Hygiene/grooming							
UB bathing							
UB dressing							
LB dressing							
Wet tub/shower							
Toilet transfer							
Toileting skills							
Functional mobility							
Personal device care							

IADL Status							
Kitchen survival skills							
Meal preparation							
Shopping							
Laundry							
Light housekeeping							
Community mobility							
Financial mgmt							
Care of others							

Work/Leisure/Social participation

Figure 12-2 Sample occupational therapy evaluation form. *ADL,* Activities of daily living; *CGA,* contact guard assist; *dep,* dependent; *DOB,* date of birth; *DX,* diagnosis; *HICN,* health insurance carrier number; *IADL,* instrumental activities of daily living; *indep,* independent; *LB,* lower body; *LUE,* left upper extremity; *max,* maximum assist; *min,* minimum assist; *mod,* moderate assist; *OT,* occupational therapy; *ROM,* range of motion; *RUE,* right upper extremity; *sup,* supervised; *UB,* upper body. *(From Pendleton H, Schultz-Krohn W [eds]:* Pedretti's Occupational Therapy: Practice Skills for Physical Dysfunction, *ed 6, St. Louis, 2006, Mosby.)*   *Continued*

| Vocational: |
| Avocational: |
| Leisure participation: |
| Social participation: |

Client Factors:

Functional cognition	
Perceptual status	
Memory	
Vision/hearing	
Pain	

ROM:
  RUE:
  LUE:	

Motor control:
  RUE:
  LUE:	

Strength:
  RUE:
  LUE:	

Muscle tone	
Coordination/bilateral integration	
Body system function	

Performance Skills: Patient/family goals:

Posture
  Sit:
  Stand:	

Mobility	
Endurance/effort	

Short-term goals:	Long-term goals:
OT intervention plan:	Frequency/duration:

_____
Therapist's Signature   Date

Figure 12-2, cont'd

Evaluation is seen as a critical decision-making role requiring a depth of understanding of many factors; as a result, the final responsibility of evaluation rests with the OT. The OTA, though not responsible for the complete evaluation, may be delegated responsibility for certain evaluation procedures and thus may contribute to an evaluation under an OT's supervision. The OTA communicates the results of all evaluation procedures to the OT. As with the screening process, service competency for tasks performed by an OTA needs to be established. Indeed, within any given setting, an OTA may become very proficient in specific phases of evaluation. The overall evaluation, or the process of compiling all of the information to form a composite picture of the client, however, is the responsibility of an OT.

The evaluation requires that the OT gather accurate and useful information to identify the needs and problems of the client to plan intervention. The techniques used during the evaluation process can be classified into three basic procedures: (1) interview, (2) skilled observation, and (3) formal evaluation procedures.[7,12]

INTERVIEW

The **interview** is the primary mechanism for gathering information for the occupational profile. Interviewing the client and his or her significant others provides more data. The interview is a planned and organized way to collect pertinent information. Because the focus of occupational therapy is *occupation* and the activities in which a person engages throughout the day, gathering information related to the individual's occupations is a primary concern to the OT practitioner. The practitioner asks questions regarding the client's function in daily activities before the onset of the problem that resulted in the occupational therapy referral. The interview is also used as a means of developing trust and rapport with the client.[13]

In some instances, the client is asked to fill out a checklist or questionnaire (focusing on the person's interests and activities) before the interview. For example, the interest checklist (Figure 12-3) developed by Matsutsuyu[10] has served as a model for others. Interest checklists enable clients to self-report on hobbies and interests. Another technique for addressing a client's interests is the activity configuration, in which the client charts how his or her time is spent each day. After completing the chart, the client compiles a list of all the different activities in which he or she participates. Each activity is classified according to the area of performance (e.g., activities of daily living, instrumental activities of daily living, education, work, play, leisure, and social participation) and is rated according to whether the activity is one he or she *has* to do or *wants* to do and how adequately the activity is performed. From the data gained, the practitioner can determine how the person spends his or her day and in what types of activities he or she is involved.

The interview should take place in a setting that is quiet and allows for privacy.[13] Ideally, the interview should be relaxed and comfortable for both the interviewer and the client. The skill of interviewing involves blending the formal accumulation of information with informal person-to-person communication. Three stages of an interview can be identified: initial contact, information gathering, and closure.

Initial Contact

At the point of initial contact, the skilled interviewer spends the first few minutes of the interview putting the subject at ease. Often, a person is worried and anxious at a therapy interview. A client may experience stress related to the illness or trauma, or he or she may feel threatened by the prospect of entering into therapy.

The practitioner begins the interview by introducing him or herself and informing the client about the clinic, the program, and standard procedures. It is important to convey

NAME	UNIT	DATE

Please check each item below according to your interest.

	INTEREST				INTEREST		
ACTIVITY	**CASUAL**	**STRONG**	**NO**	**ACTIVITY**	**CASUAL**	**STRONG**	**NO**
1. Gardening				41. Exercise			
2. Sewing				42. Volleyball			
3. Poker				43. Woodworking			
4. Languages				44. Billiards			
5. Social clubs				45. Driving			
6. Radio				46. Dusting			
7. Bridge				47. Jewelry making			
8. Car repair				48. Tennis			
9. Writing				49. Cooking			
10. Dancing				50. Basketball			
11. Needlework				51. History			
12. Golf				52. Guitar			
13. Football				53. Science			
14. Popular music				54. Collecting			
15. Puzzles				55. Ping pong			
16. Holidays				56. Leather work			
17. Solitaire				57. Shopping			
18. Movies				58. Photography			
19. Lectures				59. Painting			
20. Swimming				60. Television			
21. Bowling				61. Concerts			
22. Visiting				62. Ceramics			
23. Mending				63. Camping			
24. Chess				64. Laundry			
25. Barbeques				65. Dating			
26. Reading				66. Mosaics			
27. Traveling				67. Politics			
28. Manual arts				68. Scrabble			
29. Parties				69. Decorating			
30. Dramatics				70. Math			
31. Shuffleboard				71. Service groups			
32. Ironing				72. Piano			
33. Social studies				73. Scouting			
34. Classical music				74. Plays			
35. Floor mopping				75. Clothes			
36. Model building				76. Knitting			
37. Baseball				77. Hair styling			
38. Checkers				78. Religion			
39. Singing				79. Drums			
40. Home repairs				80. Conversation			

Figure 12-3 Neuropsychiatric Institute (NPI) Interest Checklist. *(Courtesy University of California at Los Angeles, from Matsutsuyu JS: The interest checklist, Am J Occup Ther 23:323, 1969.)*

general information but not burden the anxious person with specific details that he or she may be afraid of forgetting.

Each OT practitioner develops his or her own interviewing style. Regardless, taking the time to create a relaxed and unthreatening atmosphere is beneficial to future therapy because the interview creates the "first impression" of the therapy process. The client who feels welcome will begin therapy prepared to become a partner in the therapy process.

Information Gathering

After an informative discussion about the center or the therapy process, the OT practitioner begins to gather information about the client. The skilled interviewer guides the conversation in a way that yields the desired data yet keeps the flow conversational, rather than cold and rote. The OT practitioner explains before beginning the interview that he or she will be taking notes. The questions are asked conversationally, while making eye contact, and are never read directly from a sheet of paper.

An unskilled interviewer may spend a great deal of time talking only to discover he or she has not collected the needed information. To ensure that the desired information is secured, the OT practitioner works from an interview outline.

Closure

Effectively putting closure on the interview is also a learned skill. The OT practitioner must remain aware of the time so that the necessary details are covered. Practice and skill are required to guide the interview in a way that allows for the collection of needed data and yet results in a pleasant, conversational experience. The interviewer should signal when the interview is about to end by summarizing the information gathered and reviewing the next steps in the process. This technique avoids the discomfort of an abrupt "time is up" ending.

DEVELOPING OBSERVATION SKILLS

Observation is the means of gathering information about a person or an environment by watching and noticing. Observation may occur through a structured series of steps introduced by the OT practitioner, or it may be intentionally left unstructured to see what takes place.[6] The OT practitioner is able to obtain a wealth of information about the client through observation. For example, the practitioner can observe the person's posture, dress, social skills, tone of voice, behavior, and physical abilities (i.e., use of the limbs and ambulation).[13]

Observation is an important professional skill. Like most skills, some people are naturally better at it than others. Whatever the degree of natural ability, the skill can be improved. The best way to improve the powers of observation is to practice using them. The key to good observation is focused attention. This can be as simple as thinking while waiting for the bus, "Now let me see how many things I notice about this place."

Practicing observation with a goal in mind helps to further develop the skills. If the long-range goal is to describe a person's appearance as completely as possible, then gather the information systematically. Concentrate on each aspect of dress separately, and try to notice as much as possible. Go beyond the general (e.g., wearing a blue shirt) to identify the detail (e.g., with a pointed collar and tiny white buttons down the front and opened at the neck; long sleeves rolled up to the elbows; tucked in neatly at the waist). Then go to another aspect.

The next level of observation skill development is to employ thought and discrimination before making the observation to gather information about what is needed. Preselect needed or desired information, and structure the observation to gather this necessary information.

A **structured observation** involves watching the client perform a predetermined activity. OT practitioners frequently use structured observation to gain knowledge of what the person can or cannot do in relation to the demands of the task. If, for example, the OT practitioner wishes to evaluate a self-care activity like shaving, the client is asked to shave the way he usually does. While observing, the practitioner learns what is needed to improve function in this task. With information that identifies the extent of the limitation, the OT practitioner can make a plan for correction or improvement. OT practitioners examine the quality of performance through observation of the process, not just by examining the end product. For example, the clinician may observe how the person responds to directions, approaches the activity, interacts with others, deals with frustration, and engages in the task during the activity. Box 12-1 presents a guide for observation.

Box 12-1   Observation Guide

1. Describe how the client performs the activity in terms of the following client factors:
   - Movement functions
   - Specific mental functions (including thought, judgement, concept formation, emotional, language, motor planning, experience of self and others)
   - Global mental functions (including consciousness, orientation, temperament and personality, energy and drive)
2. Describe the client in terms of an overall impression during activities:
   - Physical appearance
   - Reaction to testing situation
   - Response to examiner
   - Approach to tasks
   - Quality of production
   - Communications with others
3. Gather information related to specific qualities:
   - Attentiveness
   - Independence
   - Ability to follow verbal instructions
   - Ability to follow written instructions
   - Cooperativeness
   - Initiative
   - Response to authority
   - Ability to read and write
   - Timidity or aggressiveness
   - Neatness
   - Accuracy
   - Distractibility
   - Passive or active involvement
   - Ease of movement
   - Speed of performance
   - Problem solving
   - Motor skills
   - Adaptability
   - Social skills
   - Affect
   - Interactions with others

With focused attention and refinement of ability as an observer, an OT practitioner begins to observe more subtle pieces of information.

FORMAL ASSESSMENT PROCEDURES

Formal assessment procedures help determine the existing performance level of the client. Formal **assessment procedures** include test tools, instruments, or strategies that provide specific guidelines for what is to be examined, how it is to be examined, how data are to be communicated, and how the information is to be applied in clinical problem-solving. Because they have specific guidelines, formal assessment procedures can be duplicated and critically analyzed.[12]

A test is said to have **validity** if research testing shows it to be a true measure of what it claims to measure. Test **reliability** is a measure of how accurately the scores obtained from the test reflect the true performance of the client. There are several different types of reliability with which the OT practitioner must be familiar. **Test-retest reliability** is an indicator of the consistency of the results of a given test from one administration to another. **Interrater reliability** is an indicator of the likelihood that test scores will be the same no matter who is the examiner.[12] OT practitioners can place more confidence in instruments that have high validity and reliability.

A **standardized test** is one that has gone through a rigorous process of scientific inquiry to determine its reliability and validity. Each standardized test has a carefully established protocol for administering the test. Test reliability and validity rests upon the OT practitioner following the set procedures for the administration and scoring of the test. In fact, some standardized tests require that clinicians say the exact same words to each client. In addition, standardized tests may be based on **normative data,** often called *norms,* collected from a representative sample that can then be used by the examiner to make comparisons with his or her subjects. Normative data are compiled by administering the test to a large sample of subjects.[4] The Miller Assessment for Preschoolers (MAP)[11] and the Sensory Integration and Praxis Tests (SIPT)[5] are examples of standardized tests developed by OTs.

OT practitioners also use **nonstandardized tests** for measuring function. Nonstandardized tests have guidelines for administering and scoring but may not have established normative data, or reliability and validity. The administration and scoring of nonstandardized tests are more subjective and rely on clinical skill, judgment, and experience of the therapist. For example, manual muscle testing and sensory testing are nonstandardized tests.

There is a broad range of assessment instruments available to OT practitioners. OT practitioners use frames of reference to guide the selection of a test instrument as well as consideration of the client's background, diagnosis, and needs.

OT practitioners administering a test instrument must be properly prepared.[4] Before administering a test, the OT practitioner must become familiar with the procedures and know the correct way to administer items, score the test, and interpret the data. Comfort with any testing procedure is acquired through practice. Some tests even require special training or certification before they can be administered. Under the direction of an OT, an OTA may administer the test once service competency has been established.

INTERVENTION PROCESS

The aim of occupational therapy is to enable the person with a disability to function more independently in his or her environment. This requires problem-solving methods to improve occupational performance. To grasp the occupational therapy intervention process requires an understanding of how the practitioner develops goals for the client, selects activities, directs intervention to guide the client to learn ways of engaging in occupational performance, and monitors the results of the intervention.

INTERVENTION PLANNING: PROBLEM IDENTIFICATION, SOLUTION DEVELOPMENT, AND PLAN OF ACTION

The intervention plan is based on an analysis of the information accumulated during the evaluation. The initial step in developing the intervention plan is *problem identification*. The OT reviews the results of the evaluation and identifies the client's strengths and deficits in occupational performance areas, performance skills, performance patterns, client factors, and contexts. From this, the OT determines the problem areas that need to be addressed through intervention. Problem identification also includes determining a hypothesis, or the cause of the problem. Understanding the root of the problem will help the OT practitioner select the most appropriate approach to treatment.[8]

Solution development is the process of identifying alternatives for intervention and forming goals and objectives. Selecting a *model of practice* and *frame of reference* from which the OT practitioner operates is an important component of solution development. Several frames of reference are used in occupational therapy practice. Each frame of reference is based on a body of knowledge that identifies principles and processes of change (see Chapter 14 for more information on models of practice and frames of reference). The frame of reference selected provides the practitioner with guidelines for clinical reasoning and intervention planning. Exploring intervention strategies based on the different frames of reference will help the practitioner develop potential solutions.

Based on the problems and the identified frame of reference along with input received from the client, the practitioner determines a *plan of action* for intervention (expected outcomes). The first step in developing a plan of action is the creation of long- and short-term goals that address the problems identified. These goals are prioritized according to the needs of the client. Next, intervention methods that will help the client achieve the goals are determined. This involves a consideration of the tools or equipment needed, any special positioning, where the activity will take place, how it will be structured and graded, and whether it is to be performed in a group or individually.[9] The intervention methods are based on the selected frame of reference. The practitioner uses his or her knowledge of the disability and the intervention to predict which methods will likely achieve the desired results as stated in the goals. Chapter 15 discusses the types of therapeutic activities used in occupational therapy.

The outcome of this intervention planning process is a written report (or intervention plan). The written plan addresses the strengths and weaknesses of the individual, interests of the client and caregivers, estimate of rehabilitation potential, expected outcomes (short- and long-term goals) along with frequency and duration of treatment, recommended methods and media, apparent environmental and time constraints, identification of a plan for re-evaluation, and discharge planning (Figure 12-4).[2] The plan is formally entered in the client's records.

The OT is responsible for analyzing and interpreting the data from the evaluation and formulating and documenting the intervention plan.[1] The OTA contributes to this process.

IMPLEMENTATION OF THE PLAN

Intervention involves working with the client through therapy to reach client goals. Five intervention approaches are used in occupational therapy: create/promote; establish, restore; maintain; modify; and prevent (see Appendix C).[2] The following examples describe how these approaches may be implemented in practice.

□ Part A □ Part B □ Other _____ Room No. _____ □ F.F.S. □ Direct Bill Facility: _____

700 FORM OCCUPATIONAL THERAPY PLAN OF TREATMENT (Complete For Initial Claims Only) □ E.O.M. □ D/C Sum

1. Patient's Last Name	First Name	M.I.	□ M □ F	2. Provider No.	3. Provider Name

4. HIC#	5. Medical Record No.	6. Onset Date	7. SOC Date

8. DOB	9. Primary Diagnosis (Pertinent Medical DX) (ICD-9)	10. Treatment Diagnosis (ICD-9)	11. Visits From SOC

12. Functional Goals (Short Term) - In ___ weeks, patient will:
1.

2.

3.

4.

I have reviewed this Plan of Treatment and certify the need for service.
13. **PHYSICIAN SIGNATURE**   DATE   □ N/A

18. INITIAL ASSESSMENT :
Reason for Referral:

Prior Level of Function:

History/Medical Complications:

Precautions/Contraindications:

Check and document with skilled objective data, on the areas that impact function.
□ Cognition/Safety Judgment:

□ Visual Motor/Perception:

□ Neuromotor:

□ Sensorimotor:

□ Balance: Sitting Static: Dynamic:

□ Balance: Standing Static: Dynamic:

19. SIGNATURE (professional establishing POT, including credentials)   DATE

20. FUNCTIONAL LEVEL (End of Billing Period)
Skilled Interventions:

ADL Status	0 Ind	1 Sup	2 CGA	3 Min	3 Mod	3 Max	4 Total	SUP
Self Feeding								
Hygiene / Grooming								
Dressing-Upper Body								
Dressing-Lower Body								
Toileting								
Toilet Transfer								
Bathing-Upper Body								
Bathing-Lower Body								
Functional Mobility								

□ Evaluation
PLAN OF TREATMENT
□ Self Care/Home Management Training   □ Cognitive Retraining
□ Therapeutic Activities   □ Orthotics Fitting Training/UE Splinting
□ Neuromuscular Re-education   □ Other _____
□ Therapeutic Exercise   □ Other _____
□ *In Individual and/or Group Treatment*
OUTCOME (Long Term Goal) - In ___ weeks, patient will:

14. Frequency/Duration
   (e.g., 5x/wk x 4 wks)
15. Certification
   From   Through   □ N/A
16. Physician's Name

17. Prior Hospitalization
   From   Through   □ N/A

Scoring Key: *MDS ADL Self Performance: 0=Independent 1=Supervision→Supervision(SBA)*
2=Limited →C.G.A.   3=Extensive →Min, Mod, Max Assist   4=Total →Dependent
Support (SUP): 0=No Set-up   1=Set-up help only   2=1 person assist   3=2 person assist

□ ROM:

ADL Status	0 Ind	1 Sup	2 CGA	3 Min	3 Mod	3 Max	4 Total	SUP
Self Feeding								
Hygiene / Grooming								
Dressing-Upper Body								
Dressing-Lower Body								
Toileting								
Toilet Transfers								
Bathing-Upper Body								
Bathing-Lower Body								
Functional Mobility								

□ Strength:

□ Activity Tolerance:

□ Other/Comments:

Clinical Impressions:

Positive Prognostic Indicators:

Rehab Potential: □ Good □ Excellent   Patient aware of prognosis: □ Yes □ No
Admit Cond: □ Mild □ Mod □ Sev □ Dep   Patient aware of diagnosis: □ Yes □ No
Document Impairments and Reason to:
                    □ Continue Services   or   □ D/C Services
Resident/Caregiver Training:

Recommendations:

D/C Prognosis to Maintain Function: □ Good   □ Fair   □ N/A
D/C Condition: □ Goals Met   □ Improved   □ Declined   □ No Change
D/C Location: □ Home □ ALF □ LTC □ SNF □ Hospital □ Other □ Expired
21. THERAPIST SIGNATURE:
   Service Dates: From: Through:

REHABWORKS
A Division of Symphony Health Services   Modified OT 700 Form   **RW5904** OT Plan of Treatment 11/2004

Figure 12-4 Modified Medicare 700 form—occupational therapy plan of treatment. *(Courtesy RehabWorks, a division of Symphony Rehabilitation, Hunt Valley, MD. From Pendleton H, Schultz-Krohn W [eds]:* Pedretti's Occupational Therapy: Practice Skills for Physical Dysfunction, *ed 6, St. Louis, 2006, Mosby.)*

Create/Promote: The OT practitioner organizes an afternoon handwriting group for school-aged children. The practitioner recommends the group to children in his or her caseload who have difficulty with handwriting.

Establish, restore: The OT practitioner works with Galen, a 67-year-old man who has lost use of his right side since his cerebral vascular accident. The clinician works to help Galen return to his typical morning routine.

Maintain: After performing a home visit, the OT practitioner makes recommendations so 90-year-old Harry can stay at home.

Modify: The OT practitioner provides 35-year-old Karen, who has cerebral palsy, with adapted feeding equipment so that she can feed herself.

Prevent: The OT practitioner explains proper lifting techniques to a group of workers at the blanket factory with the goal of preventing injuries.

These examples are just a few of the many intervention strategies employed by OT practitioners.

Consulting is also an important part of intervention. Practitioners frequently consult with other professionals, family members, and clients regarding intervention strategies. When the OT practitioner consults others, he or she is not directly responsible for the implementation and subsequent outcome of the intervention. For example, the practitioner may consult with a teacher on how to facilitate handwriting skills in the classroom. A practitioner may consult in a work setting about ergonomically correct lifting techniques or workspace arrangements. Consultation requires advanced knowledge, the ability to communicate clearly with others, and knowledge of the context in which the consultation occurs.

Another important aspect of intervention is education.[2] OT practitioners educate the client, family, and caregiver about activities that support the intervention plan. When caregivers are responsible for implementing treatment, they need to be aware of the risks and benefits of intervention as well. Education may be formal or informal in nature. For example, the OT practitioner may provide an educational workshop to a parent group regarding a particular treatment frame of reference. The practitioner may educate the client in a session, by providing a demonstration and handout. Education must be tailored to the client's level. The OT practitioner should speak clearly and avoid the use of jargon. OT practitioners teaching clients to re-engage in occupations need to make sure that the client understands the lesson and can provide a return demonstration of the targeted techniques. The OT practitioner answers any questions and follows up at the next visit.

The interaction between the practitioner and client is an essential element of therapy, and it requires informed decision-making. A therapeutic relationship should always have the interest of the client as its central concern. The practitioner's role is to choose the interaction style that best supports the goals of the intervention plan and to help the client move toward independence. Setting the tone of interaction will be a decision made on the basis of the overall cognitive ability and attitude of the client. In Chapter 16 the development of a therapeutic relationship is described in detail.

Although the implementation of the intervention plan is the responsibility of both OT and OTA, it is the *central* responsibility of the OTA. Educational programs are designed to ensure that OTAs develop an understanding of the philosophy and skills of occupational therapy to enable them to interpret and implement intervention plans. The OTA conducts intervention under the supervision of the OT.

INTERVENTION REVIEW

As intervention is implemented, the OT practitioner re-evaluates the client's progress in therapy. The practitioner continually monitors the client's needs, circumstances, and conditions to identify whether any permanent or temporary change in the intervention plan is required. Re-evaluation may result in changing activities, re-testing, writing a new plan, or making needed referrals.

The OT practitioner assesses the client during each treatment session by monitoring the impact of intervention and evaluating whether the activity has the desired therapeutic effect. For example, if the activity becomes too easy for the client, the OT practitioner may increase the level of difficulty by adding resistance or by asking the client to sit rather than stand. As an OT practitioner becomes more experienced, the ability to monitor, evaluate, and revise will improve. Through ongoing intervention review, the OT practitioner re-evaluates the plan and how it is being carried out and achieving outcomes targeted for the client; modifies the plan as needed; and determines the need for continuation, discontinuation, or referral to another service.[2]

TRANSITION SERVICES

Transition services are the coordination or facilitation of services for the purpose of preparing the client for a change. Transition services may involve a change to a new functional level, life stage, program, or environment. The OT practitioner is involved in identifying services and preparing an individualized transition plan to facilitate the client's change from one place to another.[1] In other words, the transition plan needs to be individualized to meet the goals, needs, and environmental considerations of the individual client.

The following cases provide an example of the importance of a transition services.

Mr. G, a 75-year-old married man, was hospitalized for a total hip replacement. Because he is able to return home to a spouse willing to cook, clean, and assist him with self-care, he requires little outside assistance. His children who live nearby also will help out. His transition service plan includes training Mr. G and his spouse to safely move around the house, transfer to the toilet safely, and perform basic self-care.

Mr. W, a 75-year-old single man, was also hospitalized for a total hip replacement. However, he lives alone and has no family nearby. Mr. W will require a different transition plan. His transition plan includes a daily visit by the home health nurse, meals-on-wheels, and a home evaluation by the OT practitioner. The OT practitioner will work on mobility through the house, simple meal preparation, and home safety.

These two cases demonstrate the differences in transition services required. Some clients may need to be transferred to a lower level of care (e.g., a skilled nursing facility) before returning home. Careful planning is the key to preparing the client for the transition home.

DISCONTINUATION OF SERVICES

The last step of the intervention process is the discontinuation of the client from occupational therapy services. The client is discharged from occupational therapy when he or she has reached the goals delineated in the intervention plan, when he or she has realized the maximum benefit of occupational therapy services, or when he or she does not wish to continue services.[1] The **discharge plan** is developed and implemented to address the resources and supports that may be required upon discharge. The discharge plan includes recommendations for continued services (including occupational therapy, if necessary), equipment recommendations, and any therapy the client is required to follow after discharge. In addition, the plan may include training family members and caregivers.

The OT writes a discharge summary of the client's functional level, changes that were made throughout the course of occupational therapy intervention, plans for discharge, equipment and services recommended, and follow-up (including occupational therapy services). The OT prepares and implements the discharge plan with input from the OTA.[1]

OUTCOMES PROCESS

OT practitioners use outcome measures to determine whether goals have been met and to make decisions regarding future intervention.[2] Outcome measures provide objective feedback to the client and practitioner. Thus selecting measures that are valid, reliable, and appropriately sensitive to change is important. OT practitioners are interested in selecting measures early and using measures that may predict future outcomes.[2] Because the broad outcome of occupational therapy is engagement in occupation to support participation, measures that evaluate this outcome should be selected. OT practitioners are also interested in measuring occupational performance, client satisfaction, adaptation, quality of life, role competence, prevention, and health and wellness.[2] These outcomes and their measurement are discussed in detail in Chapter 9.

SUMMARY

The occupational therapy process is a dynamic ongoing interactive process. Generally, the process includes referral, screening, evaluation, intervention planning, implementation of the intervention plan, transition services, and discontinuation of services. Each stage requires that the OT practitioner observe carefully and listen to the client's needs. Intervention is continually monitored and adjusted as needed. As a client meets his or her goals, new goals may be developed. The OT practitioner is skillful at creating, promoting, maintaining, rehabilitating, or modifying activities for the client.

Learning Activities

1. Provide the class with a case study. Randomly assign students (or teams) with one of the five treatment approaches (e.g., create, establish, maintain, modify, or prevent). Ask students to provide examples of how this treatment approach would be used with the case. Compare and contrast the benefits of each in class.
2. Interview your classmate for a few minutes to determine the occupations in which they engage. Write a page summary of the interview. Submit a page reflection of the interview process by discussing what you could have done differently and what you did well. Ask your partner for feedback.
3. Help students improve their observation skills by writing down everything they see while watching a fellow classmate perform a simple activity (e.g., making a cup of

cocoa). After they have made a list, have them use the *Occupational Therapy Practice Framework* as a guide to examine the activity. Discuss the findings.

4. Review a journal article that examines the effectiveness of a given intervention. Summarize the intervention techniques the researchers used and the results of the study. What did you learn about occupational therapy intervention?

5. Interview an OT practitioner to find out about a particular case that the practitioner finds interesting. Find out the intervention approach and context(s) in which the intervention took place. Present this to your classmates.

Review Questions

1. What are the five general treatment approaches used in occupational therapy practice?
2. What are some techniques for successful interviewing?
3. What are the stages of the occupational therapy process?
4. Compare and contrast the roles of the OT and the OTA in the occupational therapy process.
5. What types of information is included in an occupational profile?
6. What is included in a discharge summary?

REFERENCES

1. American Occupational Therapy Association: Standards of practice for occupational therapy, *Am J Occup Ther* 59:663-665, 2005.
2. American Occupational Therapy Association: Occupational therapy practice framework: domain and process, *Am J Occup Ther* 56(6):609-639, 2002.
3. American Occupational Therapy Association: Statement of occupational therapy referral, *Am J Occup Ther* 48:1034, 1994.
4. Asher IE: *Occupational Therapy Assessment Tools: An Annotated Index,* ed 2, Bethesda, MD, 1996, American Occupational Therapy Association.
5. Ayres J: *Sensory Integration and Praxis Tests (SIPT),* Los Angeles, CA, 1988, Western Psychological Services.
6. Cook AM, Hussey SM: *Assistive Technologies: Principles and Practice,* ed 2, St. Louis, 2002, Mosby.
7. Dunn W: Assessing sensory processing enablers. In Christiansen C, Baum V (eds): *Occupational Therapy: Overcoming Human Performance Deficits,* Thorofare, NJ, 1991, Slack.
8. Early MB: *Mental Health Concepts and Techniques for the Occupational Therapy Assistant,* ed 2, New York, 1993, Raven Press.
9. Hopkins HL: Tools of practice: Section 4, problem-solving. In Hopkins HL, Smith HD (eds): *Willard and Spackman's Occupational Therapy,* ed 8, Philadelphia, 1993, JB Lippincott.
10. Matsutsuyu J: The interest checklist, *Am J Occup Ther* 23:323, 1969.
11. Miller L: *Miller Assessment for Preschoolers (MAP),* San Antonio, 1982, Psychological Corporation.
12. Opacich KJ: Assessment and informal decision making. In Christiansen C, Baum V (eds): *Occupational Therapy: Overcoming Human Performance Deficits,* Thorofare, NJ, 1991, Slack.
13. Pendleton H, Schultz-Krohn W (eds): *Pedretti's Occupational Therapy: Practice Skills for Physical Dysfunction,* ed 6, St. Louis, 2006, Mosby.

On plucking thistles and planting flowers...

How one lives life or chooses an occupation can be simple and straightforward or a long journey. As an undergraduate student, I wanted to be in premed—convinced that my calling was to be a physician. During undergraduate school, I explored two directions.

My first job was as a genetics technician in a university-based medical center. My days were spent centrifuging and fixing samples on slides, counting chromosomes, and photographing and creating karyotypes. When I closed my eyes each night, all I could visualize was chromosomes floating in emulsion. I would briefly meet people when they gave a sample in the laboratory, but I never got to know them or know what having the test meant to the greater scheme of their lives.

My second exploration was as a volunteer in an occupational therapy department in a psychiatric hospital. Suddenly, I was fascinated by people and their stories—intrigued by what went wrong and how their lives could be reorganized, allowing them to return to some sense of normalcy in their day-to-day lives. Occupational therapy seemed less scientific yet so very meaningful—listening while we were doing. I found that change and growth can be found through doing. I was a potential "agent of change"—the very meaning of the word "therapist" directed me to choose occupational therapy. The process of occupational therapy reminds me of Abraham Lincoln's words, which I have embraced: "I want it said of me by those who knew me best that I always plucked a thistle and planted a flower where I knew one would grow." I chose occupational therapy and have been plucking and planting. What a garden has grown and continues to grow each and every day!

Ann Burkhardt, OTD, OTR/L, BCN, FAOTA
Director, Division of Occupational Therapy
Associate Professor of Occupational Therapy
School of Health Professions
Long Island University
Brooklyn Campus
Brooklyn, New York

Service Management Functions

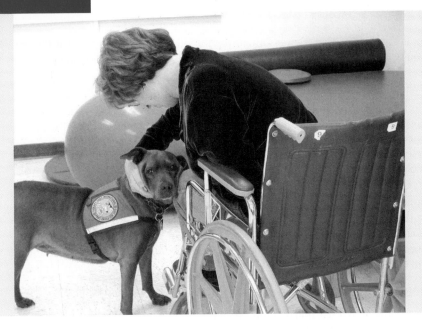

OBJECTIVES

After reading this chapter, the reader will be able to do the following:

- Explain the various service management functions
- Identify the factors that lead to a safe and efficient clinical environment
- Describe how the spread of infection is prevented in the workplace
- Explain the factors taken into consideration for scheduling staff appointments
- Define the three major categories of funding sources that reimburse for occupational therapy (OT) services
- Recognize the importance of program planning and evaluation as service management functions
- Understand the purpose of documentation
- Describe the documentation that occurs at various stages in the occupational therapy process, and identify the fundamental elements in a client record
- Understand the integration of professional development and research into practice
- State the importance of marketing and public relations as a professional responsibility

KEY TERMS

Accreditation
Diagnosis codes
Documentation
Emergency procedures
Evidence-based practice
Individualized education plan

Outcome measures
Private funding sources
Problem-Oriented Medical
  Record
Procedure codes
Program evaluation

Program process
Program structure
Public funding sources
Service management functions
SOAP note
Universal precautions

183

Service management functions include maintaining a safe and efficient workplace, documenting occupational therapy services, getting reimbursed for services, planning programs and evaluating them, integrating professional development activities and evidence-based practice into the workplace, and engaging in marketing and public relations.

MAINTAINING A SAFE AND EFFICIENT WORKPLACE

Maintaining an orderly and safe environment for the provision of occupational therapy services is important for the OT practitioner and workplace efficiency. For the safety of the client, various accrediting bodies mandate safety procedures. Because the clients have disabilities, they may require additional accommodations to make sure the intervention setting is safe for them. It is imperative that all areas in the clinic be wheelchair accessible, be free of clutter, have good lighting and ventilation, and have equipment that is properly stored and maintained.

Each person who works in the clinic setting assumes responsibility for maintaining a safe and efficient work environment. Each practitioner is responsible for reporting problems to the occupational therapy administrator or to the maintenance department. Each OT practitioner *is directly responsible* for putting away equipment and supplies that have been in use during a treatment session and for cleaning the work area. When everyone participates and cooperates in maintaining a safe and efficient work environment, the department operates more effectively and with less stress. The following sections examine in greater detail the many factors that contribute to a safe and efficient work environment.

SAFE ENVIRONMENT

Each setting must have written policies and procedures relating to the functions of maintaining a safe work environment. It is the responsibility of the OT practitioner to be familiar with these policies and procedures.

The clinical setting should have plenty of room so that staff and consumers can move without running into equipment or objects. Items that represent a potential safety hazard must be properly stored and, in some instances, placed in locked cabinets. This precaution is particularly important in psychiatric settings, where scissors, knives, and other sharp objects could be potentially used by a client to harm himself or herself or someone else. Toxic chemicals and flammable substances require careful storage in a special cabinet for flammables and should be disposed of properly. Some materials used in occupational therapy clinics may pose a physical or health hazard. The Occupational Safety and Health Administration (OSHA) requires that manufacturers of such materials evaluate the material and provide a material safety data sheet (MSDS). MSDSs provide information on the proper procedures for handling or working with a substance, including storage, protective equipment, and disposal. These procedures must be followed if a spill or other accident occurs. These MSDS sheets should be read carefully before the first use of a hazardous material, and they must be kept available in the clinic.

Many occupational therapy departments have power tools or toxic chemicals, which need to be stored and used carefully. In addition, many occupational therapy departments have kitchen facilities; safety in this area needs to be carefully considered. In particular, food needs to be handled and stored safely. All staff must be trained in the proper use of equipment and supplies that are found in the occupational therapy clinic, including the use of protective goggles when using power equipment and face masks when using toxic chemicals.[18]

Prevention of injury to the OT practitioners is also an important safety aspect in the clinic. In settings that require lifting and moving of clients from bed to wheelchair, the practitioner must use proper body mechanics to avoid injury. Injuries to the back are common and may force the practitioner to take a leave from work. Employers provide training in the proper use of body mechanics to lift and transfer clients. OT practitioners should attend these training sessions and make a concerted effort to be aware of body mechanics.

All staff must be familiar with **emergency procedures** in the case of an injury or accident in the clinic. These procedures name the person to contact for help in the case of an emergency. OT practitioners must maintain current certification in cardiopulmonary resuscitation (CPR) and training in first aid. In addition, the OT practitioner is required to know how to determine blood pressure and pulse rate, know how to manage a seizure, and know what to do if someone is choking.[18] After an injury or accident in the clinic, the practitioner must complete a report that documents what occurred, filing it in accordance with the procedures of the facility. Box 13-1 summarizes safety considerations in the occupational therapy clinic.

INFECTION CONTROL

Controlling the spread of infections is an important safety consideration in health care settings. Health care workers, including OT practitioners, are at risk for contracting infectious diseases that are transferred from person to person (i.e., hepatitis B virus [HBV], human immunodeficiency virus [HIV], and tuberculosis [TB]). Clients are also susceptible to infection from the health care worker.

The Centers for Disease Control and Prevention (CDC) is a federal agency that works to "protect people's health and safety, provide reliable health information, and improve health through strong partnerships."[13] In 1987, the CDC developed **universal precautions,** a set of guidelines designed to prevent the transmission of HIV, HBV, and other bloodborne pathogens to health care providers. Under universal precautions, blood and certain body fluids of all clients are considered potentially infectious.[12] These guidelines change as new research becomes available; therefore, it is recommended that OT practitioners remain up to date on the guidelines. Universal precautions include the use of protective

---

Box 13-1 Safety Considerations in the Occupational Therapy Setting

Sharp objects should be properly stored in a locked cabinet or drawer.
Keep flammables in a locked metal cabinet.
The clinical environment needs to be free of clutter so that staff and clients can move safely. Sharp corners on cabinets should not protrude into traffic areas. Equipment and furniture must be kept out of traffic areas.
Bathroom areas that are used by clients must have securely anchored grab bars.
The emergency call system should be readily available, and all staff must understand emergency procedures.
Flooring must be nonslip, and the staff must alert others to anything that changes this condition (i.e., water).
All staff are required to have proper training in the safe use of equipment and supplies found in the occupational therapy clinic.
In kitchen areas, foods must be safely stored and handled.
Staff need to be trained in the use of proper body mechanics when lifting or moving clients, equipment, and supplies.
Staff must be aware of who is in the clinic at all times and report suspicious persons.

barriers including gloves, gowns, aprons, masks, or protective eyewear to reduce the risk of exposure to blood and other body fluids that are potentially infectious.[12] It is recommended that OT practitioners wear protective gloves whenever working with a client during his or her activities for daily living (ADLs), such as grooming, personal hygiene, toileting, and dressing. Gloves must be changed and hands washed after contact with each client. When it is necessary for the health care worker to wear one of the other protective barriers, a notice should be placed in the client's medical record, and a sign should be posted outside the client's room to indicate the needed precautions.

The most effective method for preventing the transfer of disease is hand washing. The OT practitioner should wash his or her hands before and after each treatment, after using the toilet, and after sneezing, coughing, or coming in contact with oral and nasal areas, and before and after eating. Procedures for hand washing are provided in Box 13-2.

The responsibility for controlling the spread of infection rests with federal agencies, employers, and employees.[21] The regulations are established and monitored by the CDC and by OSHA. OSHA monitors compliance of employers and fines those settings that do not follow the regulations, whereas CDC monitors individuals' exposure to disease in the workplace.

OSHA standards define the responsibilities of the employer, which include providing education on universal precautions and on the use of protective barriers. The employer is also responsible for providing the necessary protective barriers, hand washing facilities, and supplies needed by employees. Employers are also required to provide employee health services for the purposes of mandatory annual testing for TB, HBV vaccine, and maintenance of employee health records (i.e., tests and vaccines given and any exposure to infectious disease).[21]

It is the employees' responsibilities to attend educational programs that are offered and to follow universal precautions guidelines. Employees are also required to have an annual TB test

---

Box 13-2 Techniques for Effective Hand Washing

1. Remove all jewelry, except plain band rings. Remove watch, or move it up the arm. Provide complete access to area to be washed.
2. Approach the sink, and avoid touching the sink or nearby objects.
3. Turn on the water, and adjust it to a lukewarm temperature and a moderate flow to avoid splashing.
4. Wet wrists and hands with fingers directed downward, and apply approximately 1 teaspoon of liquid soap or granules.
5. Begin to wash all areas of hands (palms, sides, backs), fingers, knuckles, and between each finger, using vigorous rubbing and circular motions. If wearing a band, slide it up or down the finger and scrub skin underneath it. Interlace fingers, and scrub between each finger.
6. Wash for at least 30 seconds, keeping hands and forearms at elbow level or below and hands pointed down. Wash longer if a patient known to have an infection was treated.
7. Rinse hands well under running water.
8. Wash as high up wrists and forearms as contamination is likely.
9. Rinse hands, wrists, and forearms under running water.
10. Thoroughly dry hands, wrists, and forearms with paper towels. Use a dry towel for each hand. Water should continue to flow from tap as hands are dried.
11. Use another dry paper towel to turn water faucet off. Discard all towels in an appropriate container.

Modified from Zakus SM: *Clinical Procedures for Medical Assistants,* ed 3, St. Louis, 1995, Mosby.

and to report any exposures to the employee health services department. It is the prerogative of the employee to decide whether to take the HBV vaccine or to sign a waiver if this option is declined.[21] Because these procedures have been established after much research and are for the safety of the health care worker, it is beneficial to the OT practitioner to comply.

ORDERING AND STORING SUPPLIES

An important part of maintaining an efficient therapy setting is having appropriate equipment and supplies on hand when needed. The amount of supplies ordered and stored at any one time varies among facilities, depending on the size of the occupational therapy department, its storage capacity, and the policies of the administration.[18]

It is necessary for effective operations to predict the supplies that may be needed over a particular period of time and to order enough supplies so that the clinic does not run out. Using an inventory system helps staff manage this information. Typically, one individual is responsible for tracking the supply inventory and ordering supplies as needed. In those facilities that employ an occupational therapy assistant (OTA), this responsibility is often part of his or her job.

SCHEDULING

To keep things flowing smoothly in the clinic, a schedule of the appointments for each practitioner needs to be maintained and displayed where it is visible by all staff members. A schedule is a useful tool for time management; it helps the OT practitioner prioritize what needs to be accomplished and serves as a plan.[16,18]

The first priority for scheduling is to identify the clients who need to be seen each day. The schedule takes into account the time needed to complete the service management functions described in this chapter. It also reflects the time needed for each OT practitioner to attend meetings or client conferences and to complete paperwork, scheduling, and billing.

The schedule for each client varies, depending on the type of facility and caseload of the each setting. For example, in some mental health outpatient programs, treatment may be performed in groups that meet only once a week. Conversely, in an outpatient setting where the practitioner treats clients with hand injuries, the client may be scheduled two or three times a week or even daily. Scheduling in outpatient settings may vary because of family schedules, other appointments that the client may have, and the availability of transportation to and from the clinic.

Third-party payers may also influence the duration and frequency of scheduled sessions. For example, Medicare requires that clients who are in acute rehabilitation be seen twice a day. If the client cannot tolerate two daily treatments, he or she should be transferred to a setting that provides a lower level of care (e.g., skilled nursing facility). Many health maintenance organizations (HMOs) limit the number of outpatient visits to the OT practitioner; typically, twelve visits is the maximum. All these factors need to be considered during the development of the intervention schedule.

The supervising occupational therapist (OT) usually decides which staff person to schedule with which client and communicates the schedule to the staff.[18] This decision-making step involves consideration of client needs, staff expertise, and cost effectiveness. Today, productivity in occupational therapy departments is highly scrutinized, as it is for all health care services. If a client can be treated by an OTA instead of an OT, this assignment will be more cost effective for the department. If there are not enough clients to complete a staff person's schedule for a day, the manager may decide to reduce the practitioner's hours. Once the schedule is in place, it is important that each practitioner manages his or her time wisely and adheres to the schedule to ensure that everything is completed as planned and the schedules of others are not affected.

DOCUMENTING OCCUPATIONAL THERAPY SERVICES

Keeping accurate records is an important aspect of service delivery. The purposes of documentation are outlined in the *Guidelines for Documentation of Occupational Therapy.*[4] **Documentation** provides a justification for initial and ongoing occupational therapy intervention. The practitioner's professional judgment and clinical reasoning are reflected in documentation. Documentation is used to communicate to other health care professionals, third-party payers, and administrators why the skilled services of an OT practitioner are needed for a particular client. Documentation also communicates to others the status of the client from an occupational therapy point of view. This facilitates effective intervention and teamwork, and it prevents duplication of services. Documentation also provides a chronological record of the client's status, the services provided, and the outcomes of those services.

Documentation to record the practitioner's activities is necessary at all stages in the occupational therapy process. Common types of documentation at the various stages of the occupational therapy process are shown in Table 13-1.[4] The *Occupational Therapy Practice Framework: Domain and Process*[5] was designed to provide standardized occupational therapy terminology to be used in documentation.

The *evaluation or screening report* contains information on the referral source and data gathered during the evaluation process.[4] Included in this report are an occupational profile of the client, an analysis of the client's occupational performance, factors that support or inhibit performance, and identification of specific areas of occupation to be targeted, along with expected outcomes. The *re-evaluation report* is a report and summary of the results of the re-evaluation.[4] Recommendations for changes to services, goals, frequency, and referral to other sources are included in the report as well.

The intervention stage includes documentation of the intervention plan, service contacts, progress reports, and a transition plan. The *intervention plan* is based on the evaluation or re-evaluation, and it documents the goals, intervention approaches, and types of interventions to be used to achieve the goals.[4] It should identify the frequency and duration of service, the service provider, and the location of service. Documentation of *service contacts*

TABLE 13-1 Types of Documentation

PROCESS AREAS	TYPES OF REPORTS
I. Evaluation	A. Evaluation or Screening Report
	B. Re-evaluation Report
II. Intervention	A. Intervention Plan
	B. Occupational Therapy Service Contacts
	C. Progress Report
	D. Transition Plan
III. Outcomes	A. Discharge/Discontinuation Report

From American Occupational Therapy Association: Guidelines for documentation of occupational therapy (2003), *Am J Occup Ther* 57(6):646-649, 2003.

is a record of the contact between the client and OT practitioner.[4] It is an ongoing log of therapy and includes date, length of time, interventions used, and the client's response. Telephone contacts, interventions, and meetings with others are also documented. An example of a daily narrative note describing a service contact (intervention session) with a client is shown in Box 13-3.

A *progress report* summarizes the intervention to date and documents the client's progress towards the goals.[4] Any new data collected are included, along with modifications to the intervention plan, and recommendations for the client to continue or discontinue services or be referred to another source. Again, the progress report will vary with the setting and the reimbursement mechanism. In some cases, a progress note is written on a weekly basis; in other cases, it is required monthly. An example of a weekly progress report is shown in Box 13-4.

A *transition plan* is written when a client is transitioning from one type of setting to another within the same delivery system. For example, a client who has spent the last 2 weeks in the rehabilitation unit following a stroke is to be transferred in 2 days to a skilled nursing facility. The transition plan would provide information to the new setting regarding the client's current status; the reason for transition; a time frame for transition, including activities to be carried out; and recommendations and rationale for occupational therapy, modifications, or assistive technology.

The *discharge/discontinuation report* is the documentation completed during the outcomes stage. This report summarizes the changes in the client's ability to participate in occupations between the initial evaluation and the discontinuation of services. Recommendations for further services and follow-up are also documented in this report.

There are many types and methods of documentation, and these differ from setting to setting. Public policy, accreditation bodies, third-party payers, and the practice setting determine documentation practices. For example, school settings in which intervention is funded by the federal and state governments require each child to have an **individualized education plan** (IEP), completed by a multidisciplinary team. The problems, goals and interventions written in a child's IEP need to reflect behaviors and skills necessary for

---

Box 13-3 Sample Narrative Daily Note

Client actively participated in eating retraining and right upper extremity strengthening program. Client ate 75% of meal with adapted utensils and required minimal assistance for cutting meat. Established treatment plan should continue.

Modified from Early MB: *Physical Dysfunction Practice Skills for the Occupational Therapy Assistant*, ed 2, St. Louis, 2006, Mosby.

Box 13-4 Sample Weekly Progress Note

Client has been treated daily for eating retraining and right upper extremity functional strengthening program. Using adapted utensils, client ate 75% of meal with minimal assistance for cutting meat. Previously, client ate 50% of meal and required moderate assistance for cutting meat. Client will eat independently with no assistive devices in 1 week.

Modified from Early MB: *Physical Dysfunction Practice Skills for the Occupational Therapy Assistant*, St. Louis, 1998, Mosby.

success in school.[24] There are also specific documentation requirements as mandated by the federal government for clients who are covered by Medicare.

One common method of documentation that is used in medical settings is the **Problem-Oriented Medical Record** (POMR). This format, developed by Dr. Lawrence Weed,[28] is a way of providing structure to documentation. It may be used for evaluation reports, treatment notes, progress notes, and discharge reports. As the name suggests, this system is based on a list of problems identified by the treatment team during the assessment of the client. Subsequent progress notes relate to the problem(s) identified in the list. The format used for writing the progress note is referred to as the **SOAP note.** S stands for *subjective* (information reported by the client); O is for *objective* (clinical findings or measurable, observable data); A represents *assessment* (OT practitioner's professional judgment or opinion); P is for *plan* (specific plan of action to be followed). In Box 13-5, a sample SOAP note documents a treatment session for a client.

A permanent record is maintained for each client who receives occupational therapy. The record needs to be organized, legible, concise, accurate, complete, grammatically correct, and objective.[4] Even though the format of the documentation will vary with the setting, there are certain fundamental elements that need to be present in all documentation (Box 13-6). The habits of good planning and regular documentation make recordkeeping easier, whatever the demands, and, ultimately, lead to better quality treatments.

GETTING REIMBURSED FOR SERVICES

To stay in business, occupational therapy departments need to produce revenue, which is produced through the collection of fees for services provided. Each OT practitioner is responsible for submitting accurate charges that are reflected in either units based on the amount of time spent with the client or a set fee based on services provided.[18] Determining charges involves a complex process, usually performed by the administration of the facility and the department. Briefly, third-party payers have different amounts that they will pay in "allowable charges" for a particular client. In essence, the charges set by the facility do not reflect what is actually paid by the third-party payer for an individual client but rather for the client population as a whole.

Occupational therapy services are reimbursed by a number of sources, which can be categorized into three groups: (1) public sources that include federal, state, and local govern-

---

Box 13-5 Sample SOAP Note

PROBLEM 1: DEPENDENCE IN WHEELCHAIR MOBILITY

S: Client stated that his hands often slip on the metal hand rims when propelling his wheelchair.

O: Friction tape was placed on rims of wheelchair to improve client's ability to grasp and propel chair. Wheelchair mobility training outside over grass and asphalt was provided. Client participated for 30 minutes in wheelchair training with only 5-minute rest period. He experienced no difficulty propelling wheelchair over varied terrain.

A: Friction tape on rims helped improve client's ability to propel wheelchair. Client's endurance for wheelchair mobility improved over yesterday.

P: Continue OT training in wheelchair mobility. Increase time and distance for wheelchair mobility. Teach client how to maneuver wheelchair in and out of doors and up and down ramps.

Box 13-6 Fundamental Elements of Documentation

1. Client's full name and case number (if applicable) on each page of documentation
2. Date and type of occupational therapy contact
3. Identification of type of documentation, agency, and department name
4. Occupational therapist's or occupational therapy assistant's signature with a minimum of first name or initial, last name, and professional designation
5. When applicable on notes or reports, signature of the recorder directly at the end of the note without space left between the body of the note and the signature
6. Countersignature by an occupational therapist on documentation written by students and occupational therapy assistants, when required by law or the facility
7. Acceptable terminology defined within the boundaries of setting
8. Abbreviations usage as acceptable within the boundaries of setting
9. When no facility requirements are listed, errors corrected by drawing a single line through an error and by initialing the correction (liquid correction fluid and erasures are not acceptable)
10. Adherence to professional standards of technology, when used to document occupational therapy services
11. Disposal of records within law or agency requirements
12. Compliance with confidentiality standards
13. Compliance with agency or legal requirements of storage of records

From American Occupational Therapy Association: Guidelines for documentation of occupational therapy (2003), *Am J Occup Ther* 57(6):646-649, 2003.

ment agencies; (2) private payers that include insurance companies; and (3) other sources that include service agencies and volunteer organizations. Each source of payment has different regulations and guidelines that identify the services for which it will pay (number of visits and equipment) and the amount of reimbursement. Because these regulations and guidelines often change, it is the responsibility of the OT practitioner to remain current. The administration of the facility and the department will also inform staff members of any changes in funding regulations.

PUBLIC FUNDING SOURCES

Public funding sources come from the federal, state, and local levels. These sources include funds provided by Medicare, Veteran's Administration, Medicaid, Maternal and Child Health programs, Department of Education, vocational rehabilitation services, and Social Security benefits. Typically, Congress authorizes funding through a specific legislation and designates a federal agency to determine the scope and criteria for the program. In each state, an agency is designated to receive the federal funds and ensure compliance with the programs mandated by the federal government.[15] The funds are then distributed to the local agencies or programs, which are responsible for ensuring that mandated services are provided. In Chapter 2, federal legislation that has mandated occupational therapy as a reimbursable service is discussed.

PRIVATE FUNDING SOURCES

Private funding sources include the individual's health insurance policy, worker's compensation, casualty insurance, and disability insurance. A growing number of individuals are paying for health care services personally because they either do not have health insurance or their plan does not provide for a specific service. Private insurance companies have a wide variety of plans that have differing benefits and restrictions. Most individuals receive the details of their health insurance policies, which stipulate whether occupational therapy services are covered and whether there are any limitations on those services (e.g., maximum number of visits, maximum amount of dollars). Funding by private health insurance companies is based on a medical diagnosis and justification that the treatment is medically necessary.

Worker's compensation benefits cover expenses incurred from work-related injuries. Worker's compensation benefits are regulated by state agencies and managed by private insurance companies. For that reason, allowable occupational therapy services vary from state to state.

OTHER FUNDING SOURCES

Sources of funding that do not fall under the categories of public or private agencies include service clubs, private foundations, and volunteer organizations. In many communities, various service clubs (e.g., Kiwanis, Rotary Club) may be a source of funding for individuals without other means. In some cases, private foundations, which are usually related to a specific disability group, will provide funding for an individual with that disability.[15] Some volunteer agencies also provide funding.

CODING AND BILLING FOR SERVICES

To receive payment for occupational therapy services, the provider (either a facility or individual) submits a claim form using the correct billing codes. Services provided in occupational therapy are either billed by diagnosis codes or procedure codes. **Diagnosis codes** are based on the client's medical condition or the medical justification for needing services. The most frequently used coding system is the *International Classification of Diseases, Ninth Revision, Clinical Modification (ICD-9-CM).*[22] Diseases are categorized in *ICD-9-CM* according to anatomical systems. Mental health providers use the *Diagnostic and Statistical Manual of Mental Disorders, Fourth Edition, Text Revision (DSM-IV-TR).*[8]

Procedure codes are based on the specific services performed by health care providers. The most commonly used procedure coding system is the *Current Procedural Terminology (CPT),* which is published and updated annually by the American Medical Association.[1] OT practitioners select the codes that most accurately define the services performed and bill to these codes by relative value units. Payers may limit the number and range of codes that a specialty may use to bill services; therefore it is critical that the OT practitioner be aware of the allowable codes for each insurer. In skilled nursing facilities, Centers for Medicare and Medicaid (CMS) require that providers of occupational therapy services document therapy minutes using the Minimum Data Set (MDS).

There are two types of claim forms commonly used in occupational therapy to bill third-party payers: (1) the Uniform Bill (UB-92; CMS-01450), which is used by hospitals, skilled nursing facilities, and home health agencies; and (2) the CMS-1500 claim form, used primarily by physicians or OTs in private practice.

OT practitioners need to educate third-party payers on a continual basis regarding the benefits of occupational therapy services, as well as be advocates for the inclusion of occupational therapy as a reimbursable service under the various policies and regulations. It is important to keep abreast of proposed changes in state and federal legislation and regulations that have the potential to affect the payment for occupational therapy services. This can be done on an individual basis and also by supporting local and national occupational therapy associations that provide lobbying efforts for the purpose of influencing legislation that may affect the profession.

PROGRAM PLANNING AND EVALUATION

Program planning and evaluation are primarily the responsibilities of the administrator, although the staff provides input into both processes. In an occupational therapy department, the administrator is involved in planning such things as space utilization, equipment needs, staff levels, effective use of staff, the annual budget, department policies and procedures, and new programs and services.

It is important as a health care profession that the effectiveness of programs be measured. This is referred to as **program evaluation,** and it involves "determining the extentto which programs are achieving the goals and objectives established for them and using that information as necessary to modify activities."[9] Program evaluation is not only important for ensuring client satisfaction, but it is also necessary for accreditation by outside agencies. **Accreditation** is a form of regulation that determines whether an organization or program meets a prescribed standard. Although it is voluntary, there is external pressure for organizations to be accredited, including the need for accreditation in order to be reimbursed by third-party payers. Many of the organizations for which OT practitioners work will likely be influenced by some type of accreditation. In health care, the two most widely known accreditation bodies are The Joint Commission (TJC) and the Rehabilitation Accreditation Commission (CARF).

TJC develops standards and accredits health care organizations in the United States. These organizations include hospitals; health care networks; and organizations that provide long-term care, behavioral care, and laboratory and ambulatory services.[17]

CARF sets standards and accredits organizations that deliver rehabilitation services, including occupational therapy. CARF's standards and guidelines are separated into three areas: behavioral health, employment and community services, and medical rehabilitation. The CARF accreditation process is aimed at improving the quality of services provided to individuals with disabilities.[25] CARF is also involved in research related to outcomes measurement and management.

To prepare for accreditation, a detailed program evaluation resulting in a written report of self-study is completed. Following the completion of the self-study, a team representing the accrediting body visits the facility. The program evaluation typically examines three different aspects of the services provided. The first aspect is the **program structure** of the system in which the services are delivered; for example, staff levels and expertise, equipment, budget, and range of services provided are examined. When this aspect of a program is being evaluated, the types of questions asked include: "Is there adequate staff to provide services?" "Are staff members competent in their area of service delivery, and are they current with the latest approaches?" "Does the institution have an adequate budget and equipment on hand to provide services?"

The **program process** in which the services are delivered is the second aspect and includes all of the stages described earlier in this text: referral, evaluation, and intervention. When an accreditation team evaluates this aspect of a program, individual client records are examined to determine whether certain stages occurred as they were intended and whether the procedures were acceptable. For example, "Did the client have the appropriate referral for occupational therapy?" "Was the evaluation completed in a timely manner and performed accurately?" Usually, several clients' records are randomly selected for review to determine whether the process was appropriately followed.

The last consideration in program evaluation is **outcome measures,** an aspect that evaluates the results of the intervention after the service has been provided. There are a number of tools that are used to measure outcomes. One of the more popular tools is the Functional Independence Measure (FIM™) instrument.[27] The FIM™ instrument measures an individual client's functional ability for 18 items across the domains of self-care, motor, and cognitive.[27] The person is given a separate score for each item and also a total score. The FIM™ and similar measures are used to score a client at different points in the rehabilitation process (e.g., at time of referral and at discharge), and they provide a fairly objective measure of how the individual is progressing. Individual client data are not looked at in program evaluation, but rather a compilation of client data. For example, the program could compile data over the last fiscal year that portrayed the average percentage of change in client scores from time of admission to time of discharge. Or it could compile data that showed what percentage of discharged clients received scores at the highest level of independence in self-care. For an occupational therapy service in an acute rehabilitation unit or skilled nursing facility, this type of data is useful for measuring performance outcomes.

By examining these three aspects as a part of program evaluation, the institution's administration and staff can address specific problem areas in the self-study. After problem areas are identified, corrective measures can be taken. Program evaluation is an ongoing process that helps ensure that quality services are provided by the occupational therapy program. The conclusions made from a program evaluation provide valuable information to the practitioner, the consumer, the accrediting agency, and the third-party payer, each of whom has an interest in the quality of the services provided. Program evaluation may also add to the evidence base of the profession.

INTEGRATING PROFESSIONAL DEVELOPMENT ACTIVITIES AND EVIDENCE-BASED PRACTICE INTO THE WORKPLACE

In Chapter 6, we discussed the need for practitioners to maintain competence in the field through participation in educational programs and other professional development activities. OT practitioners can participate in educational opportunities at their workplace through inservice presentations. For example, an OT practitioner working in the school district may provide an inservice presentation to teachers and aides on how to properly feed a child with swallowing difficulties, or an OT practitioner who has attended a workshop on a special treatment technique may spend an hour presenting the information he or she learned to the occupational therapy staff. Inservice presentations are an effective way to train staff members, both internally and externally, as well as a good public relations tool for the occupational therapy department.

Another way that OT practitioners can be involved in professional development in the workplace is by supervising Level I or Level II fieldwork students. OTs and OTAs with a minimum of 1 year of work experience (not including their own fieldwork experience) are eligible to supervise students. Clinical internships are critical to the continuation of the profession, and practitioners who mentor the next generation provide a valuable service. Not only is fieldwork an important component of the student's training, but it is also a valuable and rewarding experience for the supervisor, who learns and grows professionally from the mentoring experience.

Throughout this text, the importance of evidence-based practice has been emphasized. The credibility of occupational therapy practice depends upon the use of best evidence in practice and continued research related to occupational therapy outcome studies. Consumers, practitioners and third-party payers want to know that occupational therapy services are being provided based on the best available evidence regarding their effectiveness (best outcome in least amount of time).[10,20]

All OT practitioners are required to have a certain degree of education in research practices. The standards for accredited educational programs for both the OT and OTA, developed by the Accreditation Council for Occupational Therapy Education (ACOTE) of the American Occupational Therapy Association (AOTA), speak to the need for the student to be able to read and understand current research that affects practice. The standards common to both professional levels state that the student will do the following[6,7]:

- Articulate the importance of professional literature (OTA)/research (OT) for practice and the continued development of the profession
- Be able to use professional literature to make informed practice decisions
- Know when and how to find and use informational resources, including appropriate literature within and outside of occupational therapy

The *Standards of Practice for Occupational Therapy*[3] also addresses the responsibilities of OT practitioners in research. Specifically, Standard I.9 states: "An occupational therapy practitioner is knowledgeable about evidence-based research and applies it ethically and appropriately to the occupational therapy process."[3] But what is evidence-based practice, and how does one incorporate evidence into clinical practice?

Evidence-based practice is "finding, appraising, and using contemporaneous research findings as the basis for clinical decisions."[26] This research evidence is used by the OT practitioner in conjunction with clinical knowledge and reasoning to determine the interventions that are effective for a particular client.[19] There are four steps in evidence-based practice: (1) forming a clinical question that can be researched; (2) searching the literature for best evidence on the question; (3) appraising the evidence for validity, impact, and applicability to practice; and (4) applying the evidence to practice.[14] Applying the research to practice does not always entail changing the intervention approach. It may mean providing clients with more specific, detailed, and current information about the efficacy of the approaches used.[11] In some situations, the research may provide information on interventions to facilitate the client's outcomes.[11]

Several information resources are available on the World Wide Web that can assist the OT practitioner in retrieving research findings. AOTA has two resources on its website that are a good place to start for the novice investigating evidence-based practice. AOTA's *Evidence Briefs* is a series of evidence-based literature reviews of occupational therapy effectiveness with particular health conditions (e.g. brain injury, attention deficit hyperactivity disorder, substance use).[2] Each brief presents a summary of a selected article that outlines the study's key features and provides answers to fundamental questions: "Why research this topic?" "What did the researchers do?" "What do the findings mean?" and "What are the study limitations?" A structured abstract also accompanies each brief. The other resource is the *Evidence-Based Practice (EBP) Resource Directory*.[2] This directory provides links to Internet sites related to the use of evidence-based practice in occupational therapy. Another information resource on the Internet is the website of the American Foundation for Occupational Therapy (www.aotf.org). Students and practitioners are urged to use these resources along with the many other resources on the Internet and through local libraries to read, critically appraise, and incorporate evidence into their daily practice.

PUBLIC RELATIONS AND MARKETING

Participation in public relations programs to increase the visibility of occupational therapy is considered a part of one's professional responsibilities. Many departments plan and implement public relations activities during the month of April, which is designated as National Occupational Therapy Month. For example, a booth set up in the facility's cafeteria that demonstrates adaptive equipment may attract a lot of attention and provide good publicity for occupational therapy. The AOTA is involved in many efforts to increase the visibility of occupational therapy and consequently has materials available for members to promote the profession. These materials include booklets, brochures, videotapes, banners, and posters.

Competition in the health care market is strong; therefore, practitioners need to be involved in marketing occupational therapy services. Marketing differs slightly from public relations in that it involves the development and implementation of a marketing plan, which is typically the responsibility of the administrator of the department. However, it is important for the practitioner to have at least a basic awareness of what is involved in marketing occupational therapy services.

The development of a marketing plan requires consideration of four target groups: (1) the clients who are served, (2) the sources who refer or have the potential to refer clients to occupational therapy, (3) the administration (or internal source of funding for the department) of the facility, and (4) the third-party payers who reimburse (or have the potential to reimburse) for occupational therapy services.[23]

Olson and Urban[23] describe five key concepts of marketing that need to be addressed when developing a marketing plan. The first concept is *product,* and the questions asked are, "What is the product or service that we are providing?" "Is this product or service needed by the community?" The second concept is *price,* and it asks whether the pricing of the service is fair and within reason for the market. The third concept is *place,* and it addresses the how, when, and where the services will be offered and who will be eligible to receive them. *Promotion* is the fourth concept, and it strives to make the product visible to the target market and considers how to promote and advertise the services that are provided. Finally, *position* is the relative place of the product among similar products in the marketplace. For example, "What unique attributes set our product apart from other similar products?" From these five key concepts, a marketing plan can be developed to promote the services that appeal to the consumer.[23]

SUMMARY

Service management functions are activities performed by the OT practitioner outside of direct service delivery to the client. These functions include maintaining a safe and efficient workplace, documenting occupational therapy services, getting reimbursed for services, planning programs and their evaluations, integrating professional development activities and evidence-based practice into the workplace, and engaging in public relations and marketing. For an occupational therapy department to operate effectively, it is important that each practitioner take the responsibility for being involved in these activities.

Learning Activities

1. Practice time management by making a weekly schedule for yourself and adhering to it. Note whether you seem to get more accomplished when using the schedule.
2. Visit any occupational therapy department. After leaving the facility, ask yourself, "How would I feel about working in this setting?" Prepare written notes about the environment of the department. Is the storage adequate? Does there appear to be an adequate amount of equipment and supplies? Does the clinic appear cluttered, or is it neat with everything safely put away? Are there any obvious safety hazards that you noticed during your visit?
3. Interview either an OTA or an OT about the types of service management functions they perform. Compare notes with your classmates. Is there a significant difference between what OTs and OTAs do? Is there any difference across the spheres of practice?
4. In a group of two or three students, come up with several public relations activities that you could use to promote National Occupational Therapy Month. Select one of the activities and perform the activity at your school or the local mall.
5. Visit a local occupational therapy department, and discuss with the staff OT practitioners the type of documentation used by their facility. If the facility allows it, ask to see examples of documentation (e.g., assessment reports, progress notes, treatment plans, and discharge summaries).

Review Questions

1. What are the various service management functions in which the OT practitioner participates?
2. What are some factors for safety in the clinic?
3. What are universal precautions?
4. What does each of the areas of the SOAP method of documentation mean?
5. Why is research important in practice?
6. How is program evaluation used in practice?

REFERENCES

1. American Medical Association: *Current Procedural Terminology 2006,* Chicago, 2006, American Medical Association.
2. American Occupational Therapy Association: Evidence-based practice resources. Retrieved August 23, 2006, from http://www.aota.org/members/area15/index.asp.
3. American Occupational Therapy Association: Standards of practice for occupational therapy, *Am J Occup Ther* 59(6):663-5, 2005.
4. American Occupational Therapy Association: Guidelines for documentation of occupational therapy (2003), *Am J Occup Ther* 57(6):646-649, 2003.
5. American Occupational Therapy Association: Occupational therapy practice framework: domain and process, *Am J Occup Ther* 56(6):609-639, 2002.
6. American Occupational Therapy Association: *Standards for an Accredited Educational Program for the Occupational Therapist,* Bethesda, MD, 1998, American Occupational Therapy Association.
7. American Occupational Therapy Association: *Standards for an Accredited Educational Program for the Occupational Therapy Assistant,* Bethesda, MD, 1998, American Occupational Therapy Association.
8. American Psychiatric Association: *Diagnostic and Statistical Manual of Mental Disorders, Fourth Edition, Text Revision (DSM-IV-TR),* Arlington, VA, 2000, American Psychiatric Association.
9. Bair J, Gray M (eds): *The Occupational Therapy Manager,* Rockville, MD, 1985, AOTA.
10. Canadian Association of Occupational Therapists, the Association of Canadian Occupational Therapy University Programs, the Association of Canadian Occupational Therapy Regulatory Organizations, and the President's Advisory Committee: Joint position statement on evidence-based occupational therapy (1999). Retrieved August 23, 2006, from http://www.caot.ca.
11. Case-Smith J: Continuing competence and evidence-based practice, OT Practice Online, 2004, American Occupational Therapy Association. Retrieved August 23, 2006, from www.aota.org/featured/area3/links/cc-040504.asp.
12. Centers for Disease Control and Prevention: Fact sheet: universal precautions for prevention of transmission of HIV and other bloodborne infections, released 1987, updated 1996. Retrieved August 20, 2006, from http://www.cdc.gov/ncidod/dhqp/bpuniversalprecautions.html.
13. Centers for Disease Control and Prevention: Vision, mission, core values, and pledge. Retrieved August 20, 2006, from http://cdc.gov/about/mission.htm.
14. Centre for Evidence Based Medicine, University Health Network: Practising evidence-based medicine, Toronto, 2004, Centre for Evidence Based Medicine, University Health Network. Retrieved August 23, 2006, from http://www.cebm.utoronto.ca/practice/.
15. Cook AM, Hussey SM: *Assistive Technologies: Principles and Practice,* St. Louis, 1995, Mosby.
16. Early MB: *Mental Health Concepts and Techniques for the Occupational Therapy Assistant,* ed 2, New York, 1993, Raven Press.
17. Joint Commission on Accreditation of Healthcare Organizations: Facts about the JCAHO. Retrieved July 17, 2006, from www.jointcommission.org/AboutUs.
18. Jones RA: Service operations. In Ryan SE (ed): *Practice Issues in Occupational Therapy: Intraprofessional Team Building,* Thorofare, NJ, 1993, Slack.
19. Law M, Baum C: Evidence-based occupational therapy, *Canad J Occup Ther* 65(3):131-135, 1998.
20. Lieberman D, Scheer J: AOTA's evidence-based literature review project: an overview, *Am J Occup Ther* 56(3):344-349, 2002.
21. Meriano C: Universal precautions. In Sladyk K (ed): *OT Student Primer: A Guide to College Success,* Thorofare, NJ, 1997, Slack.
22. National Center for Health Statistics: *International Classification of Diseases, Ninth Revision, Clinical Modification,* Hyattsville, MD, 2005, National Center for Health Statistics.
23. Olson TS, Urban C: Marketing. In Bair J, Gray M (eds): *The Occupational Therapy Manager,* Rockville, MD, 1985, AOTA.
24. Perinchief JM: Documentation and management of occupational therapy services. In Crepeau EB, Cohn ES, Schell BB (eds): *Willard and Spackman's Occupational Therapy,* ed 10, Philadelphia, 2003, Lippincott Williams & Wilkins.

25. Rehabilitation Accreditation Commission: Quick facts about CARF. Retrieved July 18, 2006, from www.carf.org.
26. Rosenberg W, Donald A: Evidence-based medicine: an approach to clinical problem-solving, *Br Med J* 310(6987):1122-1126, 1995
27. Uniform Data System for Medical Rehabilitation: FIM™ Instrument. Retrieved on August 23, 2006, from http://www.udsmr.org/fim2about.php.
28. Weed LL: *Medical Records, Medical Education and Patient Care*, Chicago, 1971, Year Book Medical Publishers.

My debut into the occupational therapy career happened by chance. After high school, I was trying to figure out what I wanted to do with my life. I was interested in studying psychology. However, in the country of Kenya, Africa, where I grew up, there was no psychology major at the time in any of the institutions of higher education. My sister had just completed her studies at the Kenya Medical Training College and had been awarded a diploma in radiography. She informed me that there was a program at the college called occupational therapy. She did not know much about the program, except that she saw occupational therapists doing much basket weaving and seemingly having lots of fun. However, she also knew that they studied a lot of psychology. So, I applied and got into the program.

Since graduating way back in 1985, my progress in the profession has been fortuitous. For some time, I left the profession all together and studied, and for a while I practiced counseling psychology. However, I realized that "doing" meaningful things (meaningful occupations) with clients is far more therapeutic that just talking about issues. So, I came back to the profession, hopefully much wiser and with more commitment based on insight. My experiences have led me to believe that the way to strengthen occupational therapy and ensure its survival far into the future is by therapists being very clear of their origin (which in my view is mental health), and staying true to the original principles, even while making progressive and useful innovations. That is why one of my favorites pastimes is discussing with students (future occupational therapists) occupational therapy theory and its origins, and speculating about its future development.

Moses N. Ikiugu, PhD, OTR/L
Associate Professor and Director of Research
Department of Occupational Therapy
University of South Dakota
Vermillion, South Dakota

Models of Practice and Frames of Reference

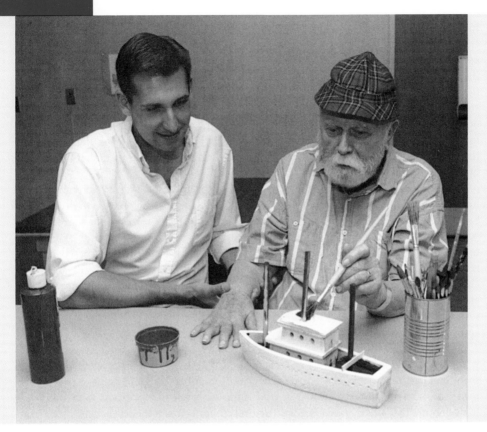

OBJECTIVES

After reading this chapter, the reader will be able to do the following:
- Define theory, model of practice (MOP), and frame of reference (FOR)
- Discuss the importance of using a model of practice and frame of reference
- Understand how research supports practice
- Identify the components of a frame of reference
- Summarize selected occupational therapy (OT) models of practice
- Identify the principles guiding selected frames of reference

KEY TERMS

Biomechanical frame of
  reference
Brain plasticity

Canadian Model of
  Occupational Performance
Cognitive disability frame of
  reference

Concepts
Evidence-based practice
Frame of reference

Continued

In Chapter 9, we described the *Occupational Therapy Practice Framework (OTPF)*.[3] The *OTPF* is a description of what occupational therapy practice entails, or occupational therapy's domain of concern. It outlines the terminology used in the profession and describes the concepts that are at the core of the profession, most specifically the concept of occupation. It is an evolving document that will change and be updated as practice changes. The contents of this document delineate generally accepted knowledge about the practice of occupational therapy, which provides standard terminology and structure of the profession for students, practitioners, consumers, and third-party payers.[3] However, the contents of the *OTPF* do not reflect the detailed information needed by practitioners that is provided by models of practice and frames of reference.

A model of practice helps organize one's thinking, whereas a frame of reference is a tool to guide one's intervention.[14,16] Basically, a frame of reference tells you what to do and how to evaluate and intervene with clients. Furthermore, frames of reference have research to support the principles guiding evaluation and intervention. Thus using a frame of reference to guide one's practice is essential to **evidence-based practice.** Evidence-based practice refers to choosing intervention techniques based upon the best possible research. This chapter will outline selected occupational therapy models of practice and frames of reference and describe how they are applied in practice.

UNDERSTANDING THEORY

A **theory** is a set of ideas that helps explain things. Research is used to support or refute theories. Occupational therapy borrows theories from other disciplines such as psychology, medicine, nursing, and social work. Theory is the analysis of a set of facts in their relation to one another.[15] There are two major structural components to theory: concepts and principles.[25,26] **Concepts** are ideas that represent something in the mind of the individual. These range from simple, concrete ideas to complex, abstract ideas. Concepts are expressed through the use of symbols and language. Children develop categories for different concepts. For example, a child learns that clothing is a category that can be divided into shoes, pants, dresses, and shirts, among others. **Principles** explain the relationship between two or more concepts.[25] For instance, once the concept of color is learned, such as blue and yellow, a child learns the principle that mixing these two colors produces green.

Theory incorporates ideas similar to what has been described and is defined as "a set of interrelated assumptions, concepts, and definitions that presents a systematic view of phenomena by specifying relationships among variables, with the purpose of explaining and predicting the phenomena."[20] It is important to realize that in practice, theories range in scope and complexity along a continuum. Theories may be broad in scope and attempt to cover many aspects of a discipline, or they may have a narrow focus and concern only a small portion of the field.[25] Figure 14-1 provides an illustration of how these concepts fit together.

Students frequently resist theory. There is a desire to "get in there and do something" and not to discuss why it is done. One may ask, "Why is it important to know about and

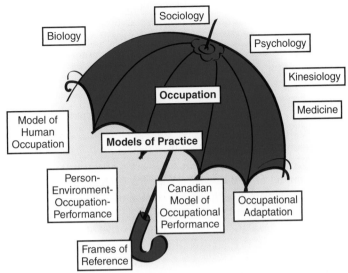

Figure 14-1 The umbrella of occupation: a conceptual diagram of the relationship between theories, occupation, models of practice, and frames of reference. *(From MacRae N, O'Brien J: OT 301 Foundations of occupational therapy, unpublished lecture notes, 2001, University of New England.)*

use theory in occupational therapy practice?" Not applying theory to practice is similar to taking a trip without a road map. The trip will be disorganized and lack structure. The traveler may eventually find a way to the final destination but may not know exactly how he or she got from point A to point B. Consequently, it will be difficult to give directions to anyone else or to replicate the journey in the future. It is necessary to develop an appreciation for theory, because only when an individual knows the reason something is done can he or she do it well; only when a person knows the theory on which various practices and techniques are based will he or she be innovative and employ good clinical reasoning.

Parham states the importance of theory: "Theory is a key element in problem setting and in problem solving. It is a tool that enables the practitioner to 'name it and frame it.' Both language and logic are needed to identify a problem (name it) and to plan a means for altering the situation (frame it). Theory provides these by giving us words or concepts for naming what we observe and by spelling out logical relationships between concepts."[17] Theory allows the OT practitioner to structure and organize his or her intervention.

Additional reasons for using theory include (1) to validate and guide practice, (2) to justify reimbursement, (3) to clarify specialization issues, (4) to enhance the growth of the profession and the professionalism of its members, and (5) to educate competent practitioners.[25] More importantly, however, a theoretical base serves as a unifying foundation for the profession and helps tie together its unique aspects.

Theories specific to occupational therapy practice originated in science-based disciplines such as biology, chemistry, physics, psychology, and occupational science. The practitioner may use a number of theories during intervention and combine parts of theories. To do so, however, the practitioner must be knowledgeable about the theories that are in use to ensure that they are compatible with one another. Theories used in occupational therapy include those developed by Mosey, Kielhofner, Ayres, Reilly, Llorens, and Fidler. It is beyond the scope of this introductory text to describe the various theories used. It is recommended that the reader refer to the text by Walker and Ludwig[25] for an overview of the work of each theorist.

How does the practitioner apply theory to practice? Theory is linked to clinical practice through models of practice and frames of reference, the means by which theory relates to intervention.

MODEL OF PRACTICE

The terms *model of practice, conceptual model, practice model,* and *frame of reference* have been used interchangeably in texts. In this text, we will distinguish between model of practice and frame of reference. However, this is just one way to organize the content.

A **model of practice** takes the philosophical base of the profession and organizes the concepts for practice. As such, occupational therapy models of practice help OT practitioners organize their thinking around occupation,[14] which is the central unifying feature of the occupational therapy profession. A model of practice provides practitioners with terms to describe practice, an overall view of the profession, tools for evaluation, and a guide for intervention.[9,14,16]

By reading and critically analyzing current literature, practitioners who use a model of practice to guide their practice find a depth of information, which allows them to better understand practice and intervention to the benefit of clients. Using a model of practice ensures a systematic examination of the client and is an important step in providing evidence-based practice.

The **Model of Human Occupation** (MOHO)[10] is perhaps the best-researched model of practice in occupational therapy. Kielhofner and colleagues have published extensively on all aspects of this model, and thus this model provides well-supported evidence to support its use in practice. The Model of Human Occupation views occupation in terms of volition, habituation, performance, and environment. Volition refers to the person's motivation, interests, values, and belief in skill. Habituation refers to one's daily patterns of behaviors, one's roles (the rules and expectations of those positions), and one's everyday routine. Performance refers to the motor, cognitive, and emotional aspects required to act upon the environment.[10] Environment refers to the physical, social, and societal surroundings in which the person is involved. Each system is divided into components with many well-researched instruments to operationalize the terms for practice.[10] Working with the assessment tools or tests designed to operationalize the concepts of the model for practice helps practitioners understand the concepts more fully.

The **Canadian Model of Occupational Performance** (CMOP)[11,23] has also generated a wealth of research to support its design. The core of this model is spirituality, which is defined broadly as anything that motivates or inspires a person.[11,23] The person, environment (which includes institutions), and occupations are the other parts of the model. This model emphasizes client-centered care,[11,23] which refers to understanding the client's desires and wishes for intervention and outcome. Getting to know the client is crucial to this model. The *Canadian Occupational Performance Measure*[12] is a semistructured interview based on this model and provides practitioners with a tool to organize their thoughts.

The **Person-Environment-Occupation-Performance** (PEOP) model[7] developed by Christiansen and Baum provides definitions for each term and describes the interactive nature of the human being. This model provides generic, broad terms for each area (e.g., person, environment, occupation, performance). *Person* includes the physical, social, and psychological aspects of the individual. *Environment* includes the physical and social supports, and those things that interfere with the individual's performance. *Occupation* refers to the everyday things people do and in which they find meaning. *Performance* refers to the actions of occupations.[7]

Occupational adaptation, articulated by Schkade and Schultz, proposes that OT practitioners examine how they may change the person, environment, or task so the client may engage in occupations. In this model, occupation is viewed as the primary means for the individual to achieve adaptation. Individual adaptation is seen as both a state of being and a process that can be examined at a given time, over a specified time period, or over a lifetime.[21] This model focuses on the person, the occupational environment, and the interaction. It supports compensatory techniques if necessary.

Other models of practice exist in occupational therapy practice, such as the ecological model by Dunn and spatiotemporal adaptation by Gilfoyle and Grady.

CASE APPLICATION

The following case studies provide an overview of the use of the different models of practice.

Raven is a 37-year-old woman who was hospitalized with a brain aneurysm, which affected her speech, right-sided movement, and cognitive abilities. Raven is unable to remain standing for long periods of time, and she needs frequent breaks during seated activities. Raven experiences difficulty with memory and poor concentration.

The occupational therapist (OT) meets with Raven on her first day on the rehabilitation unit. The following comparison describes the type of information she will collect about Raven.

Model of Human Occupation

Volition: Raven enjoys family events, singing, and cooking. Raven lives close to her family and sees her mother, three children, and many other family members daily. Furthermore, the family attends church services on Sunday and then gathers at Raven's for a potluck supper. She is active in the church choir.

Habituation: Raven works 5 days a week from 8 AM to 5 PM in a local grocery store, where she is the assistant manager. She attends her grandchildren's school events and periodically helps her daughters with child care and transportation. Raven attends church Wednesday evenings and Sundays.

Performance: Prior to her aneurysm, Raven was able to complete all occupations without difficulty. Currently, she is unable to use her right side, slurs her speech, has difficulty maintaining a conversation, and becomes easily confused. Raven is unable to remain active for over 20 minutes, showing obvious signs of fatigue.

Environment: Raven lives in a small apartment building in the city with her husband. She has been married for 20 years. They live on the third floor. The building has elevators, but Raven is afraid to use them. Raven's family members live close by and frequently visit her. She holds many family gatherings at her house.

Canadian Model of Occupational Performance

Spirituality: Raven attends church Wednesday nights and Sundays. She is active in her church and enjoys the family camaraderie of the church. Raven sings in the choir and defines herself as a very devoted Christian.

Person: Raven is a 37-year-old married woman who suffered an aneurysm and is in a rehabilitation hospital. She is unable to use her right side, slurs her speech, and shows poor memory and concentration.

Environment: Raven works for the institution of a grocery chain. As such, she must follow institutional policy and procedures. She has medical insurance. She also follows the church's institutional policies.

Occupations: Raven enjoys spending time with family; she is active in the church and a member of the choir. Raven works at a local grocery store. She attends her grandchildren's school events when possible.

Person-Environment-Occupation-Performance

Person: Raven lives with her husband. She has been married for 20 years. She has many family members whom she sees regularly. Raven enjoys family events, singing, and cooking.

Environment: Raven lives in a small apartment building in the city. She lives on the third floor. Raven's family live close by.

Occupations: She works 5 days a week from 8 AM to 5 PM in a local grocery store. Raven attends church and sees her family frequently. Raven attends her grandchildren's events.

Performance: Raven slurs her speech and has difficulty using her right side. She fatigues easily.

Occupational Adaptation

Occupation: Raven works as an assistant manager at a grocery store. She takes care of her family and is involved in the church. She enjoys socializing with others. Currently, she is unable to engage in these occupations, due to right-sided weakness, slurred speech, and fatigue.

Adaptation: The OT practitioner changes the demands of the occupation of socializing, by allowing Raven to sit in a chair and visit with family members for short periods of time. The OT practitioner provides Raven with short projects in which she can participate with her grandchildren when they visit. This helps Raven continue her nurturing occupations, while helping her gain function.

Conclusion

The above case study applications illustrate the subtle discrepancies of each model of practice. Although the information gathered may be similar, the focus differs. Readers should explore the complexities, definitions, and explanations of each of the terms because they provide more insight into how to analyze human occupation. Furthermore, readers are encouraged to examine the available assessment tools and measures that more specifically define the concepts of the various models. For example, the volitional questionnaire designed under the Model of Human Occupation (MOHO) examines one's interests, values, and personal causation. Understanding this assessment tool helps practitioners more completely understand the concept of volition to better serve their clients.

FRAMES OF REFERENCE

Williamson states that "Frames of reference are produced from the body of knowledge of the profession and address a specific aspect of the profession's domain of concern."[26] A specific area of practice is the focus of a frame of reference, which describes a process for change in the client and identifies principles for moving a client along a continuum from dysfunction to function. Depending on the focus of intervention, the practitioner may use several frames of reference at one time or use them sequentially over time.[26]

One of the most efficient and practical ways to conduct evidence-based practice is to examine frames of reference, which apply theory and put principles into practice. As such, frames of reference provide practitioners with specifics about how to treat specific clients. A **frame of reference** includes a description of the population, theory regarding change, function and dysfunction, principles of intervention, role of the practitioner, and evaluation instruments. The parts of a FOR are listed in Box 14-1 and are described in the following sections.

POPULATION

The frame of reference identifies the types of diagnoses that would benefit from the intervention. For example, clients who experience decreased strength and endurance are typically treated using the biomechanical FOR. Research has supported the use of repetitive exercise in strengthening muscles. Practitioners using a biomechanical FOR do not have to conduct their own research on how to strengthen muscles; instead, they use the research from this FOR, which states that providing repetitive movements, increasing the weight, and providing gradual resistance are all techniques that improve strength.[18,19,24]

CONTINUUM OF FUNCTION AND DYSFUNCTION

The FOR defines behaviors that are characteristic of function and dysfunction according to the principles. The therapist evaluates these behaviors, which vary according to the frame of reference, during the assessment process. For example, using the biomechanical FOR, function includes strength, endurance, and range of motion (ROM) that is adequate to perform occupations. Dysfunction is measured in limitations to strength, range of motion, and endurance.[18,19,24]

Conversely, behavioral frames of reference define function as the absence of abnormal behaviors, and dysfunction is the presence of behaviors that interfere with function. According to a behavioral frame of reference, abnormal behaviors may be socially unacceptable behaviors or any other behavior defined by the team as interfering with function.

Research has provided guidelines to determine "typical" function. Thus, the practitioner is able to use the available research to determine if occupational therapy services are warranted. This is evidence-based practice.

THEORIES REGARDING CHANGE

The FOR will describe the theory and hypotheses regarding change. For example, many of the neurological frames of reference (e.g., neurodevelopmental theory [NDT], sensory integration [SI], motor control) are based upon the theory of **brain plasticity,** which refers to the phenomenon that the brain is capable of change and through activity one may get

---

Box 14-1 Necessary Parts of a Frame of Reference

- Population
- Continuum of function/dysfunction
- Theory regarding change
- Principles
- Role of the practitioner
- Assessment instruments

improved neurological synapses, improved dendritic growth, or additional pathways. Therefore intervention is aimed at improving neuronal firing and generating improved brain activity through repetition. Understanding the theory regarding change is important to providing evidence-based intervention.

PRINCIPLES

The FOR defines the underlying principles behind the evaluation and intervention. These statements, which relate back to the theoretical base, describe how an individual is aided to make changes and progresses from a state of dysfunction to one of function. Understanding the principles of the FOR allows practitioners to use clinical reasoning to determine whether the FOR may benefit their client (although it may not be originally intended for that population). The principles are based upon theory and researched using multiple studies and scientific data. OT practitioners may have to critique the rationale if the FOR does not provide adequate evidence to support its claims. The FOR should be clear about the principles surrounding the techniques. For example, the principle of strengthening is that by repetitive muscle contractions, more fibers are recruited and the muscle is able to lift more.[19] Practitioners benefit from knowing that the principle behind strengthening is the recruitment of more muscle fibers.

ROLE OF THE PRACTITIONER

The role of the practitioner is based upon the principles and theory of the FOR. These statements provide a guide as to how the practitioner will interact with the client and the environment. This is based upon research evidence that supports the expectation that if an OT employs a certain technique the client's function will improve. Subsequently, OT practitioners can be assured when using a FOR that it worked for someone else. However, a careful analysis is still required to determine whether the technique is well founded or supported. Evidence-based practice suggests that the OT practitioner examine the rigor of the study, which includes the methodology, rationale, results, and design. Examining the research of a FOR helps the practitioner fully understand the intricacies of the FOR and as such the role of the practitioner. For example, studies examining sensory integration practice must explain to the reader the procedures that were used to conduct sensory integration therapy.[4,6] Often, researchers provide sensorimotor therapy rather than sensory integration therapy. A closer look at the sensory integration theory allows the reader to determine whether the researchers conducted sensory integration therapy. This helps practitioners critique the research more adequately. Practitioners should not change practice or base practice on weak findings.

Importantly, the FOR describes how the practitioner should interact with the client. For example, practitioners using a behavioral frame of reference are to reward positive behaviors and ignore negative ones. The behavioral FOR provides insight into the type of cues that may be provided to clients. The neurodevelopment FOR requires that the practitioner touch the client throughout the movement and facilitate a normal movement pattern.[5,22] Thus knowledge and investigation into the FOR provide practitioners with a wealth of information for practice.

ASSESSMENT INSTRUMENTS

The FOR also provides the OT practitioner with a variety of instruments to operationalize the principles. For example, Allen's Cognitive Levels was designed to identify the level of cognitive functioning for clients and to be used with the cognitive disability frame of reference.[1,2]

The Sensory Integration and Praxis Tests, Miller Assessment for Preschoolers, Adult Sensory Profile, and clinical observations are based upon SI principles and designed to assist the therapist in determining how the client would benefit from the FOR.[4,6] Numerous instruments have been developed to examine a client's functioning in relation to the principles of a specific FOR.

WHY USE A FRAME OF REFERENCE?

In reality, how is a FOR used? Students frequently return from fieldwork convinced that their supervisor did not use a FOR. However, if that is the case, did the supervisor develop the principles of range of motion by himself or herself? In fact, the principle of gradual stretch to elongate the muscle fibers was developed under the biomechanical FOR. Many researchers evaluated the changes in muscle tension through passive stretch before developing the principle. The research entailed examination of EMG function on numerous clients. Today, range of motion is a standard occupational therapy intervention; few practitioners stop to think about the theory behind it. However, if range of motion is not working for a client, the OT practitioner may find it helpful to review the principles and previous research. This is all part of critically analyzing the research and explaining what OT practitioners do, and it is considered essential to evidence-based practice.

If OT practitioners do not use a FOR, then how do they justify their practice? They are basing their results on someone's work. Certainly, they are not coming up with the entire practice on their own. OT practitioners also need to articulate what they are doing, even if the practice is a traditional one. As occupational therapy moves to a master's level, professionals are being asked to justify their practice and to contribute new knowledge. It is not sufficient to do things just because someone says you should do it this way. Instead, OT practitioners must become critical consumers of research so they can critique and analyze current practices.

APPLICATION OF TWO FRAMES OF REFERENCE

Several frames of reference can be found in occupational therapy, and they vary in breadth and depth. For illustration purposes, two different frames of reference are described using the above components. The first is the **biomechanical frame of reference.** This frame of reference is derived from theories in kinetics and kinematics (sciences that study the effects of forces and motion on material bodies).[24]

On the function-dysfunction continuum, the biomechanical frame of reference is used with individuals who have deficits in the peripheral nervous, musculoskeletal, integumentary (e.g., skin), or cardiopulmonary system. These individuals, however, have a central nervous system that is intact.[18,19,24] The deficits may cause posture and mobility problems, impairment in range of motion and strength, and decreased endurance. Disabling conditions that may benefit from the biomechanical approach include rheumatoid arthritis and osteoarthritis, fractures, burns, hand traumas, amputations, and spinal cord injuries.

The practitioner evaluates the client's range of motion, muscle strength, and endurance through the use of a variety of tools. Through exercise, activity, and physical agent modalities, change in the person's range of motion, strength, and endurance can be demonstrated.[8]

Another frame of reference used for illustration purposes is the **cognitive disability frame of reference** proposed by Claudia Allen. This frame of reference is based on the premise that cognitive disorders in those with mental health disabilities are caused by neurobiologic defects or deficits related to the biologic functioning of the brain.[1,2] Its theoretical base is derived from research in neuroscience, cognitive psychology, information processing, and biologic psychiatry.[8]

Along the function-dysfunction continuum, function exists when an individual is able to process information to perform routine tasks demanded by the environment.[8] Dysfunction results when the person's ability to process information is restricted in such a way that carrying out routine tasks is impossible. Allen defines six cognitive levels, which are organized in a hierarchy along a continuum. Level 1 represents the individual who has a profound disability in information processing, whereas level 6 represents the normal ability to acquire and process information. Each cognitive level defines the information processing behaviors indicative of function-dysfunction. Two specific tools used by practitioners to evaluate an individual's level of functioning are the Allen Cognitive Level (ACL) Test and the Routine Task Inventory Test.[8] The cognitive disability frame of reference proposes that change occurs because of (1) the capacity of the client and (2) the environment. Change in the capacity of the client may be influenced by medical intervention and psychotropic medications, as well as occupational therapy intervention, which teaches the client how to perform routine tasks (cognitive levels 4 and 5). Occupational therapy intervention can also produce change in the environment through modification of task procedures, amount of assistance offered, directions, and setting.[8] Environmental changes may allow the client to experience greater success in performing activities.

USING MULTIPLE FRAMES OF REFERENCE

Although organizing one's thoughts around one model of practice makes sense in occupational therapy, there are many FORs for different clientele. OT practitioners may use multiple FORs, depending on the setting and clientele. The practitioner must examine the theory, principles, and techniques used according to the FOR before deciding if the FOR would work with a given client and setting. If the practitioner is going to modify the FOR, the practitioner must be mindful of the reasons why and critically examine the rationale. Using a FOR in a different way may result in less dramatic changes, but may be more practical in certain situations.

Sometimes, a practitioner may decide to combine FORs. For example, combining a sensory integration and behavioral frame of reference may work with some clients. However, the OT practitioner must carefully observe how this blend is working and understand the principles behind each FOR to determine if the blending is appropriate.

Some FORs do not fit together, and using them together may result in less progress toward the stated goals.

EVALUATING FRAMES OF REFERENCE

The OT practitioner is responsible for evaluating the client's progress towards his or her goals. If progress is slow or not being made, the OT practitioner re-examines the goals and the FOR. A careful examination of the techniques provided by the FOR may reveal other techniques to help the client reach the goals. Furthermore, the FOR may provide more insight into the role of the practitioner. The practitioner may change how he or she is working with the client, or modify some techniques. It may be necessary to consult with a more experienced practitioner (e.g., an NDT–certified practitioner may suggest different techniques).

The practitioner will want to explore the principles of the FOR to understand the reasoning behind the lack of progress. Could something else be going on that has been missed? The practitioner may want to re-examine the literature to determine if others have found this FOR successful with the given population. If so, what techniques were used? How did the service differ from what the therapist is currently doing? It may be that the practitioner needs more time or needs to treat the client with more intensity.

When the FOR is not working, the OT practitioner may decide to change FORs. Again, he or she may consider the principles, goals, role of the therapist, and the client's motivations. Changing the FOR may provide the right momentum to spur progress.

CASE APPLICATION

> George is a 34-year-old man who experienced a head trauma from a motor vehicle accident. He currently walks with a wide-based gait and shows uncoordinated movement patterns. He leans to the right and drags his left leg. George has poor lip closure (right facial droop) and difficulty chewing some foods. George has a poor right-handed grasp. He shows impaired long-term and short-term memory. Frequently, George is tearful during the session and he has difficulty reading other's cues.

The following examples show how the OT practitioner might view this case from different frames of reference.

Behavioral: Work on George's ability to complete activities and engage in social conversation without inappropriate affect or comments. The practitioner provides positive reinforcements when positive behavior is noted.

Biomechanical: Improve George's strength and endurance through repetitive activity. The OT practitioner provides George with activities that are increasingly difficult. The sessions focus on strength, endurance, and range of motion.

Cognitive-behavioral: Help George identify his own goals and behaviors in hopes that through self-reflection he may make the changes. The OT practitioner allows George to complete an activity and discusses how it went afterwards and how they would improve his behavior next time. The theory behind this frame of reference is that clients will make more significant changes when they are able to cognitively acknowledge them.

Developmental: Identify the highest level motor, social, cognitive skills in which George can engage, and facilitate improvements in function from that starting point. Grade activities so that he can achieve them, but is slightly challenged. Help "close the gap" in the areas in which he is unable to perform.[13]

Motor control: Work on George's impaired motor skills through activities in the natural environment. Allow George to make mistakes and learn from them. The motor control frame of reference suggests that the practitioner provide verbal and physical cues as necessary. Practice should take place in short sessions with frequent breaks.

Neurodevelopmental: Work on George's motor skills by inhibiting abnormal muscle tone and facilitating normal movement patterns. The OT practitioner requests that George complete activities while the practitioner facilitates the movement at selected "key points of control" (i.e., hand, shoulders, and waist).

Perceptual motor training: Work with George on improving his memory, cognitive skills, safety awareness, and visual perception through a variety of table top activities. Perceptual motor training may include many computer-type games and strategies.

Sensorimotor: Work on improving George's motor skills through practice of occupations. The OT practitioner sets up activities in which George practices his coordination.

The above examples provide a brief summary of how intervention differs when using selected frames of reference. The OT practitioner relies on clinical reasoning, experience, judgment, current research, and a thorough understanding of the occupational profile of the client, including the contexts in which the occupations occur. Together, this information forms the basis for the occupational therapy intervention.

SUMMARY

Models of practice help organize one's thinking, whereas frames of reference tell practitioners what to do in practice. Organizing one's practice around the concepts of occupation is central to the profession. Thus, selecting a model of practice developed by OTs provides the best assurance that the practitioner is "thinking" like an OT. This is helpful in educating the public, clients, and consumers about the profession.

Frames of reference are important in ensuring that practitioners are using evidence-based practice. By critiquing the research on the effectiveness of the selected frame of reference, practitioners are able to fully understand the principles, intervention procedures, and techniques. This helps practitioners adapt the frame of reference if necessary for clients and diagnoses in which the research has not been conducted so that other clients may benefit. Practitioners with knowledge of the subtleties of the frames of reference are able to skillfully work with clients. Articulating the rationale behind one's intervention techniques is important in today's health care environment. Furthermore, understanding the frames of reference helps OT practitioners better serve clients.

Learning Activities

1. Use a selected model of practice to analyze yourself. Summarize your findings in a report format.
2. Compare and contrast two models of practice in a short paper.
3. Have each member of the class present findings from at least three intervention studies on a given frame of reference. Discuss the effectiveness of this FOR on a selected population.
4. Ask students to provide their rationale for selecting a specific FOR for a given population. Use at least three research studies to justify the selection.
5. Identify the theory for change, principles, and intervention strategies for a specific frame of reference. Present the findings in class.
6. Visit an occupational therapy department and determine which models of practice and frames of reference are used at this setting. Ask to observe an OT practitioner during a treatment that implements one of the frames of reference.

Review Questions

1. What is a theory, model of practice, and frame of reference?
2. Why is it important to use a model of practice? Frame of reference?
3. What are the parts to a frame of reference?
4. How does research on frames of reference support occupational therapy practice?
5. What are some occupational therapy models of practice? Describe them in general terms.

REFERENCES

1. Allen CK: Activity, occupational therapy's treatment method, *Am J Occup Ther* 41:563, 1987.
2. Allen CK: *Occupational Therapy for Psychiatric Diseases: Measurement and Management of Cognitive Disabilities,* Boston, 1985, Little, Brown.
3. American Occupational Therapy Association: Occupational therapy practice framework: domain and process, *Am J Occup Ther* 56(6):609-639, 2002.
4. Ayres JA: *Sensory Integration for the Child,* Los Angeles, 1979, Western Psychological Services.
5. Bobath B: Sensorimotor development, *NDT Newsletter* 7:1, 1975.
6. Case-Smith J: *Occupational Therapy for Children,* ed 5, St. Louis, 2005, Mosby.
7. Christiansen CH, Baum CM (eds): *Occupational Therapy: Enabling Function and Well-being,* Thorofare, NJ, 1997, Slack.
8. Crepeau EB, Cohn ES, Boyt Schell BA (eds): *Willard and Spackman's Occupational Therapy,* ed 10, Philadelphia, 2003, Lippincott Williams & Wilkins.
9. Kielhofner G: *Conceptual Foundations of Occupational Therapy,* Philadelphia, 1997, FA Davis.
10. Kielhofner G: *A Model of Human Occupation: Theory and Application,* ed 3, Baltimore, 2002, Williams & Wilkins.
11. Law M, Cooper B, Stewart D, et al: The person-environment-occupation model: a transactive approach to occupational performance, *Canad J Occup Ther* 63(1):9-23, 1996.
12. Law M, Baptiste S, Carswell A, et al: *Canadian Occupational Performance Measure,* ed 2, Toronto, 1994, Canadian Association of Occupational Therapists Publication.
13. Llorens LA: *Application of a Developmental Theory for Health and Rehabilitation,* 1976, Rockville, MD, 1976, American Occupational Therapy Association.
14. MacRae N, O'Brien J: OT 301 Foundations of occupational therapy, unpublished lecture notes, 2001, University of New England.
15. Mish F (ed): *Merriam-Webster's Collegiate Dictionary®,* ed 10, Springfield, MA, 1994, Merriam-Webster.
16. O'Brien J, Solomon J: Scope of practice. In Solomon J, O'Brien J: *Pediatric Skills for Occupational Therapy Assistants,* ed 2, St. Louis, 2006, Mosby.
17. Parham D: Toward professionalism: the reflective therapist, *Am J Occup Ther* 41:555, 1987.
18. Pedretti LW, Paszuinielli S: A frame of reference for occupational therapy in physical dysfunction. In Pedritti LW, Zoltan B (eds): *Occupational Therapy: Practice Skills for Physical Dysfunction,* ed 3, pp. 1-17, St. Louis, 1990, Mosby.
19. Pendleton H, Schultz-Krohn W (eds): *Pedretti's Occupational Therapy: Practice Skills for Physical Dysfunction,* ed 6, St. Louis, 2006, Mosby.
20. Reed KL: Understanding theory: the first step in learning about research, *Am J Occup Ther* 38:677, 1984.
21. Schkade JK, Schultz S: Occupational adaptation: toward a holistic approach in contemporary practice, Part I, *Am J Occup Ther* 46:829-837, 1992.
22. Schoen S, Anderson J: Neurodevelopmental treatment frame of reference. In Kramer P, Hinojosa J (eds): *Frames of Reference for Pediatric Occupational Therapy,* Baltimore, 1993, Williams & Wilkins.
23. Townsend E, Brintnell S, Staisey N: Developing guidelines for client-centered occupational therapy practice, *Canad J Occup Ther* 57:69-76, 1990.
24. Trombly CS, Radomski MV: *Occupational Therapy for Physical Dysfunction,* ed 5, Philadelphia, 2002, Lippincott Williams & Wilkins.
25. Walker KF, Ludwig F (eds): *Perspectives on Theory for the Practice of Occupational Therapy,* ed 3, Austin, TX, 2004, Pro-Ed.
26. Williamson GG: A heritage of activity: development of theory, *Am J Occup Ther* 36:716, 1982.

Occupational therapy provides me with the unique opportunity to observe and to share my knowledge and my experiences in order to affect the well-being of another person. The potential to observe makes life interesting. It provides an opportunity to stand aside, note, and experience reality within its context, be it beautiful or painful. Observation further provides an opportunity to stand still and acknowledge. It provides the occupational therapist with an opportunity to apply activity analysis—the main method of occupational therapy—to detect function or dysfunction of task performance, as well as the performance components; but task performance is the focus of the human being. Observation thus allows the occupational therapist to view the human through activities or tasks, these tasks being crucial forces responsible for shaping the human being. In other words, an occupational therapist is an observer with a powerful tool, "activity analysis." Through observation, the therapist can assess performance, set goals, treat the individual with the set goals in mind, and critically evaluate its impact, all by applying different forms of clinical reasoning.

The human being evolves around task performance. The human is shaped by what he or she performs, and life is meaningless without the ability and the motivation to perform at whatever small capacity. The smallest gains can be as rewarding and worthwhile for those involved as are the bigger accomplishments or achievements for others.

Occupational therapy has further allowed me to share my knowledge regarding occupational performance that could, in some instances, affect the quality of life of those involved. It has provided me with an opportunity to challenge limitations at different levels of performance, in a very exciting way, as some of these limitations have been at a level that I would have thought would be impossible to influence. Limitations have the potential to develop maturity in life, and many limitations not only bring about frustrations and negative aspects but the inner beauty of the person involved and the unknown potentials that may flourish and thereby enhance maturity.

Task performance is, therefore, the force that molds the human being into an occupational being. It is a privilege to be an occupational therapist and to be involved with that powerful driving force.

Guorún Árnadóttir, MA, BOT
Private Practitioner
Reykjavík, Iceland

Intervention Modalities

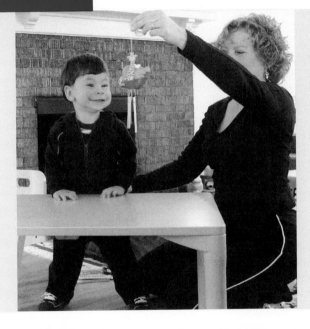

OBJECTIVES

After reading this chapter, the reader will be able to do the following:

- Identify the principal tools of occupational therapy (OT) practice
- Describe the difference between preparatory, purposeful, simulated, and occupation-based activity
- Explain the purpose of activity analysis, and describe its application to occupation
- Understand the role of the OT practitioner in the use of physical agent modalities
- Understand the role of the OT practitioner in splinting and in assistive technology

KEY TERMS

Activity analysis
Activity synthesis
Adapting
Assistive devices
Grading
Media

Methods
Modality
Occupation-based activity
Orthotic device
Physical agent modalities
Preparatory methods

Purposeful activity
Simulated activity
Sensory input
Splint
Therapeutic exercise

OT practitioners use a variety of modalities as tools of the trade. A **modality** includes both the method of intervention as well as the medium. The steps, sequences, and approaches used to activate the therapeutic effect of a medium are the **methods.**[12] The supplies and equipment used are the **media.** For example, an OT practitioner might use the medium of a scooter board to treat a child. The OT practitioner may ask the child to use the scooter board in different ways to activate different therapeutic responses. One method may be to ask the child to ride the board on his stomach down an incline in order to promote extension in the prone position. Another method may have the child lying on his back and pulling himself on a rope using hand over hand, with the purpose being to work on the flexor muscles.

During intervention, the OT practitioner considers the whole modality, that is, both the medium and the method. Through the selection and use of modalities, OT practitioners aim to reach the goals identified in the client's intervention plan. Selecting the modality to use and the time to use it becomes a skill that is developed through a review of literature, experience, and practice. For the student entering the field, this can be challenging, and therefore OT students must become familiar with the modalities of the profession early and understand how they are used in practice.

This chapter describes occupational therapy intervention modalities as outlined in the *Occupational Therapy Practice Framework (OTPF)*.[2] The *OTPF* identifies the four categories of intervention as: (1) therapeutic use of self, (2) therapeutic use of occupations and activities, (3) consultation process, and (4) education process. In this chapter, we focus on therapeutic use of occupations and activities, which include preparatory methods, purposeful activity, and occupation-based activity. Therapeutic use of self is described in Chapter 16, and consultation and education are described in Chapter 9.

Therapeutic use of occupations and activities includes the use of preparatory, purposeful, and occupation-based activity. OT practitioners help clients reach their goals by using specially designed activities. In using these activities therapeutically, the OT practitioner needs to consider context, activity demands, and client factors as they relate to the goals of the client.[2]

PREPARATORY METHODS

Preparatory methods are used in conjunction with or in order to prepare the client for purposeful activity and occupational performance. They include sensory input, therapeutic exercise, physical agent modalities, and orthotics/splinting.[2] These methods address the remediation and restoration of problems associated with client factors and body structure, with the long-term purpose of supporting the client's acquisition of performance skills needed to resume his or her roles and daily occupations.

SENSORY INPUT

Providing **sensory input** to help a client resume functional movement is considered a preparatory activity. For example, the OT practitioner may stimulate a muscle through vibration in an attempt to activate muscle fibers for contraction and subsequent movement. Using sensory input such as deep pressure may help inhibit abnormal muscle tone in order for the client to engage in purposeful movement.[14] Many of these techniques were originated by Margaret Rood, and they help clients prior to the actual activity. Thus providing sensory input to change muscle tone or sensory sensitivity is considered preparatory activities.

Sensory input may be provided as a technique to help clients relearn movements that may be lost due to illness, disease, or trauma. Although the goal of sensory input is improved function, the techniques do not require the client to engage in activity. Generally, the sensory input is provided to the muscle fibers directly. Therefore, OT practitioners use sensory input as an adjunct to purposeful and occupation-based activity.

THERAPEUTIC EXERCISE

Therapeutic exercise, a modality from the biomechanical frame of reference, is the "scientific supervision of exercise for the purpose of preventing muscular atrophy, restoring joint and muscle function, and improving efficiency of cardiovascular and pulmonary function."[13] By understanding the principles of therapeutic exercise, the practitioner is able to apply biomechanical principles to purposeful activity. Therapeutic exercise is most effectively used as an intervention for lower motor neuron disorders that result in weakness and flaccidity (e.g. spinal cord injuries, poliomyelitis, Guillain-Barré syndrome), or orthopedic conditions such as arthritis.[6]

The general goals of therapeutic exercise are to (1) increase muscle strength, (2) maintain or increase joint range of motion and flexibility, (3) improve muscle endurance, (4) improve physical conditioning and cardiovascular fitness, and (5) improve coordination. The OT practitioner selects an appropriate therapeutic exercise from available options on the basis of the client's needs, goals, capabilities, and precautions related to his or her condition.[6] Although a description of each therapeutic exercise is beyond the scope of this entry-level text, Table 15-1 provides a summary of the types of therapeutic exercise used for each of the general goals.

The advantage of therapeutic exercise is that the practitioner can target specific muscle groups and motor movements by asking the client to perform particular exercises. The amount of resistance and number of repetitions can be controlled. The disadvantage of using therapeutic exercise is that it does not involve the whole person, whereas purposeful and occupation-based activity provides a holistic approach to intervention by requiring the individual to use many different performance components (e.g., gross and fine motor, visual, emotional). Therapeutic exercise should not be used exclusively but may be used to prepare a client for purposeful activity and occupational performance.

PHYSICAL AGENT MODALITIES

Physical agent modalities (PAMs) are considered preparatory methods. PAMs are used to bring about a response in soft tissue and are most commonly used by OT practitioners for treating hand and arm injuries or disorders. PAMs use light, sound, water, electricity, temperature, and mechanical devices to promote changes in function.[1] Thermal modalities that involve heat transfer to an injured area (i.e., warm paraffin baths, hot packs, whirlpools, or ultrasound) are used to decrease pain and joint stiffness, increase motion, increase blood flow, reduce muscle spasms, and reduce edema.[6] Another thermal modality is the use of cold transfer (i.e., cold packs and ice). Cold transfer is used in the treatment of pain, inflammation, and edema. Electrical modalities include media such as transcutaneous electrical nerve stimulation (TENS), functional electrical stimulation (FES), and neuromuscular electrical stimulation devices (NMES), and are used to reduce edema, decrease pain, increase motion, and re-educate muscles.[6]

The use of PAMs in occupational therapy is controversial.[6,9,15] After debate and discussion, the American Occupational Therapy Association (AOTA) developed a position statement on the use of PAMs that states, "Physical agent modalities may be used by occupational therapists (OTs) and occupational therapy assistants (OTAs) as an adjunct to or in preparation for

TABLE 15-1 Summary of Types of Therapeutic Exercise

General Goal	Type of Exercise	Description of Exercise
Increase muscle strength	Active assisted	Client moves body part as much as he or she can and is assisted to complete movement by practitioner or therapeutic equipment.
	Active range of motion	Client actively moves body part through complete range of motion without assistance or resistance.
	Resistive	Client moves body part through available range of motion against resistance; resistance may be applied manually, by special therapeutic equipment, or through the use of weights; the amount of resistance increases as the person's strength increases.
Maintain or increase joint range of motion and flexibility	Passive range of motion	Client is not able to move the body part, so movement is provided by an outside force such as a practitioner or a therapeutic device (e.g., continuous passive motion device); no muscle contraction takes place.
	Active range of motion	See above.
Improve muscle endurance	Low load, high repetition program	Practitioner determines client's maximum capacity for a strengthening program, then reduces the maximum resistance load and increases the number of repetitions.
Improve physical conditioning and cardiovascular fitness	Sustained rhythmic, aerobic	Examples include jogging, bicycle riding, swimming, and walking.
Improve coordination	Coordination training	Repetitious activities and exercises that require smooth, controlled movement patterns (e.g., placing pegs in holes, stacking blocks, picking up marbles).

intervention that ultimately enhances engagement in occupation." The use of PAMs solely as intervention without application to occupational performance is not considered occupational therapy.[1] PAMs are not to be used by entry-level practitioners; rather, the practitioner needs to complete specialized postprofessional training and provide evidence that he or she has the theoretical background and technical skills needed to use PAMs. With proper application, the use of PAMs in occupational therapy allows the practitioner to provide a comprehensive treatment program for the client.[6]

ORTHOTICS AND SPLINTING

Any "apparatus used to support, align, prevent, or correct deformities or to improve the function of movable parts of the body"[7] is considered an **orthotic device,** or orthosis. Orthotic devices can be prefabricated or custom made and involve assessing the client, determining the most appropriate orthotic device, designing the device, and evaluating the fit. OT practitioners train clients in the use of the orthosis, monitor the wearing schedule, and evaluate the client's response to the orthosis. Orthoses include braces made for the lower extremities and trunk. These types of orthoses are usually made from high-temperature thermoplastic materials that are molded over a plaster model of the body part. These materials are very strong and durable, and they require special tools for cutting ands shaping. Typically, orthoses made from these types of materials are fabricated by an orthotist. Seating and positioning systems, which support, align, and help to prevent deformities, are also considered orthoses. OT practitioners may be involved with other team members in the evaluation of a client and the fabrication of a seating and positioning system. However, the subject of seating and positioning is beyond the scope of this text.

A splint for the upper extremity is another type of orthosis and one that is commonly made by OT practitioners. A **splint** is "an orthopedic device for immobilization, restraint, or support of any part of the body."[4] A splint may be rigid or flexible. Three primary purposes of a splint are to (1) restrict movement, (2) immobilize, or (3) mobilize a body part.[5] The OT practitioner is expected to recognize when there is a need for a splint, select a design that is correct for the problem, fabricate the splint, and educate the client in its proper use and care.

There are two main classifications of splints—static splints and dynamic splints. The *static splint* has no moving components; as the name implies, it remains in a fixed position. Static splints are used to protect or rest a joint, diminish pain, or prevent shortening of the muscle.[5] Figure 15-1, *A,* shows an example of one type of static splint called a resting pan splint. The *dynamic splint* has one or more flexible components that move. The purpose of the dynamic splint is to increase passive motion, enhance active motion, or replace lost motion.[5] The movable components (elastic, rubber band, or spring) are attached to a static base. Figure 15-1, *B,* shows an example of a dynamic splint.

Both static and dynamic splints can be purchased ready made or custom fabricated by the OT practitioner. Custom-made splints are easily fabricated using low-temperature plastics, which become flexible and moldable when heated in hot water or with a heat gun.

The OT is responsible for evaluating the client and recommending the type of splint. Either the OT or the OTA may fabricate the splint. The OT practitioner must consider how the splint fits, both initially and throughout its use. The OT practitioner is responsible for assuring that the attachments that hold it in place are comfortably located and that the device keeps the body part aligned in the correct position. The client must be educated

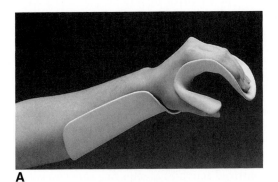
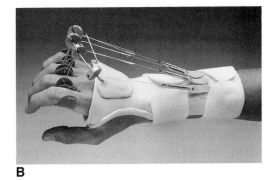

A **B**

Figure 15-1 Static splint: resting pan splint (**A**). Dynamic splint: forearm-based four-digit outrigger with dynamic extension assist supplied by springs (**B**). *(From Pedretti LW:* Occupational Therapy: Practice Skills for Physical Dysfunction, *ed 4, St. Louis, 1996, Mosby.)*

about the wearing of the splint—how to correctly put it on and take it off, the amount of time the splint should be worn, and how to keep the affected area and the splint clean. At each therapy session, the practitioner looks for pressure areas and signs of distress, such as redness, swelling, or reported discomfort.

Splinting requires an in-depth knowledge of body structure, motion analysis, and disability precautions, as well as knowledge of the client. Although functional considerations are the primary concern, the practitioner must also keep in mind cosmetic and psychological factors. Client cooperation and support are essential, for the best-designed splint will not help the client who refuses to wear it.

PURPOSEFUL ACTIVITY

The uniqueness of occupational therapy practice is the use of purposeful activity in intervention. **Purposeful activity** is defined as "goal-directed behaviors or tasks that comprise occupations. An activity is purposeful if the individual is an active, voluntary participant and if the activity is directed toward a goal."[3,10] Examples of purposeful activity may include making a clay pot versus pinching clay (preparatory) or making a sandwich versus strengthening one's grip using resistive putty (preparatory).

Purposeful activity has both *inherent* and *therapeutic* goals. The inherent goal is the end product of the activity. For example, the inherent goal of a leather lacing kit may be to make a leather coin holder. The inherent goal of cooking is to prepare something to eat. The significance of this is that the client focuses on the outcome of the activity rather than the performance of individual components such as the motor movement required to complete the activity. The result is that the client becomes absorbed in the activity itself, and performance is more automatic and natural.[2,3,10]

The OT practitioner also has therapeutic reasons for asking the client to participate in a selected activity. For example, the practitioner may use the leather lacing activity for the therapeutic purpose of improving the individual's fine motor or sequencing skills. The therapeutic goals of the cooking activity may be to increase safety awareness, improve self-esteem, or demonstrate problem-solving skills. OT practitioners are urged to explain the therapeutic purpose of the activity to the client if it is not readily apparent.

Research has demonstrated that clients will conduct more repetitions when the activity is purposeful. Purposeful activity requires client involvement and is geared toward prevention, maintenance, or improvement of function. Purposeful activity may include activities of daily living (ADLs) and instrumental activities of daily living (IADLs), vocational activities, social activities, sports, crafts, games, or construction activities.

SIMULATED OR CONTRIVED ACTIVITY

In some situations, the use of a purposeful activity is not possible or practical. The clinical environment may not have the required materials and equipment for the activity; the client may not yet have the skills or stamina needed, or there might not be enough time to complete the activity. In these instances, the practitioner uses **simulated** or contrived **activities**. Fisher describes contrived activities as requiring some aspect of pretending.[10] For example, a contrived activity may be imitating the movement required to spread peanut butter on a sandwich, with no actual materials. Clothing fastener boards that simulate dressing tasks such as buttoning or zipping, or the use of manipulation boards (Figure 15-2, *A*) that simulate different types of hand grips for tasks such as opening a door lock, turning on a water faucet, or switching on a light are other examples of contrived activities. The inclined sanding board (Figure 15-2, *B*), which has a long history in occupational therapy and is used to exercise muscles of the arm, simulates sanding of wood; however, there is no actual end product.[10] There are various table-top media used to train cognitive and perceptual skills that also fall into this category.

The use of contrived activities as a part of treatment should be carefully considered. Contrived activities are valuable when resources are limited or when retraining motor, perceptual, and cognitive skills, but they should only be a part of a comprehensive intervention plan that also includes purposeful and occupation-based activities. They may not result in generalization. Furthermore, practitioners should be careful not to design activities that are too contrived and lose the purpose of the activity.

OCCUPATION-BASED ACTIVITY

The aim of occupational therapy services is to help clients engage in occupations.[2,3,10] For example, the student role may be central to one's identity. The **occupation-based activities** the student engages in are to read literature, study for exams, and write papers. These activities make up the occupation and therefore are necessary. For another person, being a student may not be central to his or her identity. Consider the client who attends school only because he "has to go." For this student, school is a task or activity that must be completed but is not central to his or her identity.

Although OT practitioners realize that we all engage in tasks that may not be central to our identity, finding those occupations in one's life is key. Therefore the goal of occupational therapy is to help people find those meaningful occupations and return to them.

The constellation of occupations in which a person engages varies, although many of the tasks we complete are the same. It is this fine analysis of the many facets of occupations that makes the profession so unique.

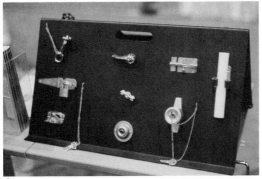
A

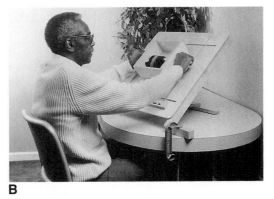
B

Figure 15-2 Manipulation board simulates the different hand grasps used in everyday activities (**A**). Inclined sanding board simulates sanding wood on an inclined plane and is used to exercise elbow and shoulder musculature (**B**). *(B Courtesy S & S Worldwide, Adaptability, 1995.)*

ACTIVITY ANALYSIS

To understand the many facets of occupations and how activities are selected and implemented to achieve the client's goals for occupational performance, the OT practitioner must first understand and be able to analyze activities. **Activity analysis** is the process by which the steps of an activity and its components are examined in detail to determine the demands on the client.[2,3,8,9] Through the process of activity analysis, the practitioner determines the requirements to perform a given activity successfully. With experience in analyzing activities, the OT practitioner is able to quickly identify the factors required for performing an activity and assess its therapeutic value.

There are different ways to approach the analysis of activities. One way is to base the activity analysis on the frame of reference being used. The frame of reference identifies the areas that need to be examined. For example, when using a biomechanical frame of reference, the clinician analyzes range of motion, type of muscle contraction, and strength required to complete the activity.[6] Using a developmental frame of reference, the clinician would analyze activities to determine how they might meet age-specific developmental goals.

Another approach to analysis of activities is an occupation-based approach.[10] The approach to activity analysis used for the purposes of this text is an occupation-based approach using the *OTPF* described in Chapter 9. The *OTPF* encourages the OT practitioner to look at activities in relationship to how they affect the whole person, not just one component.

The practitioner first determines the contexts in which the activity typically occurs and identifies what is needed to perform it (activity demands) including the physical space, tools, equipment, materials, time, cost required, and social demands. Social demands are also part of the context of the activity and include the rules of a game, number and expectations of other participants, and cultural expectations that may be associated with it.[2] Next, the practitioner breaks down the activity into the steps involved and describes any sequencing or timing requirements of the activity. For example, making a cake requires some attention to the sequence (e.g., mix the dry ingredients before adding the wet ones) and most certainly requires attention to how long the cake is baked. The practitioner then needs to analyze each step of the activity to determine the required actions, body functions, and body structures.[2]

Let's examine a simple task such as answering the door. To analyze the activity we need to think about the way that it is *typically* completed. Imagine that a woman is sitting in a chair and needs to respond to a caller who comes to the door. First, the woman hears the knock at the door. She identifies the specific door from which the sound is coming and determines where the door is located. The woman stands and walks to the door. She reaches out with her arm, while opening her hand, and grasps the doorknob. She turns the knob and pulls the door open. She sees the caller and says, "Hello." What performance skills are needed for the woman to complete this simple task? What body actions and body structures are necessary? She must have global and specific mental functions to be oriented, to recognize the sound of the knock as a signal that indicates the caller's arrival, and to have the level of arousal and ability to sequence the steps necessary to greet the caller; the sensory function of hearing so that she hears the sound of the knock and auditory perception to distinguish the door from which the sound is coming; vision and visual perception to see the door and a clear path to it; motor skills and body functions to rise out of the chair;

equilibrium and postural control to navigate across the room, and range of motion and strength in her upper extremity to turn the door knob and pull the door open. Furthermore, she needs communication and interaction skills to greet the caller appropriately and to manage the potential feelings. Maybe it is late at night, she is home alone, and she is afraid to answer the door, or perhaps she is expecting someone or something and is excited that they have arrived. Everyday activities like this require a number of steps and many complex components that most of us take for granted.

ACTIVITY SYNTHESIS

OT practitioners select activities to meet therapeutic goals. Therapeutic activity is used to assist the client in mastering a new skill, restoring a deficit, compensating for a functional disability, maintaining health, or preventing dysfunction.[3] Prescribing purposeful or occupation-based activity does not rest solely on the analysis of the activity. It also requires that the OT practitioner has completed an occupational profile and an occupational performance analysis of the client (see Chapter 12). The focus of the evaluation is on the functioning level of the client, and it involves identification of the person's deficits for which compensation must be found and the assets from which strength can be drawn. The OT practitioner uses what he or she knows about an activity through an activity analysis and compares it to the current performance of the client.[11] Having analyzed the activity and evaluated the client, the OT practitioner identifies gaps in performance and bridges those gaps by grading or adapting the activity or the environment in order to provide the "just right challenge" for the client. This is referred to as **activity synthesis.** An example of the use of activities to reach the client's occupational performance goals is shown in Box 15-1.

Grading involves changing the process, environment, tools, or materials of the activity to increase or decrease the performance demands of the client.[3] Grading an activity is used when the therapeutic goal is to improve or restore function and when the practitioner wants to challenge the client to a certain level. For example, if the practitioner thinks the client is not maximally challenged while sanding a piece of wood for a project, the sand paper can be changed to provide greater resistance, or the wood can be positioned on an incline. When the client is experiencing difficulty performing the activity, the OT practitioner may decrease the requirements. Perhaps on a particular day, the client is feeling tired as a result of having slept poorly the night before. He does not feel capable of completing his shaving routine while standing. The practitioner may decrease the requirements of the activity by allowing him to sit while shaving or by requiring him to shave only one side of his face while the practitioner shaves the other. The goal of the practitioner when determining how a specific activity will be graded is to find the "just right challenge" for the client. Table 15-2 summarizes the ways in which activities may be graded.

Adapting of the activity or the environment may allow the client to perform an activity at the highest possible level of function. "Adaptation is the process that changes an aspect of the activity or the environment to enable successful performance and accomplish a therapeutic goal."[3] Adaptation may involve modification of the environment and the use of assistive technologies or alternative strategies.[6,8,14]

Assistive devices range from *low-* to *high-technological devices.* Typically, devices that are considered low technology do not have electronic components. These devices, such as those designed for self-feeding (shown in Figure 15-3, *A*), have been a part of occupational therapy for many years. High-technological devices, however, were introduced

Box 15-1 Case Application of Activity Synthesis

Frances is a 72-year-old woman who lives with her daughter in a small ranch home in the country. Frances loves to garden and cook. She especially enjoys making cookies for her grandchildren. Frances was recently hospitalized with complications from her diabetes and heart condition. She has poor endurance now and exhibits some confusion. Frances works slowly. The OT practitioner, Leah, will be treating Frances daily while Frances remains in the rehabilitation unit.

Leah begins the evaluation by asking Frances what types of things she did prior to the hospitalization.

Prior Occupations: Frances enjoyed gardening and cooking (cookies for her grandchildren). Her daughter made the meals. Frances dressed and bathed herself. She helped with light housekeeping, but her daughter was primarily responsible for housework. Frances enjoyed conversation with family members and spending time watching TV, playing card games, and doing puzzles. Frances did not drive.

The daughter will be home for 3 weeks after her mother is discharged and is concerned that her mother will be bored if not able to garden or cook.

The OT decides to work on helping Frances return to cooking (cookies) and gardening. Furthermore, the OT will make sure Frances is able to perform self-care activities. The following activity analysis examines the factors involved in Frances' gardening.

Performance Pattern: During the summer months, Frances spends at least 1 hour a day caring for her flower garden. She waters the plants and weeds them.

Contexts:
- *Cultural.* Frances' mother enjoyed gardening and always had fresh flowers on the table. Frances has passed this on to her daughter. Frances likes to discuss flowers with other gardeners who share her love of this hobby.
- *Physical.* The garden is located in the country close to the house. The garden consists of many flower plants. It is situated on flat terrain with large flat slate providing the walking path. The garden is shaded by surrounding trees.
- *Social.* Frances enjoys gardening by herself, but also enjoys showing others (e.g., her neighbors and grandchildren) the beautiful flowers.
- *Personal.* Frances is a 72-year-old woman who enjoys showing others her garden and likes to be active.
- *Spiritual.* Frances gets inspiration and motivation from her garden.
- *Temporal.* Frances enjoys summer when she can be outside in her garden.

Performance skills:
- *Motor skills.* Frances must be able to walk outside on a smooth (slate rock) path (approximately 20 feet) and bend to pick up weeds. She must be able to carry a watering can and have enough strength to dig in the dirt as needed. She must be able to get up.
- *Process skills.* Frances must be aware of the differences between plants and weeds. She must realize when the plants need water and determine how to take care of the plants.
- *Communication/interaction skills.* Frances must be able to interact with others who stop by to see her flowers. She must request assistance as needed from her daughter.

Activity demands: Gardening requires working with plants, garden tools, and the environment. One must bend and reach, pull weeds, and carry garden tools. The gardener must first gather supplies, walk to the garden, and begin to care for the plants. One must identify plants from weeds and acknowledge when the job is completed.

Client factors: The OT has decided to focus on the neuromusculoskeletal and movement-related functions. Upon evaluation, the OT learned Frances has full range of motion throughout. Frances has difficulty maintaining her posture and fatigues quickly. She currently exhibits poor muscle strength in her arms, trunk, and legs. Endurance is limited to 20 minutes of seated

Continued

Box 15-1   Case Application of Activity Synthesis—cont'd

activity. Frances fatigues after walking 10 feet and walks with a wide-based unsteady gait. She is able to pick up objects with both hands, but shows limited hand strength. Eye-hand coordination is adequate for fine-motor tasks.

The OT practitioner may approach Frances' difficulties from many angles and design activities to meet her goal to return to gardening.

Using a biomechanical approach to address Frances' poor endurance, the OT works in the clinic on tabletop activities including making a flower collage by tearing out pictures and pasting them on the page. The OT practitioner engages in conversation with Frances about gardening. Once Frances is able to tolerate 30 minutes of seated activity, Leah will increase the demands by engaging Frances in an indoor gardening activity such as planting seeds in small pots or transplanting several plants. These activities can be graded so that Frances stands for the tasks as tolerated until her endurance is sufficient.

TABLE 15-2   Grading of Activity

Areas of Grading	Examples of Grading
Strength	Increase/decrease the repetitions
	Increase/decrease amount of resistance
Range of motion	Increase/decrease movement required
	Provide assistance in moving the extremity
Endurance and tolerance	Increase/decrease time on task
	Do activity sitting versus standing
Coordination	Decrease size of objects being manipulated
	Increase/decrease the number of objects being manipulated
	Change the texture or properties of the object
Perceptual Skills	Increase/decrease the time to complete skills
	Increase/decrease the object size (e.g., puzzle)
	Increase/decrease the complexity
	Increase/decrease the extraneous stimulation
Cognitive skills	Increase/decrease number of steps given in a task
	Provide more or less problem-solving to the task
	Require the client do more or less of the task without asking questions
	Increase/decrease the novelty of the task
	Increase/decrease the familiarity of materials and directions
Social skills	Move from an individual activity to a group activity
	Increase/decrease the behaviors expected
	Increase/decrease the familiarity with the social setting or people
	Increase/decrease the intensity of the conversation
	Increase/decrease the goal of the social event

to occupational therapy more recently and include those with electronic components. Examples of high-technological devices are augmentative communication equipment, electronic aids for daily living, and power wheelchairs. Figure 15-3, *B*, shows an example of an augmentative communication device. The use of devices to aid function is an integral part of the profession and can provide the necessary adaptations so that a client can achieve.

Training a client to perform an activity in an alternative way is another type of adaptation. OT practitioners educate clients daily on a host of topics, including strategies to improve function. For example, an OT practitioner may teach a client techniques for dressing or bathing with one hand after an injury. In some situations all that is needed is training in these types of strategies and the client can forgo the of assistive devices.

OT practitioners must also be alert to the need for modifications to a person's environment that could facilitate function. The primary environments (e.g., home, work, and school) in which an individual functions should be evaluated for accessibility. The OT practitioner evaluates the accessibility of the environment, makes recommenda-

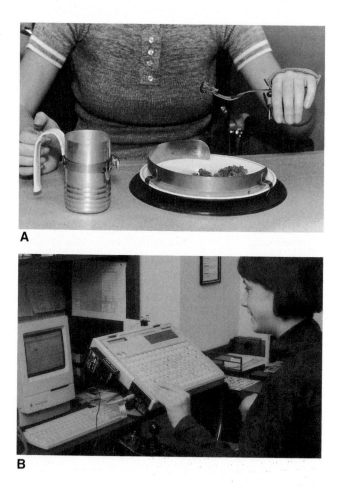

A

B

Figure 15-3 Low- and high-technology assistive devices. **A,** Self-feeding using several low-tech assistive devices to compensate for absent grasp: universal cuff, plate guard, nonskid mat, and clip-type cup holder. **B,** This individual uses her augmentative communication device to access the computer. *(A From Pedretti LW: Occupational Therapy: Practice Skills for Physical Dysfunction, ed 4, St. Louis, 1996, Mosby. B Courtesy Prentke Romich Company, Wooster, OH.)*

tions for modifications, and follows up to ensure that the recommended modifications have been properly made and are effectively used by the client. Examples of environmental modifications include the installation of ramps into buildings, installation of grab bars for bathroom safety, and arrangement of furniture in the home or at work.

The following examples illustrate the difference between grading and adapting.

Juan was involved in a motor vehicle accident resulting in a spinal cord injury. He has lost the ability to grasp objects. The OT practitioner realizes that this deficit cannot be overcome; however, Juan wants to be able to feed himself independently. The practitioner performs an activity analysis to be aware of the demands of self-feeding and realizes that the ability to perform hand grasp is needed to hold the utensil. Consequently, if Juan is to be independent in self-feeding, a way must be found around his inability to grasp by adapting the activity. To do this, the practitioner begins by having Juan try a utensil-holding appliance cuff (called a universal cuff), which slips on his hand, thus eliminating the need to grasp the fork or spoon (see Figure 15-3, *A*). Juan is able to eat using the device, although initially it is challenging for him. Juan and the OT practitioner decide that they can work together on a training program with this device to achieve the goal of self-feeding. Within a week, Juan is using the universal cuff at all of his meals to feed himself independently. This is an example of adapting the activity to compensate for lack of hand grasp.

In another treatment setting, the OT practitioner is working with Sandra, who has a mental illness. She is withdrawn and avoids social contact. The OT practitioner analyzes the available group activities to determine which may be best for the client. The practitioner uses clinical judgment and decides not to begin with a cooking group because it is a highly social activity. Instead, the practitioner chooses a craft activity that is simple, undemanding, and can be performed in an area of the room where Sandra can be among others but need not interact with them. As Sandra improves and becomes more comfortable with social interaction, the activity is graded to make it more challenging. Specifically, the OT practitioner begins by asking Sandra to work independently on a craft activity at the same table as other clients. Gradually, the OT practitioner increases the amount of interaction and sharing of supplies. The goal is that eventually Sandra will be able to participate in a group that is preparing a meal. The practitioner uses activity analysis to determine the demands of the activity, recalling Sandra's strengths (fine motor skills) and weaknesses (poor social interactions). To meet the goal, the OT practitioner grades the activity by selecting one with low social demands, gradually increasing the level of social contact until the client is able to relate to others without being threatened.

Every OT practitioner must be able to assess the demands of an activity at many levels, to integrate the information with knowledge of the client's needs and abilities to select appropriate activities, and to grade and adapt activities as needed.

SUMMARY

There is a wide range of therapeutic modalities used in occupational therapy to achieve the goals of the client—specifically, therapeutic use of self (Chapter 16), therapeutic use of activities and occupations, consultation (Chapter 9), and education (Chapter 9). OT practitioners educate clients daily on a host of issues. For example, the OT practitioner may teach a client how to dress or bath using one hand after an injury. Often, OT practitioners provide alternative techniques for performing occupations. Therapeutic use of activities and occupations includes the use of preparatory, purposeful, and occupation-based activity. Preparatory activities are used to prepare the client for purposeful activity or occupations and include sensory input, therapeutic exercise modalities, physical agent modalities, and splints. Purposeful activity has an inherent goal in addition to the therapeutic goal. Occupation-based activity includes the performance of activities of daily living, instrumental activities of daily living, work and school tasks, play or leisure tasks, and social participation by the client, and is the ultimate goal of occupational therapy intervention. Activity analysis is learned through practice and becomes second nature to the experienced OT practitioner. Activity synthesis includes knowing how to grade activities and when and how to provide adaptations and assistive technology.

Learning Activities

1. Select a simple activity, and identify all of the requirements for performance of the activity. Exchange lists with classmates, and identify any requirement omitted from the other's list.
2. Find and read an article on splinting (with picture or design) from *American Journal of Occupational Therapy* or another professional source. Report on the article to your class or to a small group of students from your class.
3. Gather available resources on assistive devices. This can be done two ways:
   a. In your community, research companies that provide assistive devices and study the types of equipment and services they provide.
   b. Select one particular category of assistive devices (e.g., feeding equipment, augmentative communication devices, power wheelchairs), and search the Internet for companies that produce or sell these devices. In a report, summarize the information that you find.
4. Critique the benefits of purposeful activity in occupational therapy.
5. Review the literature on the use of PAMs in occupational therapy.

Review Questions

1. Define and describe preparatory, purposeful, and occupation-based activity.
2. What is the difference between purposeful and occupation-based activity?
3. What is meant by grading and adapting activities?
4. What are the roles of the OT and OTA in splinting?
5. What are PAMs, and how are they used in occupational therapy?

REFERENCES

1. American Occupational Therapy Association: Physical agent modalities: a position paper, *Am J Occup Ther* 57:650-651, 2003.
2. American Occupational Therapy Association: Occupational therapy practice framework: domain and process, *Am J Occup Ther* 56(6):608-639, 2002.
3. American Occupational Therapy Association: Position paper: purposeful activity, *Am J Occup Ther* 47(12):1081, 1993.
4. Anderson KN (ed): *Mosby's Medical, Nursing, and Allied Health Dictionary,* ed 4, St. Louis, 1994, Mosby.
5. Belkin J, English CB: Hand splinting: principles, practice, and decision making. In Pedretti LW (ed): *Occupational Therapy: Practice Skills for Physical Dysfunction,* ed 4, St. Louis, 1996, Mosby.
6. Breines EB: Therapeutic occupations and modalities. In Pendleton HM, Schultz-Krohn W (eds): *Pedretti's Occupational Therapy Practice Skills for Physical Dysfunction,* ed 6, St. Louis, 2006, Mosby.
7. Centre for Cancer Education, University of Newcastle upon Tyne: On-line medical dictionary, 1998. Retrieved August 28, 2006, from http://cancerweb.ncl.ac.uk/cgibin/omd?query=orthotic&action=Search+OMD.
8. Crepeau EB, Cohn ES, Boyt Schell BA (eds): *Willard and Spackman's Occupational Therapy,* ed 10, Philadelphia, 2000, JB Lippincott Williams & Wilkins.
9. Dutton R: Guidelines for using both activity and exercise, *Am J Occup Ther* 43:573, 1989.
10. Fisher AG: Uniting practice and theory in an occupational framework, *Am J Occup Ther* 52(7):509-521, 1998.
11. Moyers P: Introduction to occupation-based practice. In Christiansen CH, Baum CM, Bass-Haugen J: *Occupational Therapy: Performance, Participation, and Well-Being,* ed 3, Thorofare, NJ, 2005, Slack Inc.
12. Reed KL: Tools of practice: heritage or baggage, *Am J Occup Ther* 40:597, 1986.
13. Thomas CL (ed): *Taber's Cyclopedic Medical Dictionary,* ed 18, Philadelphia, 1997, FA Davis.
14. Trombly CS, Radomski MV: *Occupational Therapy for Physical Dysfunction,* ed 5, Philadelphia, 2002, Lippincott Williams & Wilkins.
15. West WL, Wiemer RB: Should the representative assembly have voted as it did, when it did, on occupational therapists' use of physical agent modalities? *Am J Occup Ther* 45:1143, 1991.

There is a mystique in occupational therapy that is hard to put into words. When we treat a client and affect something relevant to that person, the magic of our profession comes to light. Whether we are splinting a finger injury, demonstrating an adapted key holder, or instructing in time management, what matters is that the interaction is meaningful to the client. We treat the entire person, not just the isolated injury or diagnosis printed on the referral form. We treat people's illness experiences, not just their illness. We probe clients' real-life needs and help them recover their abilities to participate in daily routines. We acknowledge the value of the "blissful ordinariness"[5] of a day and help clients return to it. We listen as they tell us about the mundane details of their lives that are disrupted by their injury or illness. We help find ways to return to these activities, and in doing so, we validate the importance of ordinary things in their lives. And when our treatment process is successful, patients return to their "blissful ordinariness" with greater awareness of its value. The mystique of occupational therapy is not easy to articulate. What looks so simple on the surface is actually very complex and powerful. Often, clients understand this intuitively. In these instances, words may not be needed.

Cynthia Cooper, MFA, MA, OTR/L, CHT
Director of Hand Therapy
NovaCare Rehabilitation
Phoenix, Arizona

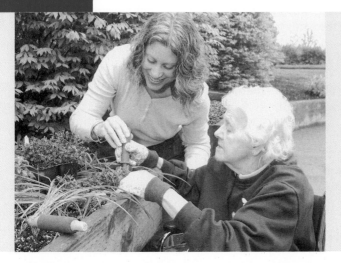

OBJECTIVES

After reading this chapter, the reader will be able to do the following:
- Explain the uniqueness of the therapeutic relationship
- Identify the stages of loss
- Describe how the "use of self" is used as one of the tools of therapy
- Understand the importance of self-awareness for effective therapeutic relationships
- Identify the three "selves" recognized in self-awareness
- Explain the skills needed for developing effective therapeutic relationships
- Demonstrate the necessary skills for "taking charge" of a group

KEY TERMS

Active listening
Clarification
Empathy
Group
Group dynamics

Ideal self
Nonverbal communication
Perceived self
Real self
Reflection

Restatement
Self-awareness
Therapeutic relationship
Therapeutic use of self
Universal stages of loss

People interact with one another on a daily basis without thinking much about it, but what is human interaction? At the simplest level of understanding, the term means an exchange among people—an interaction with one another. This exchange is complex because each person lives in two worlds—an outer world of objects, actions, and situations; and an inner world of thoughts, feelings, and desires. Each world affects and is affected by the other. In therapy, when the focus is on the person's outer world, technical skills are employed. When the focus is on the person's inner world, human interaction skills are used.

Human communication is complex, in and of itself, and the interaction between an occupational therapy (OT) practitioner and a client requires more than the skills used in everyday human interactions. The interaction between a practitioner and a client is the **therapeutic relationship,** in which the OT practitioner is responsible for facilitating the healing and rehabilitation process. The effective practitioner knows that the relationship established with each client is an important element of therapy. Regardless of the individual's cognitive, physical, or psychosocial deficits, the OT practitioner needs to have proficient communication skills to develop rapport with each person, ensuring that the client will actively participate in reaching his or her maximum potential.

PSYCHOLOGY OF REHABILITATION

From the beginning of one's study in the field of occupational therapy, the psychology of rehabilitation must be embraced. People who have suffered catastrophic trauma or illness have great emotional and physical needs. Usually, the physical needs receive attention from many areas of treatment, but the emotional needs are frequently overlooked. Because of the intent of the profession and the nature of treatment, OT practitioners are in a unique position to give attention to these needs. Historically, all occupational therapy literature emphasizes treating the whole person, and most treatment is individualized and personal, with close body contact and ongoing practitioner–client interaction.

In psychology classes, OT students will likely study the stages of death and dying, first identified by Elisabeth Kübler-Ross.[4] These **universal stages of loss** are recognized as *denial, anger, bargaining, depression,* and *acceptance.* The majority of clients in occupational therapy experience some or all of these stages. The OT practitioner's ability and willingness to recognize these stages will provide the client the opportunity to work through them.

Daniel Goleman's book *Emotional Intelligence* is a groundbreaking study of the critical role emotions play in a person's life. He states, "The design of the brain means we very often have little or no control over *when* we are swept by emotions, nor over *what* emotion it will be. But we can have some say in *how long* an emotion will last." He continues, "A universal trigger for anger is the sense of being endangered . . . not just an outright physical threat, but also, as is more often the case, by a symbolic threat to self-esteem or dignity." Therefore anger is so often a part of a client's experience, and so too is depression. "The sadness that loss brings has certain invariable effects: it closes down our interest in diversions and pleasures, fixes attention on what has been lost, and saps our energy for starting new endeavors."[3] The OT practitioner's sensitivity to the emotional impact of the stages of loss will make a significant difference between a merely adequate and a truly competent practitioner.

THERAPEUTIC RELATIONSHIP

It is in light of the psychology of rehabilitation that the importance of the therapeutic relationship is recognized. Although some aspects of therapeutic interaction may appear like a friendship, the relationship is, by design, distinctly different. Friendships are expected to be reciprocal; that is, each person contributes to and receives from the relationship in more or less equal measure. Each expects a balance of rewards and responsibilities. The therapeutic relationship, however, is unique because it is designed to benefit the one being served. The OT practitioner is fully aware that the purpose of the interaction is to meet the needs of the client. Yet, it is often true that the practitioner receives "reward," albeit not by intention or design.

In every therapy session, the OT practitioner is expected to be aware of the client's needs and, using technical and interaction skills, to select responses or courses of action that benefit the one being served. Although technical skills employed by the OT practitioner are important, his or her interaction skills in the therapeutic relationship often make the difference between a successful and an unsuccessful therapy experience. As with any other therapeutic tool, an OT practitioner must constantly assess interaction skills and make judgments about when to use what, and to what degree. Just as technical skills can become mechanical and rob therapy of its value and purpose, so too can a "professional personality" develop and rob a relationship of its usefulness and meaning.

In *Patient–Practitioner Interaction*, Davis states, "Superior skill in the technology of the profession must be balanced with the art of relating to those who request our services in such a way that healing is facilitated rather than interfered with." Davis' reference to "the art of relating" is also termed the **therapeutic use of self,** which entails being aware of oneself and of the client and being in command of what is communicated.[1]

Taylor (in press) has developed the Intentional Relationship Model, which systematically describes therapeutic use of self and the development of modes of interacting with clients for their benefit. The Intentional Relationship Model defines the six primary interpersonal modes (or styles) used in therapeutic relationships: advocating, collaborating, empathizing, encouraging, instructing, and problem-solving. Taylor postulates that the intentional relationship works best when therapists are aware of their modes of interacting and are able to shift modes as needed.[9] This model provides exercises to develop skill and awareness in therapeutic use of self.

The OT practitioner must be aware of what is said and what is not said and keep both in proper balance in order for the client–practitioner relationship to be truly useful. Early lists 10 qualities that must be developed by the practitioner, who employs therapeutic use of self as a tool. These are active listening, empathy, genuineness, immediacy, respect, self-disclosure, sensitivity, specificity, trust, and warmth.[2] These qualities are needed to establish and sustain a therapeutic relationship. Later in this chapter, these qualities are described in detail.

The context in which a therapeutic relationship takes place may be a one-on-one interaction or a group treatment setting. A **group** is defined as more than two people interacting with a common purpose. Occupational therapy treatment often occurs in groups, particularly in mental health settings. Other examples in which group treatment occurs are children's groups for diagnostic categories, geriatric groups, family support groups, and life-skill groups for the developmentally delayed. The establishment of a therapeutic relationship needs to be a consideration in both didactic (one-on-one) and group-treatment situations.

SELF-AWARENESS

Occupational therapy regards *therapeutic use of self* as an important element in therapy. Through the *use of self,* the OT practitioner consciously builds a relationship with the client to promote intervention goals and to pursue a higher level of client function. To facilitate another person's healing and to develop an effective therapeutic relationship, the OT practitioner must have **self-awareness.** Self-awareness is knowing one's own true nature; it is the ability to recognize one's own behavior, emotional responses, and effect on others. Throughout recorded history, some form of the admonition "Know thyself" can be found. All wisdom begins with self-knowledge.

Self-awareness may appear so obvious that one may expect it to happen automatically, often disregarding the fact that it takes effort. Of course, experience does yield some measure of self-awareness, just as some knowledge about trees comes from just having them around. However, when trees are the *focus* and are systematically studied, greater knowledge is gained. True knowledge requires disciplined pursuit of specific awareness.

People often have the mistaken fear that too much focus on oneself will foster egoism. Egoism is seeing all things only from one's own point of view, considering only one's own wants and needs in all circumstances and situations. Most people have been correctly taught that egoism is a character trait to avoid. Although an appropriate development stage of early childhood, egoism is inappropriate for mature adults. Self-awareness, however, is very different from egoism.

The contrast between egoism and self-awareness can be illustrated by the following simple example: A 3-year-old boy walks into a room of people watching television and stands in front of the screen without regard for the fact that he is blocking everyone's view. This behavior displays egoism. The child is aware only of what he wants. Conversely, self-awareness enables an adult to be conscious of the relative nature of self and others. Self-awareness causes an adult to look around, to become aware of blocking the view of others, and to adapt his or her behavior.

Self-awareness is essential for mature, healthy interaction, and it is often poorly developed because of the defenses erected to protect against unpleasant truths. To develop better self-awareness, consider the nature of the self.

Each person is composed of three selves: the ideal self, the perceived self, and the real self. Each is an aspect of the total self. The **ideal self** is what an individual would like to be if free of the demands of mundane reality. This aspect is the "perfect self," with only desirable qualities and with all wants and wishes fulfilled. The ideal self is an unrealistic goal, not an obtainable reality. The ideal self that resides in the inner world has access to all intention, feeling, and desire but remains little known to others. Each person feels the need to defend the ideal self (though perhaps subconsciously) when others do not acknowledge it.

The **perceived self** is the aspect that others see; it is what they perceive without the benefit of knowing a person's intentions, motivations, and limitations (i.e., as defined only by outward behavior). This perceived self is not the true self, however, because it comes from the perspective (and also the biases) of the one perceiving. The behavioral or perceived self exists in the outer world, and reports from others regarding the perceived self (comments on behavior) are often received as criticism. The reports are not in agreement with the ideal self's perceptions; consequently, there is denial of what others report as a person's behavior or his or her effect.

The **real self** is a blending of the internal and external worlds involving intention and action plus environmental awareness. The real self includes the feelings, strengths, and limitations of the person, as well as the reality in which the person exists (his or her environment). The inclusion of the perceived self, along with recognition of the limits of the ideal self, allows the emergence of the real self, which processes awareness and determines what behavioral adjustments are needed.

It is possible to be unaware of any or all of these aspects of self. Such a lack of awareness is the result of building defenses against unpleasant truths and denying that behavioral changes are needed. The results are distorted self-perceptions that are destructive to "real" relationships. When busy defending the ideal self and denying the perceived self, the real self is kept from emerging. The process of gaining self-awareness involves making an effort to realistically acknowledge shortcomings of both the internal and external worlds so a person can live from the real self. A self-aware person is able to distinguish among the three aspects and is able to realistically acknowledge his or her own shortcomings and limitations without self-condemnation.

Self-awareness is the process of opening up to the real self—the blend of all aspects. Individuals working on self-awareness examine both how they see themselves and how others see them. The self-aware individual can contrast the ideal self with the perceived self and know that he or she is, of necessity, different. There are many ways to develop self-awareness. Simply being aware of the multifaceted self is a step toward self-understanding. Keeping a journal—writing down feelings and reactions—is a rich source of self-knowledge. By being open to how he or she is seen by others, an individual can gain access to information and new perspectives. Participation in group interaction is another way to develop self-awareness because the central purpose of a group is to give and receive feedback about the perceived self.

When a person lives predominately in the real self, he or she is ready to reach out and help others find their real selves, balancing strengths and weaknesses to embrace their humanness realistically. Self-respect is gained by being aware of and making conscious choices about behavior and by accepting the range of emotional responses experienced in the unexpected turns of life—by living in reality. A person relates successfully to others in proportion to his or her self-knowledge. Developing self-awareness is a lifelong undertaking that will reap rich rewards in all relationships but especially in the therapeutic relationships encountered as an OT practitioner.

SKILLS FOR EFFECTIVE THERAPEUTIC RELATIONSHIPS

Sustaining the therapeutic relationship is a skill. Warmth, caring, and empathy must be balanced with analysis, judgment, and a demand for performance. When the OT practitioner is too detached, technical, or critical, his or her relationship with the client may be damaged by coldness and alienation. When the practitioner is too friendly and "chummy," the therapy may be clouded by a failure to use clinical judgment to select the most beneficial course of action.

In addition to self-awareness, there are a number of skills and qualities needed to establish and maintain therapeutic relationships. The most essential are the abilities to develop trust, demonstrate empathy, understand verbal and nonverbal communication, and use active listening.[1,2,10] The OT practitioner must also be skilled in leading a group.

DEVELOPING TRUST

Foremost to establishing a therapeutic relationship is the ability to develop the trust of the client, whose confidence in the OT practitioner is necessary for a therapeutic relationship to be effective. Trust and acceptance will facilitate the relationship and motivate the client to be interested in the therapy and treatment.

As a part of gaining an individual's trust, the OT practitioner must be genuine about who he or she is. Sincerity and honesty without pretense will facilitate the development of trust between the practitioner and client. Opening up to the client in treatment and disclosing personal information is beneficial. In the therapeutic relationship, the OT practitioner asks the client to divulge personal facts; the relationship can be strengthened if the practitioner also discloses some personal information to the client.[2] However, self-disclosure needs to be done with care and consideration; as always, the timing needs to be appropriate. Self-disclosure is most appropriate when the client asks for it; it should never be offered when the client is in the middle of a crisis or expressing thoughts.[2] The amount and type of information disclosed also need to be considered. It is not advisable, for example, for the OT practitioner to give his or her address or phone number to a client. Additionally, it is not appropriate for the practitioner to transfer all his or her problems and emotions onto the client. Disclosure of information by the therapist should be for the client's benefit not the therapist's.[2]

UNDERSTANDING VERBAL AND NONVERBAL COMMUNICATIONS

Not all communication is verbal, and effective interaction between the OT practitioner and client requires that the practitioner understand not only what is overtly communicated but also what the client expresses nonverbally. Frequently, thoughts and emotions are expressed through **nonverbal communication,** including facial expressions, eye contact, tone of voice, touch, and body language. The effective practitioner is sensitive to and watchful for nonverbal forms of communication.

In many instances, the client will verbally express one thought while communicating an entirely different message with facial expressions or body language. An example of this is the client, Mr. Bertrand, who is in therapy working to increase his shoulder range of motion after an injury. The OT practitioner is moving Mr. Bertrand's arm through its available range of motion and asks him if it hurts. Mr. Bertrand responds with a "no" answer to the OT practitioner, while expressing a nonverbal wincing of his face. The OT practitioner should not ignore the facial expression, which communicates that Mr. Bertrand is experiencing pain, and he or she needs to choose whether to confront the discrepancy between the client's verbal and nonverbal responses. This confrontation will depend on the nature of the relationship and the degree of trust.[8]

In some instances, the nature of the client's disability may make it difficult for him or her to verbally communicate or understand verbal communication. In these situations, both the OT practitioner and client rely on nonverbal forms of communication. Being attuned to the client's facial expressions and body language is extremely important.

The OT practitioner must also be aware of the nonverbal behavior that he or she uses. In therapeutic relationships, it is usually desirable for the OT practitioner to convey friendliness and interest. This can be demonstrated by nonverbal behaviors such as smiling, touching, leaning toward the client, and making eye contact. The OT practitioner needs to use body language carefully, however, and match it to the particular needs of the client.[2] Obviously, it is not appropriate to smile when the individual is sharing feelings of how life has changed for the worse. Touching the person may also indicate that the practitioner cares and is there to help. However, some people may be uncomfortable being touched.[2] Different cultures, societies, and age groups vary in terms of the boundaries they have for being touched. In addition, individuals with central nervous system dysfunction may not tolerate being touched. The OT practitioner needs to be alert and sensitive to these possibilities and respect each person's individual differences regarding touch.

DEVELOPING EMPATHY

Empathy toward the client is another quality that needs to be developed. In the therapeutic relationship, empathy is the ability of the OT practitioner to place himself or herself in the client's position and understand what he or she is experiencing. Empathy is not to be confused with pity or identification. To express pity for the client is to feel sympathy with condescension. Pity is demeaning to the individual and conveys the attitude the practitioner is better than the client. Equally as undesirable is identification with the client, which means the OT practitioner feels at one with him or her and, as a result, loses sight of the differences. In identifying with a client, the practitioner may forget that the individual has different values and feelings; the values and needs of the practitioner may become confused with those of the client in such a way that they become less important to the therapy process.[1]

Empathy toward another individual does not mean that therapeutic objectivity is lost.[1] When empathetic, the practitioner understands and is sensitive to the thoughts, feelings, and experiences of the client without losing objectivity. Empathy is important to the development of trust in the therapeutic relationship because the client who sees that the OT practitioner empathizes with his or her experience is more willing to communicate and participate in treatment.[2]

USING ACTIVE LISTENING

A critical skill for maintaining an effective therapeutic relationship is **active listening.** The practitioner actively listens to the client without making judgments, jumping in with advice, or providing defensive replies. With active listening, the receiver paraphrases the speaker's words to ensure that he or she understands the intended meaning. Active listening should not only be used with the client, but also in the practitioner's interactions with family and friends. Caution must be taken, however, against allowing active listening to become no more than a repetition of the client's words (also known as "parroting").

Davis[1] describes active listening as having three processes: restatement, reflection, and clarification. Using **restatement** in the therapeutic relationship, the receiver of the message (the practitioner) repeats the words of the speaker (the client) as they are heard. To illustrate restatement, the client says, "I am angry that I had this stroke. I just retired, and my wife and I planned to travel and see the world." A restatement would be, "You are angry because your stroke may prevent you from traveling with your wife?" Restatement is used only in the initial phases of active listening; its primary purpose is to encourage the person to continue talking.[1]

Reflection is a response wherein the purpose is to "express in words the feelings and attitudes sensed behind the words of the sender."[1] Using reflection in the therapeutic relationship, the OT practitioner verbalizes both the content *and* the feelings that are implied by the client. An example of the use of reflection is the client saying, "I've been trying to dress myself for weeks now; I just can't do it." A reply from the practitioner may be, "You're frustrated and feeling defeated because you can't dress yourself?" Using reflection, the OT practitioner demonstrates to the client that he or she is hearing the emotions behind the words, not just the words.[1] If the practitioner has not correctly identified the emotions, reflection is posed as a question, which gives the client an opportunity to clarify what he or she is really feeling.

During **clarification** in the therapeutic relationship, the client's thoughts and feelings are summarized or simplified.[1] For example, the client may say, "When my doctor referred me to occupational therapy, I thought you would be the person who would help me get the use of my arm back. I've been coming to therapy for weeks now, and I still don't have full functioning in my arm. What am I supposed to do? Will I ever be able to use my hand again?" Clarification may sound something like, "When you came to occupational therapy, you expected to immediately get the function back in your arm. Now you realize that the return of arm and hand function is going to take longer than expected and is more than a matter of someone just fixing it?" Clarification is used when the OT practitioner wants to help the client look closer at the thoughts and feelings experienced.

All of these active listening skills can be acquired with practice. The practitioner starts by using restatement, reflection, and clarification in his or her interactions with the client's family and friends. Recording statements made by family and friends, as well as the appropriate responses, is also helpful.

GROUP LEADERSHIP SKILLS

Another skill to consider is group leadership. Because group treatment is one technique of the profession, the OT student must expect to study group dynamics—how groups interact and function.

In the 1960s and 1970s, groups became a popular phenomenon. There were therapy groups, training groups, sensitivity groups, and encounter groups. This widespread interest led to critical examination of the group process. People have always gathered in groups, but the idea of analyzing the different elements of groups and using them as a treatment or learning approach is a contemporary discovery. As people interact in groups around shared concerns, patterns of behavior emerge. The awareness and understanding of these patterns allow the OT practitioner to guide and direct the interactions in positive, goal-oriented directions.

Task groups in occupational therapy can be generally categorized as therapeutic groups, peer support groups, focus groups, and consultation and supervision groups.[7] Table 16-1 describes these small task groups. Most occupational therapy groups are therapeutic groups that involve structure, activity, and goals for client change. Common group activities include cooking, arts and crafts, exercise, activities of daily living, and reality orientation. The goals of the group and the techniques used depend, in large part, on the setting (inpatient or outpatient) in which the group meets. Other variables to consider include the size and composition of the group, client population, the frame of reference, and the duration and frequency of the group meetings.[7]

Some people are natural group leaders, yet group leadership is a skill that can also be learned. Group leadership involves incorporating the principles of the therapeutic use of self, as well as developing an awareness of group dynamics. **Group dynamics** refers to "the interacting forces within a small human group; the sociological study of these forces."[6] Group leadership skills can be acquired only through involvement and practice; awareness of the basic structures and processes provides the starting point for understanding the experience.

Studying group processes requires becoming a group participant and examining all aspects of the process. The "doing" and "understanding" are different. This study calls for

TABLE 16-1 Types of Small Task Groups Used in Occupational Therapy

Type of Group	Description
Therapeutic groups	Primary aim of group is individual change; OT practitioner uses therapeutic tasks that are designed to restore or develop functioning in occupational performance areas and client factors; other purposes may include prevention and support of existing strengths. Group size is typically 6 to 10 individuals.
Peer support groups	Primary purpose is to provide support for individuals who have a diagnosis, medically related problem, or disability in common; group may also involve the partners, families, and caregivers of the individuals; involvement of the OT practitioner varies from active involvement as leader to consultative role as facilitator. Group size can be large or small, depending upon the format.
Focus groups	Objective of these small groups is to find out about the attitudes and opinions of the members; gaining popularity in occupational therapy as a means of investigating a theme to generate research hypotheses or organizing a discussion around a specific topic.
Consultation and supervision groups	Use of group format for peer support, consultation, and supervision of OTAs, aides, and caregivers; seen as an increasing need as large occupational therapy departments diminish and more practitioners work independently in private and community-based practices.

Adapted from Schwartzberg SL: Group process. In Crepeau EB, Cohen ES, and Schell BAB (eds): *Willard and Spackman's Occupational Therapy*, ed 10, Philadelphia, 2003, Lippincott Williams & Wilkins.
OTA, Occupational therapy assistant.

examination of the skills needed by both leaders and group members. Leaders need to know how to exhibit leadership, convey knowledge about groups to group members, carry out organizational tasks, structure sessions, and guide members' performance. As group members, participants must be aware of task assignments (the specific responsibilities of the individuals), the importance of active listening, and the various roles that members assume as they interact in different ways.

The group leader needs to effectively take charge because when a group lacks confidence in the leader's ability to lead, confusion often results. If an individual sounds and looks as if he or she is in charge, confidence will be communicated to group members, and they will support the activity. Assuming a leadership role is not becoming a dictator, but it means appearing confident and clearly structuring the process so people know what is expected of them. As group interaction progresses, leadership can and does shift within the group— as part of the dynamics—but the OT practitioner is ultimately responsible for the form and structure. A group's success is highly dependent on early and clear leadership.

Box 16-1 provides guidelines for exercising leadership in the earliest stages of group formation and task identification. It is important to be aware of these points before entering a formal course on group dynamics; they will be useful in any situation of leadership. (See Learning Activities, question 5, for ways to practice the skill.)

Box 16-1 Taking Charge of a Group

1. Plan and practice or rehearse the activity to know what is needed.
2. Anticipate! Think how people might interpret the instructions.
3. Carry a written list of all the points to remember.
4. Stand to address the group.
5. Get everyone's attention before talking (expect it, and it will happen).
6. Regulate voice appropriately (loud and clear, as needed).
7. Tell in sequence. Keep words to a minimum, and demonstrate "first," "next," and so on.
8. Tell the group what to do when the task is complete.
9. Indicate the end of instructions and the beginning of the activity.

APPLICATION OF THERAPEUTIC USE OF SELF TO OCCUPATIONAL THERAPY

To illustrate how the therapeutic use of self is applied in occupational therapy, several examples are presented.

Jack is an OT practitioner in a public school setting who has a personality that can be described as moderately cheerful and easygoing. Although his approach serves many children, successful interaction with the following two clients requires a style change.

Amanda is an overly indulged, whining child who acts out her feelings. As Jack works with Amanda—if he is truly conscious of the use of self as a therapeutic tool and of the importance of building a therapeutic relationship—he quickly realizes that his usual easygoing, cheerful manner may be detrimental to therapy, especially because the child sees him as a "pushover" for her manipulative behavior. He elects to employ a stern, almost detached, no-nonsense approach. His plan for Amanda involves clearly defined expectations with rewards and consequences spelled out.

The first time the child "tests" him with a tantrum, he calmly allows the behavior to run its course and then unemotionally repeats his expectations of her. By using this approach, Jack convinces the child that he means what he says and is not going to be influenced by her manipulations. Once this relationship is established, he gradually relaxes and resumes his usual approach yet remains prepared to return to the no-nonsense approach if needed.

Nicole is a child who is fearful, shy, and compliant. As Jack works with Nicole, he again considers the child's personality and assesses her needs. He concludes that the client does not require the no-nonsense approach; she needs to have fun and exercise choice-making. Jack approaches therapy with a "have-fun-and-be-silly" playtime attitude. Each time there is a media change, he presents her with several alternatives and expects her to choose. He allows her to share in planning when appropriate and listens to her concerns.

These two examples illustrate how a practitioner effectively works one-on-one, builds therapeutic relationships, and uses interaction as a tool to promote better function. Whether a practitioner works one-on-one or in a group, with children or adults, the same principles apply. The effective OT practitioner builds the relationship on the uniqueness of the client, applying the therapeutic use of self according to client needs.

Additional examples are examined that involve a second OT practitioner working with adults.

The OT practitioner, Jennifer, is intent, serious, and competent; she makes good technical treatment choices, and usually her approach is matter-of-fact and informative.

The client, Mr. Butler, is 40 years of age and talks constantly, but his monologues have little content. He agrees to his therapy plans, but never quite finishes the activities; he appears to be lazy and unmotivated.

Mr. Butler has had several OT practitioners and has developed a reputation for being difficult. The practitioner has studied the client ahead of time to determine the best therapeutic relationship. She realizes that her normal approach—direct, informative, and matter-of-fact—may not be effective; as a result, she decides on another approach. She schedules 1-hour, one-on-one sessions in an individual treatment room, rather than the usual half-hour time blocks. During this hour, she also schedules other clients to overlap each end of the hour, leaving him as her "only" client for approximately 10 minutes, 20 minutes into the hour.

Jennifer meets with him, speaks in a friendly manner, and explains that she is aware that he works slowly and has allowed more time for treatment—but she must schedule others at the same time. She writes a checklist for his activities and informs him that she will regularly look in on him. Jennifer explains that although his schedule allows 1 hour, he can leave when the planned activities are completed. Because he is alone in the small treatment room, there is no one with whom he can talk.

As the treatment plan is implemented, Jennifer regularly checks the client. After 20 minutes, she remains with him only when he has completed most of the activities, in which case she uses the remaining 10 minutes (of the usual half-hour session) to pleasantly talk about nontherapeutic things.

Mr. Viejo is a young adult who is sullen and angry. He was in an automobile accident that has left him in a wheelchair. In therapy, he either refuses to cooperate or deliberately sabotages treatment plans. Jennifer's approach to Mr. Viejo is entirely different. When he comes for treatment, she schedules no other clients. She designs a step-by-step plan, explains it in detail (identifying its purpose and goals) but exerts no pressure on him to accept the plan or engage in the activities. She says she will spend time with him each day, regardless of whether he engages in therapy. She reads articles about his condition and sometimes shares the material with him. She encourages him to talk about what he is experiencing inside and is careful NOT to say she understands how he feels. Instead, Jennifer asks the client to describe what it is like to have his life changed so drastically, using active listening techniques to restate, reflect, and clarify what he says. She also asks him what he would like to accomplish in therapy and agrees to revise the plan to include his goals for treatment.

In each case, the OT practitioner considers the needs of the client. Mr. Butler sabotages his own program by passive resistance—he agrees to work but wastes therapy time with no evidence of inner conflicts, only an unwillingness to accept responsibility for his program. Through effective planning and scheduling, the OT practitioner removes the opportunity for the client to waste therapy time. She extends the treatment time to facilitate the expectation that he will complete the activities and rewards his efforts by chatting in the manner he enjoys when he does so.

Mr. Viejo is actively resistant to therapy and has not sufficiently dealt with the denial and anger of becoming paralyzed at a young age. In response, the OT practitioner gives the client her full attention—making no demands. She explains the treatment plan and makes it clear that she is ready to work when the client is ready. She also encourages him to share his therapy goals so they can be included in the plan. In sharing reading materials on his condition, she signals a willingness to discuss any aspect of the trauma the client desires. The client believes he has lost control of his life; therefore, the OT practitioner does not take more of his sense of control by forcing him into therapy for which he is not ready. She accepts his hostility and anger by simply being there. She is aware that often a person needs the patience of another who is willing to wait and listen.

SUMMARY

Important in therapy is the interaction between the client and OT practitioner—the therapeutic relationship. The effective practitioner is prepared to engage high quality interaction skills by developing self-awareness. This awareness, called the therapeutic use of self, enables the OT practitioner to adapt his or her manner of relating to result in the greatest benefit to the client. To the OT practitioner, the use of the self is as important in the therapy process as technical skills and knowledge. In addition to self-awareness, several other skills are needed by the OT practitioner to sustain an effective therapeutic relationship. These skills include understanding verbal and nonverbal communication, developing empathy and trust, practicing active listening, and leading a group treatment session. The clients in occupational therapy come from different backgrounds and have different needs; consequently, the OT practitioner must learn how to adapt his or her approach to each individual.

Occupational therapy is an individual and personal form of treatment that focuses on the whole person. The OT practitioner's use of self creates a therapeutic relationship—an atmosphere supportive of improving the client's overall functioning.

Learning Activities

1. Make a list of desirable qualities for use in therapeutic relationships. Seek out a written description for each quality. Write a one- or two-sentence description for each, and make a self-rating scale.
2. Working with a partner, agree to monitor each other's communication (verbal and nonverbal) in a specific situation (i.e., class discussion, visit to a clinic, at lunch table). Each person is to keep a "personal reaction log" on the events and a "report log" of the other's behavior. At the end of the monitored time, share the logs and compare the personal reactions against the reported behavior.
3. If a videotape library is available, watch videotapes of people with impairments, disabilities, or problem behaviors. Write a description of the therapeutic relationship you would develop in each case, should that person become your client. Include a rationale for your choice of therapeutic relationship.
4. Select a partner. Each person is to write four to five verbal messages that a client may say to an OT practitioner. Switch your messages with those of your partner. On a separate piece of paper, each person is to write an appropriate active listening response to each message. When finished, ask your partner to read his or her messages one at a time as you give your response. Share feedback to the responses with each other (i.e., How did it feel getting the response from your partner? Did the response demonstrate active listening?).

5. Practice taking charge of a group. The object is to "own" the activity and demonstrate leadership. This can be accomplished in small groups of six to ten in the following manner:
   - On slips of paper equal in number to the people, write simple activities (e.g., write a word on the board, form a line and walk around the desk, etc.).
   - Each member should draw one slip and not let the others know the content.
   - Given planning time, each member then leads the group in the identified activity.
   - After the activity, provide written feedback about leadership qualities displayed.

Review Questions

1. What are the characteristics of a therapeutic relationship?
2. What are Kübler-Ross' stages of loss?
3. Provide an example of how "use of self" is a tool of therapy.
4. Describe what is meant by the ideal self, the perceived self, and the real self.
5. How can an OT practitioner develop trust with a client?
6. What is empathy, and how can it be developed?

REFERENCES

1. Davis CM: *Patient–Practitioner Interaction: An Experiential Manual for Developing the Art of Health Care,* ed 3, Thorofare, NJ, 1998, Slack.
2. Early MB: *Mental Health Concepts and Techniques for the Occupational Therapy Assistant,* ed 3, Philadelphia, 2000, Lippincott Williams & Wilkins.
3. Goleman D: *Emotional Intelligence,* New York, 1995, Bantam Books.
4. Kübler-Ross E: *On Death and Dying,* New York, 1969, Macmillan.
5. McEwan I: *The Innocent,* New York, 1990, Doubleday.
6. Mish F (ed): *Merriam-Webster's Collegiate Dictionary®,* ed 11, Springfield, MA, 2004, Merriam-Webster.
7. Schwartzberg SL: Group process. In Crepeau EB, Cohen ES, and Schell BAB (eds): *Willard and Spackman's Occupational Therapy,* ed 10, Philadelphia, 2003, Lippincott Williams & Wilkins.
8. Schwartzberg SL: Therapeutic use of self. In Hopkins HL, Smith HD (eds): *Willard and Spackman's Occupational Therapy,* ed 8, Philadelphia, 1993, JB Lippincott.
9. Taylor RR: *The Intentional Relationship: Use of Self and Occupational Therapy,* Philadelphia, in press, FA Davis.
10. Tufano R: Therapeutic communication. In Sladyk K (ed): *OT Student Primer: A Guide to College Success,* Thorofare, NJ, 1997, Slack.

I found out about occupational therapy when I was 13 years of age, and it immediately appealed to me. I learned that occupational therapy helps people perform activities that make life worth living—cooking a good dinner, eating food, playing a game with friends, or completing a project. What could be more important? I was right; occupational therapy is about the power of engagement in occupations. It is one of the best-kept secrets of our American health care system. Over the years, I have found working directly with clients tremendously rewarding—and challenging—but it is also extremely gratifying to plan programs, educate student therapists, and conduct research. I have been an occupational therapy practitioner for 31 years; at this stage in my career, I find that I help shape the future of the profession by contributing to our knowledge base through research, a particularly rewarding and fun part of being a practitioner. I keep coming back to the insight I had when I was 13 years of age—occupations have a powerful influence on who we are as individuals and who we will become as we grow older. What could be more fascinating than exploring how occupation works? What could be more exciting than working with a group of people who share the commitment to understand occupation and how it can be used to help people lead healthy, fulfilling lives?

L. Diane Parham, PhD, OTR, FAOTA
Associate Professor
Occupational Science and Occupational Therapy
University of Southern California
Los Angeles, California

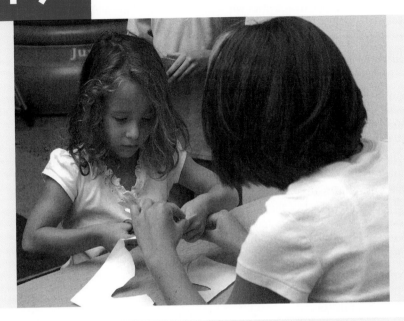

OBJECTIVES

After reading this chapter, the reader will be able to do the following:

- Explain the nature of clinical reasoning
- Understand the three elements of clinical reasoning
- Describe the thought processes and strategies of clinical reasoning that are used by occupational therapy (OT) practitioners
- Compare the clinical reasoning skills of the novice with those of the expert
- Identify ways the OT practitioner can develop clinical reasoning skills

KEY TERMS

Advanced beginner
Artistic element
Clinical reasoning
Competent practitioner
Conditional reasoning

Ethical element
Expert
Interactive reasoning
Narrative reasoning
Novice

Pragmatic reasoning
Procedural reasoning
Proficient practitioner
Scientific element

Juan is a 2-year old boy with developmental delays. Corinne, the occupational therapist (OT), is scheduled to see him for an evaluation and intervention planning session. What does she know about this child's diagnosis? What are his strengths and weaknesses? How will she determine the type of therapy he needs? How will she pick a frame of reference? What type of activities will be most useful? How will she measure his success? What issues is the family experiencing? Will she relate to the family? Will they be able to trust her and follow through with her suggestions? How will she organize the information?

There are many questions to contemplate when working with a client. Figuring out how to address client issues and intervene requires **clinical reasoning,** which is the thought process that therapists use to design and carry out intervention. It involves complex cognitive and affective skills; that is, it involves both thinking and feeling. Knowledge of clinical reasoning helps therapists become better practitioners who better serve their clients. All OT practitioners use clinical reasoning throughout each step of the occupational therapy process.

OT practitioners use clinical reasoning to make decisions about intervention.[6] Consumers and employers search for practice that is based upon evidence (i.e., supported through research). Because OT practitioners may have to critically analyze research, make decisions regarding services, and work with individual clients, evidence-based practice requires clinical reasoning, a foundational skill for practitioners. This chapter provides an overview of the clinical reasoning process.

ELEMENTS OF CLINICAL REASONING

Clinical reasoning is a complex, multifaceted process. Rogers characterizes three elements of clinical reasoning: the scientific, the ethical, and the artistic.[6] There is no particular order in which these elements are applied by the OT practitioner. The **scientific element** addresses the question, "What are the possible things that can be done for this client?" The answer to this question is found in the evaluation and assessment procedures used to determine strengths and weaknesses of the client, the writing of a plan to guide and direct the change process, and the selection of therapeutic modalities that result in successful occupational performance outcomes. The scientific element demands careful and accurate assessments, analysis, and recording.

Aiko is a 7-year old girl diagnosed with Williams' syndrome. Marie, the OT working in the school system, investigates this syndrome and reviews literature on the issues these children face. She decides that she needs to evaluate Aiko's muscle tone, musculoskeletal functions, endurance, visual-motor integration skills, and fine motor abilities, and she believes that she will be able to work with Aiko on improving her ability to function in the classroom by providing modifications.

By determining the child's strengths and weaknesses in light of the medical condition, the OT in this example used scientific reasoning to plan the child's intervention. Frequently, clinicians start the clinical reasoning process using scientific reasoning because this type of reasoning allows the clinician to gather all the facts prior to determining the plan.

The **ethical element** poses the question, "What *should* be done for this client?" The answer must take into account the client's perspective and his or her goals for intervention. Each individual has different views on what is health, what is important in life, and how things are accomplished. When the OT practitioner understands and respects the client's perspective, an intervention plan that preserves the client's values can be developed.[6] It is the OT practitioner's responsibility to supply information to the client so that he or she can participate in making decisions regarding intervention goals and methods. The OT practitioner considers all the scientific information, but ultimately, the decision of what should be done is an ethical one based on the individual's particular needs, goals, culture, environment, and lifestyle.[6]

> Mark, a 79-year-old man, wants to return home after his cerebral vascular accident (stroke). The team does not feel this would be the best solution for him because he has limited access to others. Mark refuses to discuss options related to living elsewhere. The OT practitioner conducts a home evaluation and reports on safety issues that may prevent him from returning home. The OT practitioner provides a list of suggestions so the team may explore other options. The OT practitioner must decide whether to support Mark's choice to return home. The OT discusses her role with the client and explains that she will try to support his choice if at all possible.

This example illustrates one of many ethical dilemmas OT practitioners may face. In this case, the clinician uses clinical reasoning to investigate all areas that might interfere with Mark's living alone. This information can help the team develop alternative ethical solutions. Ethically, she is contributing to the desires of the client without letting the team down.

The **artistic element** of clinical reasoning is evident in the skill used by the OT practitioner when he or she guides the treatment process and selects the "right action" in the face of uncertainties inherent in the clinical process.[6] The therapeutic process involves integrating and blending many separate components—the deficiencies to be addressed, the client's interests and wishes, the medium or activity to be used, and the interpersonal climate that is to support the therapy process. The therapeutic relationship and the way in which the OT practitioner interacts with the client play a major role in the artistic element. The therapeutic process is indeed an art, for there is no pre-existing formula for success. To the student and entry-level practitioner, the artistic element may seem the most difficult to grasp and pursue.

> Missy (the occupational therapy assistant [OTA]) jokes in therapy with Brian, a 77-year-old veteran who has had his right leg amputated just below the knee. Brian does not want to come to occupational therapy today, and Missy looks him gently in the eyes, smiles, and kids, "Brian, you say that every day. Come on, let's go." Missy does not take no from him, and Brian smiles as he follows her to therapy.

Missy has developed a rapport with Brian, and the art of this interaction is evident as Missy reads Brian's words as kidding. Missy knows she has connected with Brian and can afford to joke with him. This same scenario may be interpreted as refusal for therapy and handled differently for another client. The art of therapy is reading the client's cues within the context of the setting and the client–therapist relationship. Artistic reasoning requires skill in the therapeutic relationship, reflection, and self-awareness (see Chapter 16).

THOUGHT PROCESS DURING CLINICAL REASONING

Clinical reasoning is a cognitive thought process in which many diverse bits of information are gathered together (evaluation), many outside factors are considered (e.g., life space, prognosis, and desires), the demands of activities are analyzed (activity analysis), time investment choices are made (plan), and a progressive approach in terms of identifiable goals is organized (intervention). The clinical reasoning used throughout the therapy process requires the analysis of data, the use of specific knowledge bases, and the synthesis of awareness. The OT practitioner must actively think and process information, not just remember something once learned. The process demands the use of critical thinking—the ability to think independently.

Rogers and Holm[7] describe an information-processing view of cognition that is used during the occupational therapy evaluation to form an occupational therapy intervention plan. During the different steps in the approach, the OT practitioner's mind works with specific processing capabilities to gather, organize, analyze, and synthesize information.[7] Box 17-1 summarizes these steps.

In the first step, the OT practitioner forms a *preassessment image* of the client, an outline that will be used for further assessment of the client. To form this image, the OT practitioner gathers initial information. Two important factors that the practitioner will consider are the diagnosis and the age of the client. The OT practitioner asks himself or herself, "What am I going to consider in regard to this client?" "What do I know about this condition (in general and how it affects this person)?" Another important factor to consider is the client's life roles and functional status before he or she was referred to occupational therapy. All of this information about the client is linked to the practitioner's model of practice and frame of reference to construct the preassessment image.

Using the preassessment image, the OT practitioner begins the *cue acquisition* step. This second step involves gathering the data regarding the client's functional status and occupational roles. Although the practitioner may not choose to use all data, the data used are called *cues*.

After cue acquisition, the practitioner proceeds to the third step, *hypothesis generation*. With this step, the practitioner organizes the data that have been gathered and makes tentative assumptions, which will serve as the basis for therapeutic action.

Box 17-1　Steps in the Thought Process of Clinical Reasoning

1. *Formation of preassessment image:* Practitioner gathers initial information regarding the client, including information on diagnosis, age, and prior level of function. The practitioner asks, "What am I going to consider in regard to this client?" "What do I know about this condition (in general and how it affects this person)?"
2. *Cue acquisition:* Practitioner gathers the data regarding the client's functional status and occupational roles.
3. *Hypothesis generation:* Practitioner organizes the data that have been gathered and makes tentative assumptions, which will serve as the basis for therapeutic action.
4. *Cue interpretation:* Practitioner gathers further cues and continues the search for data. Each cue is compared with the hypothesis being considered to determine relevancy. The practitioner interprets whether the cue confirms the hypothesis, does not confirm the hypothesis, or does not contribute in either way to the hypothesis.
5. *Hypothesis evaluation:* Practitioner examines the data that have been collected and weighs the evidence for and against each of the diagnostic hypotheses. The hypothesis with the most supporting evidence is selected and forms the basis for intervention.

In evaluating a female client's ability to feed herself, the OT practitioner notices that the client is having difficulty and does not eat all of the food on her plate (cues). The practitioner's hypothesis in this situation is that the difficulty is the result of a left-sided neglect caused by the client's stroke. There can be one or more hypotheses; the practitioner can also surmise that the client's difficulty is due to the fact that she must use her nondominant hand to feed herself, which makes it hard to get the food on the utensil and tires her out easily.

The process continues with step four, *cue interpretation*. Further cues are gathered as the practitioner continues the search for data. Each cue is compared with the hypothesis being considered to determine if there is relevancy. The practitioner interprets whether the cue confirms the hypothesis, does not confirm the hypothesis, or does not contribute in either way to the hypothesis.[6]

Eventually, the OT practitioner completes the initial collection phase and begins the fifth step, an examination of the data that has been collected. Rogers and Holm[7] refer to this as the *hypothesis evaluation* step. The practitioner weighs the evidence for and against each of the diagnostic hypotheses. The hypothesis with the most supporting evidence is selected, and it forms the basis for intervention.

The outcome of this process is an occupational therapy diagnosis that describes the occupational performance deficits of the client. The diagnosis also provides information on the likely cause of the deficit, the signs and symptoms that led the practitioner to the diagnosis, and the pathological condition that caused the deficit.[7] Through this thought process, the OT practitioner has gone from sensing that there is a problem to defining the problem.

The clinical reasoning thought processes is also used to determine what intervention options are available. The OT practitioner asks, "What approaches will be most effective in this situation, and how long might it take for them to achieve the desired results?" Each time an OT practitioner treats a client, he or she searches long-term memory to retrieve scientific knowledge and practical experience that relate to the situation of the current client.[6] The practitioner may change the approach if its similarity to the current situation is minimal or if the outcome was not totally successful. The practitioner may compare a number of intervention situations to determine the most suitable approach for the current client.

The actual therapy session represents many levels of analysis and synthesis. The results of the intervention are closely monitored and evaluated by the practitioner to determine whether the modalities that were selected achieved the intended goal(s). The practitioner continues to process his or her knowledge about the disorder, a holistic view of the client, his or her skill and ability as the practitioner, and the modalities to be used to facilitate change and enhance the client's occupational performance. It is important that the OT practitioner collaborate with the client throughout the process to confirm that therapy is proceeding on a track that is meaningful to the client.

CLINICAL REASONING STRATEGIES

Therapists who understand and employ a range of clinical reasoning strategies are able to adapt their interventions to meet individual clients' needs. Several types of clinical reasoning strategies are described in Table 17-1.

Research conducted by Mattingly and Fleming discovered that OT practitioners used three distinct strategies, or tracks, for clinical reasoning[2,4]: the procedural, the interactive,

TABLE 17-1   Strategies Used by Occupational Therapy Practitioners in Clinical Reasoning

Strategy	Description
Procedural reasoning	Strategy used by the OT practitioner to focus on the client's disease or disability and determine what will be the most appropriate modalities to use to improve the client's functional performance. Central tasks include problem identification, goal setting, and treatment planning.
Interactive reasoning	Strategy used by the OT practitioner when he or she wants to understand the client as a person; takes place during face-to-face interactions between the practitioner and the client.
Conditional reasoning	Involves consideration by the practitioner of the client's condition as a whole, including the disease or disability and what it means to the person, the physical context and the social context; consideration of how the client's condition may change, depending upon level of participation in treatment.
Narrative reasoning	Use of storytelling wherein practitioners tell "stories" about clients to each other. Use of story creation, wherein the practitioner envisions how the future may be for the client so that he or she may guide the intervention process.
Pragmatic reasoning	The practitioner takes into account how factors in the context of the practice setting and his or her personal context might affect intervention. Factors in the practice setting relate to the availability of resources (i.e., reimbursement or availability of equipment). Factors in the personal context of the practitioner might include repertoire of therapeutic skills and personal motivation.

and the conditional tracks. Practitioners shift easily and frequently among the three tracks, depending on what they are addressing in therapy with a specific client.

Procedural reasoning is a strategy used by the OT practitioner when he or she focuses on the client's disease or disability and determines what will be the most appropriate modalities to use to improve the functional performance. Central tasks for the OT practitioner during procedural reasoning are problem identification, goal setting, and treatment planning.[2] The problem-solving skills discussed in Chapter 12 may be employed during procedural reasoning. This track is similar to the scientific element of clinical reasoning.

> The OT practitioner working with a new client researches the diagnosis, etiology, characteristics, prognosis, and suggested interventions of a disorder. The practitioner determines the most commonly used approach for clients with this diagnosis and begins intervention based upon this.

Interactive reasoning is a strategy used by the OT practitioner when he or she wants to understand the client as a person. This type of reasoning takes place during face-to-face interactions between the practitioner and the client. OT practitioners use interactive reasoning strategies to (1) understand the disability from the client's point of view, (2) engage the client in treatment, (3) individualize the intervention setting by matching goals and procedures to the particular client and his or her life experiences and disability,

(4) impart a sense of trust and acceptance to the client, (5) relieve tension by using humor, (6) develop a common language of actions and meanings, and (7) determine whether the intervention is going well.[2]

> The OT practitioner learns that the client lives at home with his wife of 20 years and three teenage children. The client hopes to return to his job as a certified public accountant (CPA); he enjoys biking with his family and hiking in the country. The OT practitioner uses this information along with the information about the diagnosis, prognosis, etiology, and intervention strategies when designing the intervention plan.

Interactive reasoning takes into account the client's goals and environment. Thus the OT practitioner uses procedural reasoning to form a foundation for intervention, and he or she personalizes the intervention through interactive reasoning.

The third type of strategy used by OT practitioners is **conditional reasoning.** Conditional reasoning has several aspects.[2] During conditional reasoning, the practitioner first considers the client's condition as a whole, including the disease or disability and what it means to the person—the physical context and the social context. Next, the OT practitioner pictures how the client's condition may change. A change in the client's present condition is dependent on his or her active involvement in treatment. This imagined condition is dependent on the practitioner's ability to motivate the client to participate in intervention, as well as to share the same vision for improvement of his or her condition.[2] With these images in mind, the practitioner implements intervention and mentally checks along the way to compare the changes observed in the client with the client's future goals.[2]

> Anna, the OT practitioner, evaluates Sam's progress in therapy and decides to change the focus of intervention from remediation to compensation. Anna believes that Sam has worked hard in therapy, but based upon the severity of his condition and the progress to date, Anna decides that compensation techniques will enable Sam to return to his occupations earlier.

Anna used conditional reasoning to change the focus of the intervention and to allow Sam to return to his occupations.

Another clinical reasoning strategy described in the literature is called **narrative reasoning.** Mattingly describes two different ways in which OT practitioners use narrative reasoning—storytelling and story creation.[3] In storytelling, OT practitioners tell "stories" about clients to each other. Storytelling helps practitioners reason how particular clients may be experiencing their disabilities and how intervention might proceed. Storytelling may take place informally over lunch or more formally in a case study presentation at a staff meeting.

OT practitioners also create stories. The practitioner envisions how the future may be for the client so that he or she may guide the intervention process. This technique is similar to conditional reasoning. In another aspect of story creation, OT practitioners create experiences for clients to make the activities meaningful.

Nick, the OT practitioner, is treating Carlos, a 63-year-old client who has had a stroke. Nick and Carlos are working toward improving movement in Carlos' affected arm and hand so that he can return to his occupation as a car mechanic. Nick has asked Carlos to make a tile mosaic trivet. Nick creates a vision for Carlos by explaining to him that making a tile mosaic trivet requires concentration, design, problem solving, and fine motor skills in his affected arm, which are also skills Carlos needs when working as a mechanic. Nick explains to Carlos that working hard to complete this project is a step toward returning to his job as car mechanic.

Part of storytelling is explaining to the client how this activity relates to other meaningful activities and how completing the project can help him or her overcome his or her disability. In summarizing the use of narrative reasoning, Mattingly states, "Narratives make sense of reality by linking the outward world of actions and events to the inner world of human intention and motivation."[3]

Pragmatic reasoning is another strategy that has been suggested by Schell and Cervero as contributing to the clinical reasoning process. Pragmatic reasoning takes into consideration factors in the context of the practice setting and in the personal context of the OT practitioner that may inhibit or facilitate intervention. Factors related to the context of the practice setting include reimbursement and the availability of equipment and space.[8] For example, reimbursement must be considered during clinical reasoning in situations where the client has a need for occupational therapy services but does not have the insurance coverage or ability to pay for services. Availability of resources, such as equipment and space, often impact a practitioner's clinical reasoning. The practitioner cannot plan an intervention unless the treatment setting has the necessary equipment or space for it.

The OT practitioner must also consider personal factors, including his or her repertoire of therapeutic and negotiation skills and personal motivation. The practitioner makes decisions regarding intervention based upon his or her knowledge and experience. Therefore, all practitioners are obligated to become as informed as they are able to benefit clients.

FROM NOVICE TO EXPERT: DEVELOPMENT OF CLINICAL REASONING SKILLS

Clinical reasoning is not a skill that can be taught; it is developed over time with practical experience. Slater and Cohn describe variations in clinical reasoning at five different stages of career development: novice, advanced beginner, competent, proficient, and expert.[9] As would be expected, differences have been noted when comparing the clinical reasoning skills of the novice practitioner to those of the expert practitioner (Table 17-2).

The focus of the **novice** practitioner (stage 1) is on the learning of the procedural skills (e.g., assessment, diagnostic, and treatment planning procedures) necessary to practice.[2,9] The novice practitioner feels most comfortable with performing and refining the techniques and procedures learned in school. Novice practitioners do not feel comfortable using interactive reasoning strategies. At stage 2, the **advanced beginner** is learning to recognize additional cues and beginning to see the client as an individual.[9] However, the advanced beginner still does not see the whole picture.

Slater and Cohn describe the **competent practitioner** (stage 3) as being able to see more facts and to determine the importance of these facts and observations.[9] The practitioner

TABLE 17-2 Development of Clinical Reasoning Skills

Stage of Development	Name	Type of Functioning
1	Novice	Uses procedural or scientific reasoning, knowledge from coursework
2	Advanced beginner	Recognizes additional cues and begins to see client as an individual
3	Competent	Sees more facts, understand client's problems, individualizes treatment, may lack creativity and flexibility
4	Proficient	Views situations as whole instead of in isolated parts, able to develop a vision of where the client should go, able to modify easily
5	Expert	Recognizes and understands rules of practice, uses intuition to know what to do next, uses conditional reasoning

at this stage has a broader understanding of the client's problems and is more likely to individualize treatment. However, flexibility and creativity are still lacking. The **proficient practitioner** (stage 4) is able to view situations as a whole instead of as isolated parts.[9] The practical experience of the proficient practitioner allows him or her to develop a direction and vision of where the client should be going. If the initial plans do not work, the proficient therapist is easily able to modify them.

Expert practitioners (stage 5) recognize and understand rules of practice; however, for this group of practitioners the rules shift to the background.[9] The expert practitioner often uses intuition to know what to do next. "This intuitive judgment is based on correct identification of relevant cues at a particular time in the patient's therapy; and a variety of medical, physical, and psychosocial factors are considered."[9] Expert practitioners use both procedural and interactive skills without difficulty.[2] Conditional reasoning is also carried out more easily by the expert practitioner, who can rely on past clinical situations to help process imagined outcomes for the client.

Rogers relates some of the differences in clinical reasoning to the way in which novice and expert practitioners remember information and solve problems.[6] Novices record information in individual cues; experts use chunking to sort and record information. Chunking is a strategy that is used to remember several units of information. For example, it is easier to remember a phone number if it is divided into chunks instead of trying to remember individual numbers (e.g., 501-555-9487 instead of 5015559487). Expert practitioners use the technique of chunking to categorize information about clients according to how it applies to practice.[6]

Without the experience of the expert, how can the student or novice practitioner enhance his or her clinical reasoning skills? The clinical reasoning process cannot be taught in customary ways, such as reading about it in a textbook, but it can be learned.[1,4] Learning clinical reasoning skills can be facilitated through coaching and role modeling.[1,5,9] It is important that the student begin to become aware of the processes and strategies used in clinical reasoning, which will facilitate the development of clinical reasoning skills. The novice practitioner can read about personal experiences of individuals with disabilities to learn to develop narrative reasoning skills.[5] The student can use case studies presented throughout his or her coursework to analyze the clinical reasoning strategies that are used or to practice developing the skills on his or her own. The novice practitioner can observe other practitioners in action or in a simulated treatment session, focusing attention on the clinical reasoning processes and strategies that are being used; he or she should consider whether the approach seems appropriate and whether he or she would do things the same way. How might the strategies used be improved? The novice practitioner can use his or her fieldwork opportunities to learn the clinical reasoning processes used by the different OT practitioners. Setting personal goals related to the development of clinical reasoning skills before fieldwork experiences may help the student focus on achieving these goals. During fieldwork, students may be encouraged to identify strategies that are successful and then seek feedback from supervisors. Discussing cases and problem solving through the clinical reasoning process with more experienced clinicians will stimulate development of clinical reasoning.

Because clinical reasoning continually develops in even expert practitioners, practitioners are encouraged to continue to seek education and knowledge and remain reflective of their own practice. Clinical reasoning skills may be further developed through new knowledge and careful analysis of one's practice skills and thinking. For example, expert practitioners may improve clinical reasoning skills by having another practitioner observe, ask questions, and provide feedback on an intervention.

In addition, conducting research through case study analysis may enhance a practitioner's clinical reasoning skills because this requires a careful examination of the intervention process. Finally, remaining current and critically examining available research enhances a practitioner's clinical reasoning skills and abilities, thereby benefiting clients.

SUMMARY

Clinical reasoning is perhaps the most important aspect of the occupational therapy process. Clinical reasoning provides the foundation for making choices and helping to improve clients' ability to function and engage in occupations.

The elements of science, ethics and art are combined in the therapy process. OT practitioners skillfully examine these areas to design intervention that will make a difference in the lives of the clients they serve. Knowledge of science provides data that is important when evaluating and intervening with clients. Science may form the basis for interventions, yet the art of therapy plays an equally important role. The art of therapy involves designing intervention that is motivating to clients and serves their goals. The art of therapy involves the therapeutic use of self and refers to how the practitioner relates to clients, including listening and mannerisms. Finally, ethical considerations may influence the actions of the client and OT practitioner, thereby determining the course of the intervention and outcomes.

OT practitioners use a variety of strategies throughout the therapy process to effectively deal with the scientific, artistic, and ethical elements. These reasoning strategies include procedural, interactive, conditional, narrative, and pragmatic reasoning. The strategies are seldom used in isolation, and in fact, expert practitioners are able to intertwine the strategies to provide the most effective and intuitive intervention. Novice practitioners may be limited in the strategies they use.

Practice, reflection, education, supervision, research, and critical analysis of practice provide excellent techniques for increasing a practitioner's ability to use clinical reasoning. OT practitioners must always remain mindful of the clinical reasoning strategies they are employing so that intervention remains beneficial to clients.

Learning Activities

1. When an instructor gives you an assignment or learning experience, determine which type of clinical reasoning the assignment is meant to promote.
2. View a videotape of a case study of a client in a therapy session. Analyze the clinical reasoning strategies used by the practitioner. Were the strategies effective? What would you have done differently?
3. Write a short story about someone you know who has a disability. Report how this individual's past and present may reflect on his or her possible future.[5]
4. Read a literary work about an individual who has experienced a disabling condition. Using the narrative reasoning strategy, analyze the person's experiences. In your own words, describe the person's story. Your instructor can provide suggestions for books to read.
5. Use clinical reasoning strategies to develop an intervention plan for a given case study, in which the only information you have is the client's age, diagnosis, and living situation. Discuss the findings in class. What would be the next step in your process?

Review Questions

1. What is clinical reasoning?
2. What is Rogers and Holm's clinical reasoning thought process?
3. Provide an example of scientific, ethical, and artistic elements of clinical reasoning.
4. What are the three types of clinical reasoning as described by Mattingly and Fleming?
5. What are the stages of clinical reasoning? Provide a description of each.

REFERENCES

1. Benamy BC: *Developing Clinical Reasoning Skills: Strategies for the Occupational Therapist*, San Antonio, 1996, Therapy Skill Builders.
2. Fleming MH: The therapist with the three-track mind, *Am J Occup Ther* 45:1007, 1991.
3. Mattingly C: The narrative nature of clinical reasoning, *Am J Occup Ther* 45:998, 1991.
4. Mattingly C: What is clinical reasoning? *Am J Occup Ther* 45:979, 1991.
5. Neistadt ME: Teaching strategies for the development of clinical reasoning, *Am J Occup Ther* 50:676, 1996.
6. Rogers JC: Clinical reasoning: the ethics, science and art, *Am J Occup Ther* 37:601, 1983.
7. Rogers JC, Holm MB: Occupational therapy diagnostic reasoning: a component of clinical reasoning, *Am J Occup Ther* 45:1045, 1991.
8. Schell BA, Cervero RM: Clinical reasoning in occupational therapy: an integrative review, *Am J Occup Ther* 47:605, 1993.
9. Slater DY, Cohn ES: Staff development through analysis of practice, *Am J Occup Ther* 45:1038, 1991.

Occupational Therapy Code of Ethics (2005)*

PREAMBLE

This American Occupational Therapy Association (AOTA) *Occupational Therapy Code of Ethics (2005)* is a public statement of principles used to promote and maintain high standards of conduct within the profession and is supported by the *Core Values and Attitudes of Occupational Therapy Practice*.[1] Members of AOTA are committed to promoting inclusion, diversity, independence, and safety for all recipients in various stages of life, health, and illness and to empower all beneficiaries of occupational therapy. This commitment extends beyond service recipients to include professional colleagues, students, educators, businesses, and the community.

Fundamental to the mission of the occupational therapy profession is the therapeutic use of everyday life activities (occupations) with individuals or groups for the purpose of participation in roles and situations in home, school, workplace, community, and other settings. "Occupational therapy addresses the physical, cognitive, psychosocial, sensory, and other aspects of performance in a variety of contexts to support engagement in everyday life activities that affect health, well being and quality of life."[5] Occupational therapy personnel have an ethical responsibility first and foremost to recipients of service as well as to society.

The historical foundation of this code is based on ethical reasoning surrounding practice and professional issues, as well as empathic reflection regarding these interactions with others. This reflection resulted in the establishment of principles that guide ethical action. Ethical action goes beyond rote following of rules or application of principles; rather, it is a manifestation of moral character and mindful reflection. It is a commitment to beneficence for the sake of others, to virtuous practice of artistry and science, to genuinely good behaviors, and to noble acts of courage. It is an empathic way of being among others, which is made every day by all occupational therapy personnel.

The AOTA *Occupational Therapy Code of Ethics (2005)* is an aspirational guide to professional conduct when ethical issues surface. Ethical decision-making is a process that includes awareness regarding how the outcome will impact occupational therapy clients in all spheres. Applications of *Code* principles are considered situation-specific; and, where a conflict exists, occupational therapy personnel will pursue responsible efforts for resolution.

The specific purpose of the AOTA *Occupational Therapy Code of Ethics (2005)* is to:
1. Identify and describe the principles supported by the occupational therapy profession
2. Educate the general public and members regarding established principles to which occupational therapy personnel are accountable
3. Socialize occupational therapy personnel new to the practice to expected standards of conduct

*From American Occupational Therapy Association: Occupational therapy code of ethics (2005), Am J Occup Ther 59(6):639-642, 2005.

4. Assist occupational therapy personnel in recognition and resolution of ethical dilemmas

The AOTA *Occupational Therapy Code of Ethics (2005)* defines the set principles that apply to occupational therapy personnel at all levels.

PRINCIPLE 1. OCCUPATIONAL THERAPY PERSONNEL SHALL DEMONSTRATE A CONCERN FOR THE SAFETY AND WELL-BEING OF THE RECIPIENTS OF THEIR SERVICES. (BENEFICENCE)

Occupational therapy personnel shall:

A. Provide services in a fair and equitable manner. They shall recognize and appreciate the cultural components of economics, geography, race, ethnicity, religious and political factors, marital status, age, sexual orientation, gender identity, and disability of all recipients of their services.

B. Strive to ensure that fees are fair and reasonable and commensurate with services performed. When occupational therapy practitioners set fees, they shall set fees considering institutional, local, state, and federal requirement, and with due regard for the service recipient's ability to pay.

C. Make every effort to advocate for recipients to obtain needed services through available means.

D. Recognize the responsibility to promote public health and the safety and well-being of individuals, groups, and/or communities.

PRINCIPLE 2. OCCUPATIONAL THERAPY PERSONNEL SHALL TAKE MEASURES TO ENSURE A RECIPIENT'S SAFETY AND AVOID IMPOSING OR INFLICTING HARM. (NONMALEFICENCE)

Occupational therapy personnel shall:

A. Maintain therapeutic relationships that shall not exploit the recipient of services sexually, physically, emotionally, psychologically, financially, socially, or in any other manner.

B. Avoid relationships or activities that conflict or interfere with therapeutic professional judgment or objectivity.

C. Refrain from any undue influences that may compromise provision of service

D. Exercise professional judgment and critically analyze directives that could result in potential harm before implementation.

E. Identify and address personal problems that may adversely impact professional judgment and duties.

F. Bring concerns regarding impairment of professional skills of a colleague to the attention of the appropriate authority when or if attempts to address concerns are unsuccessful.

PRINCIPLE 3. OCCUPATIONAL THERAPY PERSONNEL SHALL RESPECT RECIPIENTS TO ASSURE THEIR RIGHTS. (AUTONOMY, CONFIDENTIALITY)

Occupational therapy personnel shall:

A. Collaborate with recipients, and if they desire, families, significant others, and/or caregivers in setting goals and priorities throughout the intervention process, including full disclosure of the nature, risk, and potential outcomes of any interventions.

B. Obtain informed consent from participants involved in research activities and ensure that they understand potential risks and outcomes.

C. Respect the individual's right to refuse professional services or involvement in research or educational activities.

D. Protect all privileged confidential forms of written, verbal, and electronic communication gained from educational, practice, research, and investigational activities, unless otherwise mandated by local, state, or federal regulations.

PRINCIPLE 4. OCCUPATIONAL THERAPY PERSONNEL SHALL ACHIEVE AND CONTINUALLY MAINTAIN HIGH STANDARDS OF COMPETENCE. (DUTY)

Occupational therapy personnel shall:

A. Hold the appropriate national, state, or any other requisite credentials for the services they provide

B. Conform to AOTA standards of practice and official documents.

C. Take responsibility for maintaining and documenting competence in practice, education, and research by participating in professional development and educational activities.

D. Be competent in all topic areas in which they provide instruction to consumers, peers, and/or students.

E. Critically examine available evidence so they may perform their duties on the basis of current information.

F. Protect service recipients by ensuring that duties assumed by or assigned to other occupational therapy personnel match credentials, qualifications, experience, and scope of practice.

G. Provide appropriate supervision to individuals for whom they have supervisory responsibility in accordance with Association official documents; local, state, and federal or national laws and regulations; and institutional policies and procedures.

H. Refer to or consult with other service providers whenever such a referral or consultation would be helpful to the care of the recipient of service. The referral or consultation process shall be done in collaboration with the recipient of service.

PRINCIPLE 5. OCCUPATIONAL THERAPY PERSONNEL SHALL COMPLY WITH LAWS AND ASSOCIATION POLICIES[3] GUIDING THE PROFESSION OF OCCUPATIONAL THERAPY. (PROCEDURAL JUSTICE)

Occupational therapy personnel shall:

A. Familiarize themselves with and seek to understand and abide by institutional rules, applicable Association policies; local, state, and federal/national/international laws.

B. Be familiar with revisions in those laws and Association policies that apply to the profession of occupational therapy and shall inform employers, employees, and colleagues of those changes.

C. Encourage those they supervise in occupational therapy-related activities to adhere to the Code.

D. Take reasonable steps to ensure employers are aware of occupational therapy's ethical obligations, as set forth in this Code, and of the implications of those obligations for occupational therapy practice, education, and research.

E. Record and report in an accurate and timely manner all information related to professional activities.

PRINCIPLE 6. OCCUPATIONAL THERAPY PERSONNEL SHALL PROVIDE ACCURATE INFORMATION WHEN REPRESENTING THE PROFESSION. (VERACITY)

Occupational therapy personnel shall:

A. Represent their credentials, qualifications, education, experience, training, and competence accurately. This is of particular importance for those to whom occupational therapy personnel provide their services or with whom occupational therapy personnel have a professional relationship.

B. Disclose any professional, personal, financial, business, or volunteer affiliations that may pose a conflict of interest to those with whom they may establish a professional, contractual, or other working relationship.

C. Refrain from using or participating in the use of any form of communication that contains false, fraudulent, deceptive, or unfair statements or claims.

D. Identify and fully disclose to all appropriate persons errors that compromise recipients' safety.

E. Accept responsibility for their professional actions that reduce the public's trust in occupational therapy services and those that perform those services.

PRINCIPLE 7. OCCUPATIONAL THERAPY PERSONNEL SHALL TREAT COLLEAGUES AND OTHER PROFESSIONALS WITH RESPECT, FAIRNESS, DISCRETION, AND INTEGRITY. (FIDELITY)

Occupational therapy personnel shall:

A. Preserve, respect, and safeguard confidential information about colleagues and staff, unless otherwise mandated by national, state, or local laws.

B. Accurately represent the qualifications, views, contributions, and findings of colleagues.

C. Take adequate measures to discourage, prevent, expose, and correct any breaches of the Code and report any breaches of the Code to the appropriate authority.

D. Avoid conflicts of interest and conflicts of commitment in employment and volunteer roles

E. Use conflict resolution and/or alternative dispute resolution resources to resolve organizational and interpersonal conflicts.

F. Familiarize themselves with established policies and procedures for handling concerns about this Code, including familiarity with national, state, local, district, and territorial procedures for handling ethics complaints. These include policies and procedures created by AOTA, licensing and regulatory bodies, employers, agencies, certification boards, and other organizations having jurisdiction over occupational therapy practice.

Note: This AOTA *Occupational Therapy Code of Ethics* is one of three documents that constitute the *Ethics Standards*. The other two are the *Core Values and Attitudes of Occupational Therapy Practice*[1] and the *Guidelines to the Occupational Therapy Code of Ethics*.[2]

GLOSSARY

Autonomy—The right of an individual to self-determination. The ability to independently act on one's decisions for one's own well-being[4]

Beneficence—Doing good for others or bringing about good for them. The duty to confer benefits to others

Confidentiality—Not disclosing data or information that should be kept private to prevent harm and to abide to policies, regulations, and laws

Dilemma—A situation in which one moral conviction or right action conflicts with another. It exists because there is no one, clear-cut, right answer

Duty—Actions required of professionals by society, or actions that are self-imposed

Ethics—A systematic study of morality (i.e., rules of conduct that are grounded in philosophical principles and theory)

Fidelity—Faithfully fulfilling vows and promises, agreements, and discharging fiduciary responsibilities[4]

Justice—Three types of justice are

  Compensatory—Making reparation for wrongs that have been done

  Distributive—The act of distributing goods and burdens among members of society

  Procedural—Assuring that processes are organized in a fair manner and policies or laws are followed

Morality—Personal beliefs regarding values, rules, and principles of what is right or wrong. Morality may be culture based or culture driven

Nonmaleficence—Not harming or causing harm to be done to oneself or others; the duty to ensure that no harm is done

Veracity—A duty to tell the truth; avoid deception

REFERENCES

1. American Occupational Therapy Association: Core values and attitudes of occupational therapy practice, *Am J Occup Ther* 47:1085-1086, 1993.
2. American Occupational Therapy Association: Guidelines to the occupational therapy code of ethics, *Am J Occup Ther* 52:881-884, 1998.
3. American Occupational Therapy Association: Association policies, *Am J Occup Ther* 52:694-695, 2004.
4. Beauchamp TL, Childress JF: *Principles of Biomedical Ethics*, ed 5, New York, 2001, Oxford University Press.
5. *Definition of Occupational Therapy Practice for the AOTA Model Practice Act*, 2004. Retrieved April 9, 2005, from http://www.aota.org/members/area4/docs/defotpractice.pdf.

AUTHORS

The Commission on Standards and Ethics (SEC):
S. Maggie Reitz, PhD, OTR/L, FAOTA, Chairperson
Melba Arnold, MS, OTR/L
Linda Gabriel Franck, PhD, OTR/L
Darryl J. Austin, MS, OT/L
Diane Hill, COTA/L, AP, ROH
Lorie J. McQuade, Med, CRC

Daryl K. Knox, MD

Deborah Yarett Slater, MS, OT/L, FAOTA, Staff Liaison

With contributions to the Preamble by Suzanne Peloquin, PhD, OTR, FAOTA

Adopted by the Representative Assembly 2005C202.

Note: This document replaces the 2000 document, *Occupational Therapy Code of Ethics (2000)* (*American Journal of Occupational Therapy,* 54, 614-616).

Prepared 4/7/2000, revised draft—January 2005, second revision 4/2005 by SEC.

Standards of Practice for Occupational Therapy*

PREFACE

This document defines minimum standards for the practice of occupational therapy. The *Standards of Practice for Occupational Therapy* are requirements for occupational therapists and occupational therapy assistance for the delivery of occupational therapy services. The *Reference Manual of Official Documents* contains documents that clarify and support occupational therapy practice.[3] These documents are reviewed and updated on an ongoing basis for their applicability.

EDUCATION, EXAMINATION, AND LICENSURE REQUIREMENTS

All occupational therapists and occupational therapy assistants must practice under federal and state law. To practice as an occupational therapist, the individual trained in the United States

- has graduated from an occupational therapy program accredited by the Accreditation Council for Occupational Therapy Education (ACOTE®) or predecessor organizations;
- has successfully completed a period of supervised fieldwork experience required by the recognized educational institution where the applicant met the academic requirements of an educational program for occupational therapists that is accredited by ACOTE® or predecessor organizations;
- has passed a nationally recognized entry-level examination for occupational therapists; and
- fulfills state requirements for licensure, certification, or registration.

To practice as an occupational therapist assistant, the individual trained in the United States

- has graduated from an associate- or certificate-level occupational therapy assistant program accredited by ACOTE® or predecessor organizations;
- has successfully completed a period of supervised fieldwork experience required by the recognized educational institution where the applicant met the academic requirements of an educational program for occupational therapy assistants that is accredited by ACOTE® or predecessor organizations;
- has passed a nationally recognized entry-level examination for occupational therapy assistants; and
- fulfills state requirements for licensure, certification, or registration.

*From American Occupational Therapy Association: Standards of practice for occupational therapy, Am J Occup Ther 59:663-665, 2005.

DEFINITIONS

Assessment. Specific tools or instruments that are used during the evaluation process.

Client. A person, group, program, organization, or community for whom the occupational therapy practitioner is providing services.

Evaluation. The process of obtaining and interpreting data necessary for intervention. This includes planning for and documenting the evaluation process and results.

Screening. Obtaining and reviewing data relevant to a potential client to determine the need for further evaluation and intervention.

STANDARD I: PROFESSIONAL STANDING AND RESPONSIBILITY

1. An occupational therapy practitioner (occupational therapist or occupational therapy assistant) delivers occupational therapy services that reflect the philosophical base of occupational therapy and are consistent with the established principles and concepts of theory and practice.
2. An occupational therapy practitioner is knowledgeable about and delivers occupational therapy services in accordance with AOTA standards, policies, and guidelines, and state and federal requirements relevant to practice and service delivery.
3. An occupational therapy practitioner maintains current licensure, registration, or certification as required by law or regulation.
4. An occupational therapy practitioner abides by the AOTA *Occupational Therapy Code of Ethics.*[2]
5. An occupational therapy practitioner abides by the AOTA *Standards for Continuing Competence*[1] by establishing, maintaining, and updating professional performance, knowledge, and skills.
6. An occupational therapist is responsible for all aspects of occupational therapy and therapy service delivery, and is accountable for the safety and effectiveness of the occupational therapy service delivery process.
7. An occupational therapy assistant is responsible for providing safe and effective occupational therapy services under the supervision of and in partnership with the occupational therapist and in accordance with the laws or regulations and AOTA documents.
8. An occupational therapy practitioner maintains current knowledge of legislative, political, social, cultural, and reimbursement issues that affect clients and the practice of occupational therapy.
9. An occupational therapy practitioner is knowledgeable about evidence-based research and applies it ethically and appropriately to the occupational therapy process.

STANDARD II: SCREENING, EVALUATION, AND RE-EVALUATION

1. An occupational therapist accepts and responds to referrals in compliance with state laws or other regulatory requirements.
2. An occupational therapist, in collaboration with the client, evaluates the client's ability to participate in daily life activities by considering the client's capacities, the activities, and the environments in which these activities occur.

3. An occupational therapist initiates and directs the screening, evaluation, and re-evaluation process, and analyzes and interprets the data in accordance with the law, regulatory requirements, and AOTA documents.

4. An occupational therapy assistant contributes to the screening, evaluation, and re-evaluation process by implementing delegated assessments and by providing verbal and written reports of observations and client capacities to the occupational therapist in accordance with law, regulatory requirements, and AOTA documents.

5. An occupational therapy practitioner follows defined protocols when standardized assessments are used.

6. An occupational therapist completes and documents occupational therapy evaluation results. An occupational therapy assistant contributes to the documentation of evaluation results. An occupational therapy practitioner abides by the time frames, format, and standards established by practice settings, government agencies, external accreditation programs, payers, and AOTA documents.

7. An occupational therapy practitioner communicates screening, evaluation, and re-evaluation results, within the boundaries of client confidentiality, to the appropriate person, group, or organization.

8. An occupational therapist recommends additional consultations or refers clients to appropriate resources when the needs of the client can best be served by the expertise of other professionals or services.

9. An occupational therapy practitioner educates current and potential referral sources about the scope of occupational therapy services and the process of initiating occupational therapy services.

STANDARD III: INTERVENTION

1. An occupational therapist has overall responsibility for the development, documentation, and implementation of the occupational therapy intervention based on the evaluation, client goals, current best evidence, and clinical reasoning.

2. An occupational therapist ensures that the intervention plan is documented within the time frames, formats, and standards established by the practice settings, agencies, external accreditation programs, and payers.

3. An occupational therapy assistant selects, implements, and makes modifications to therapeutic activities and interventions that are consistent with the occupational therapy assistant's demonstrated competency and delegated responsibilities, the intervention plan, and requirements of the practice setting.

4. An occupational therapy practitioner reviews the intervention plan with the client and appropriate others regarding the rationale, safety issues, and relative benefits and risks of the planned interventions.

5. An occupational therapist modifies the intervention plan throughout the intervention process and documents changes in the client's needs, goals, and performance.

6. An occupational therapy assistant contributes to the modification of the intervention plan by exchanging information with and providing documentation to the occupational therapist about the client's responses to and communications throughout the intervention.

7. An occupational therapy practitioner documents the occupational therapy services provided within the time frames, formats, and standards established by the practice setting, agencies, external accreditation programs, payers, and AOTA documents.

STANDARD IV: OUTCOMES

1. An occupational therapist is responsible for selecting, measuring, documenting, and interpreting expected or achieved outcomes that are related to the client's ability to engage in occupations.
2. An occupational therapist is responsible for documenting changes in the client's performance and capacities and for discontinuing services when the client has achieved identified goals, reached maximum benefit, or does not desire to continue services.
3. An occupational therapist prepares and implements a discontinuation plan or transition plan based on the client's needs, goals, performance, and appropriate follow-up resources.
4. An occupational therapy assistant contributes to the discontinuation or transition plan by providing information and documentation to the supervising occupational therapist related to the client's needs, goals, performance, and appropriate follow-up resources.
5. An occupational therapy practitioner facilitates the transition process in collaboration with the client, family members, significant others, team, and community resources and individuals, when appropriate.
6. An occupational therapist is responsible for evaluating the safety and effectiveness of the occupational therapy processes and interventions within the practice setting.
7. An occupational therapy assistant contributes to evaluating the safety and effectiveness of the occupational therapy processes and interventions within the practice setting.

REFERENCES

1. American Occupational Therapy Association: Standards for continuing competence, *Am J Occup Ther* 53:599-600, 1999.
2. American Occupational Therapy Association: Occupational therapy code of ethics (2000), *Am J Occup Ther* 54:614-616, 2000.
3. American Occupational Therapy Association: *The Reference Manual of the Official Documents of the American Occupational Therapy Association*, ed 10, Bethesda, MD, 2004, Author.

AUTHORS

The Commission on Practice:
Sara Jane Brayman, PhD, OTR/L, FAOTA, Chairperson
Susanne Smith Roley, MS, OTR/L, FAOTA, Chairperson-Elect
Gloria Frolek Clark, MS, OTR/L, FAOTA
Janet V. DeLany, DEd, MSA, OTR/L, FAOTA
Eileen R. Garza, PhD, OTR, ATP
Mary V. Radomski, MA, OTR/L, FAOTA
Ruth Ramsey, MS, OTR/L
Carol Siebert, MS, OTR/L
Kristi Voelkerding, BS, COTA/L
Lenna Aird, COTA/L, ASD Liaison
Patricia D. LaVesser, PhD, OTR/L, SIS Liaison
Deborah Lieberman, MHSA, OTR/L, FAOTA, AOTA Headquarters Liaison for the Commission on Practice
Sara Jane Brayman, PhD, OTR/L, FAOTA, Chairperson

Adopted by the Representative Assembly 2005C218.

Note: This document replaces the 1994 *Standards of Practice for Occupational Therapy*. These standards are intended as recommended guidelines to assist occupational therapy practitioners in the provision of occupational therapy services. These standards serve as a minimum standard for occupational therapy practice and are applicable to all individual populations and the programs in which these individuals are served.

Key Information from the Occupational Therapy Practice Framework*

Table C-1   Areas of Occupation

Type of Activity	Examples
Activities of daily living (ADL)	Bathing, showering
	Bowel and bladder management
	Dressing
	Eating
	Feeding
	Functional mobility
	Personal device care
	Personal hygiene and grooming
	Sexual activity
	Sleep/rest
	Toilet hygiene
Instrumental activities of daily living (IADL)	Care of others (including selecting and supervising caregivers)
	Care of pets
	Child rearing
	Communication device use
	Community mobility
	Financial management
	Health management and maintenance
	Home establishment and management
	Meal preparation and cleanup
	Safety procedures and emergency response
	Shopping
Education	Formal education participation
	Explorations of informal personal education needs or interests (beyond formal education)
	Informal personal education participation
Work	Employment interests and pursuits
	Employment seeking and acquisition
	Job performance
	Retirement preparation and adjustment
	Volunteer exploration
	Volunteer participation
Play	Play exploration
	Play participation

*All tables in Appendix C are adapted from American Occupational Therapy Association: Occupational therapy practice framework: domain and process, Am J Occup Ther 56(6):609-639, 2002.

Table C-1   Areas of Occupation—cont'd

Type of Activity	Examples
Leisure	Leisure exploration
	Leisure participation
Social participation	Community
	Family
	Peer, friend

Table C-2   Performance Skills

Skills	Examples
Motor skills	Posture
	Mobility
	Coordination
	Strength and effort
	Energy
Process skills	Energy
	Knowledge
	Temporal organization
	Organizing space and objects
	Adaptation
Communication/interaction skills	Physicality Information exchange
	Relations

Table C-3 Performance Patterns

Habits—"Automatic behavior that is integrated into more complex patterns that enable people to function on a day-to-day basis."[5] Habits can either support or interfere with performance in areas of occupation.

Type of Habit	Examples
Useful habits	
Habits that support performance in daily life and contribute to life satisfaction	Always put car keys in same place so they can be found easily
Habits that support ability to follow rhythms of daily life	Brush teeth every morning to maintain good oral hygiene
Impoverished habits	
Habits that are not established	Inconsistently remembering to look both ways before crossing the street
Habits that need practice to improve	Inability to complete all steps of a self-care routine
Dominating habits	
Habits that are so demanding they interfere with daily life	Repetitive self-stimulation such as the type occurring in autism
	Use of chemical substances, resulting in addiction
Habits that satisfy a compulsive need for order	Neatly arranging forks on top of each other in silverware drawer
Routines—"Occupations with established sequences"[2]	
Roles—"A set of behaviors that have some socially agreed upon function and for which there is an accepted code of norms"[2]	

Table C-4 Activity Demands

Activity Demand Aspects	Definition	Examples
Objects and their properties	The tools, materials, and equipment used in the process of carrying out the activity	Tools (scissors, dishes, shoes, volleyball) Materials (paints, milk, lipstick) Equipment (workbench, stove, basketball hoop) Inherent properties (heavy, rough, sharp, colorful, loud, bitter tasting)
Space demands (relates to physical context)	The physical environmental requirements of the activity (e.g., size, arrangement, surface, lighting, temperature, noise, humidity, ventilation)	Large open space outdoors required for a basketball game
Social demands (relates to social and cultural contexts)	The social structure and demands that may be required by the activity	Rules of game Expectations of other participants in the activity (e.g., sharing of supplies)

Table C-4   Activity Demands—cont'd

Activity Demand Aspects	Definition	Examples
Sequence and timing	The process used to carry out the activity (specific steps, sequence, timing requirements)	Steps—(to make tea) gather cup and tea bag, heat water, pour water into cup, etc. Sequence—heat water before placing tea bag in water Timing—leave tea bag to steep for 2 minutes
Required actions	The usual skills that would be required by any performer to carry out the activity. Motor, process, and communication interaction skills should each be considered. The performance skills demanded by an activity will be correlated with the demands of the other activity aspects (i.e., objects, space)	Gripping handlebar Choosing a dress from closet Answering a question
Required body functions	"The physiological functions of body systems (including psychological functions)"[9] that are required to support the actions used to perform the activity	Mobility of joints Level of consciousness
Required body structures	"Anatomical parts of the body such as organs, limbs, and their components [that support body function]"[9] that are required to perform the activity	Number of hands Number of feet

Table C-5   Client Factors

Client Factor	Selected Classifications from *ICF*[9] and Occupational Therapy Examples

BODY FUNCTION CATEGORIES*
Mental Functions (Affective, Cognitive, Perceptual)

Global mental functions	*Consciousness functions*—level of arousal, level of consciousness *Orientation functions*—to person, place, time, self, and others *Sleep*—amount and quality of sleep. *Note*: Sleep and sleep patterns are assessed in relation to how they affect ability to effectively engage in occupations and in daily life activities *Temperament and personality functions*—conscientiousness, emotional stability, openness to experience. *Note*: These functions are assessed relative to their influence on the ability to engage in occupations and in daily life activities *Energy and drive functions*—motivation, impulse control, interests, values
Specific mental functions	*Attention functions*—sustained attention, divided attention *Memory functions*—retrospective memory, prospective memory *Perceptual functions*—visuospatial perception, interpretation of sensory stimuli (tactile, visual, auditory, olfactory, gustatory) *Thought functions*—recognition, categorization, generalization, awareness of reality, logical/coherent thought, appropriate thought content *Higher-level cognitive functions*—judgment, concept formation, time management, problem-solving, decision-making *Mental functions of language*—able to receive language and express self through spoken and written or sign language. *Note*: This function is assessed relative to its influence on the ability to engage in occupations and in daily life activities *Calculation functions*—able to add or subtract. *Note*: These functions are assessed relative to their influence on the ability to engage in occupations and in daily life activities (e.g., making change when shopping) *Mental functions of sequencing complex movement*—motor planning *Psychomotor functions*—appropriate range and regulation of motor response to psychological events *Emotional functions*—appropriate range and regulation of emotions, self-control *Experience of self and time functions*—body image, self-concept, self-esteem

Sensory Functions and Pain

Seeing and related functions	*Seeing functions*—visual acuity, visual field functions
Hearing and vestibular functions	*Hearing function*—response to sound. *Note*: This function is assessed in terms of its presence or absence and its effect on engaging in occupations and in daily life activities *Vestibular function*—balance
Additional sensory functions	*Taste functions*—ability to discriminate tastes *Smell function*—ability to discriminate smell *Proprioceptive function*—kinesthesia, joint position sense *Touch functions*—sensitivity to touch, ability to discriminate *Sensory functions related to temperature and other stimuli*—sensitivity to temperature, sensitivity to pressure, ability to discriminate temperature and pressure
Pain	*Sensations of pain*—dull pain, stabbing pain

Table C-5   Client Factors—cont'd

Client Factor	Selected Classifications from *ICF*[9] and Occupational Therapy Examples
Neuromusculoskeletal and Movement-Related Functions	
Functions of joints and bones	*Mobility of joint functions*—passive range of motion *Stability of joint functions*—postural alignment. *Note*: This refers to physiological stability of the joint related to its structural integrity as compared to the motor skill of aligning the body while moving in relation to task objects *Mobility of bone functions*—frozen scapula, movement of carpal bones
Muscle functions	*Muscle power functions*—strength *Muscle tone functions*—degree of muscle tone (e.g., flaccidity, spasticity) *Muscle endurance functions*—endurance
Movement functions	*Motor reflex functions*—stretch reflex, asymmetrical tonic neck reflex *Involuntary movement reaction functions*—righting reactions, supporting reactions *Control of voluntary movement functions*—eye-hand coordination, bilateral integration, eye-foot coordination *Involuntary movement functions*—tremors, tics, motor perseveration *Gait pattern functions*—walking patterns and impairments, such as asymmetric gait, stiff gait. *Note*: Gait patterns are assessed in relation to how they affect ability to engage in occupations and in daily life activities
Cardiovascular, Hematological, Immunological, and Respiratory System Function	
Cardiovascular system function	*Blood pressure functions*—hypertension, hypotension, postural hypotension
Hematological and immunological system function	OTs and OTAs have knowledge of these body functions and understand broadly the interaction that occurs between these functions and engagement in occupation to support participation. Some therapists may specialize in evaluating and intervening with a specific function as it is related to supporting performance and engagement in occupations and activities targeted for intervention
Respiratory system function	*Respiration functions*—rate, rhythm, and depth
Additional functions and sensations of the cardiovascular and respiratory systems	*Exercise tolerance functions*—physical endurance, aerobic capacity, stamina, and fatigability
Voice and Speech Functions **Digestive, Metabolic, and Endocrine System Function**	
Digestive system function Metabolic system and endocrine system function	OTs and OTAs have knowledge of these body functions and understand broadly the interaction that occurs between these functions and engagement in occupation to support participation. Some therapists may specialize in evaluating and intervening with a specific function as it is related to supporting performance and engagement in occupations and activities targeted for intervention

Continued

Table C-5   Client Factors—cont'd

Client Factor	Selected Classifications from *ICF*[9] and Occupational Therapy Examples
Genitourinary and Reproductive Functions	
Urinary functions Genital and reproductive functions	OTs and OTAs have knowledge of these body functions and understand broadly the interaction that occurs between these functions and engagement in occupation to support participation. Some therapists may specialize in evaluating and intervening with a specific function as it is related to supporting performance and engagement in occupations and activities targeted for intervention
Skin and Related Structure Functions	
Skin functions	*Protective functions of the skin*—presence or absence of wounds, cuts, or abrasions *Repair function of the skin*—wound healing
Hair and nail functions	OTs and OTAs have knowledge of these body functions and understand broadly the interaction that occurs between these functions and engagement in occupation to support participation. Some therapists may specialize in evaluating and intervening with a specific function as it is related to supporting performance and engagement in occupations and activities targeted for intervention

Client Factor	Classifications (Classifications are not delineated in the Body Structure section of this table)
BODY STRUCTURE CATEGORIES†	
Structure of the nervous system	
The eye, ear, and related structures	
Structures involved in voice and speech	
Structures of the cardiovascular, immunological, and respiratory systems	OTs and OTAs have knowledge of these body functions and understand broadly the interaction that occurs between these functions and engagement in occupation to support participation. Some therapists may specialize in evaluating and intervening with a specific function as it is related to supporting performance and engagement in occupations and activities targeted for intervention
Structures related to the digestive system	
Structures related to the genitourinary and reproductive systems	
Structures related to movement	
Skin and related structures	

*Categories and classifications adapted from the *ICF*.[9]

† Categories are from the *ICF*.[9]

ICF, International Classification of Function, Disability and Health; OT, occupational therapist; OTA, occupational therapy assistant.

Table C-6   Occupational Therapy Intervention Approaches

Approach	Focus of Intervention	Examples
Create, promote (health promotion)—an intervention approach that does not assume a disability is present or that any factors would interfere with performance. This approach is designed to provide enriched contextual and activity experiences that will enhance performance for all persons in the natural contexts of life.[3]	Performance skills	Create a parenting class for first-time parents to teach child development information (performance skill)
	Performance patterns	Promote handling stress by creating time-use routines with healthy clients (performance pattern)
	Context or contexts	Create a variety of equipment available at public playgrounds to promote a diversity of sensory play experiences (context)
	Activity demands	Promote the establishment of sufficient space to allow senior residents to participate in congregate cooking (activity demand)
	Client factors (body functions, body structures)	Promote increased endurance in school children by having them ride bicycles to school (client factor: body function)
Establish, restore (remediation, restoration)—an intervention approach designed to change client variables to establish a skill or ability that has not yet developed or to restore a skill or ability that has been impaired.[3]	Performance skills	Improve coping needed for changing workplace demands by improving assertiveness skills (performance skill)
	Performance patterns	Establish morning routines needed to arrive at school or work on time (performance pattern)
	Client factors (body functions, body structures)	Restore mobility needed for play activities (client factor: body function)
Maintain—an intervention approach designed to provide the supports that will allow clients to preserve their performance capabilities that they have regained, that continue to meet their occupational needs, or both. The assumption is that without continued maintenance intervention, performance would decrease, occupational needs would not be met, or both, thereby affecting health and quality of life.	Performance skills	Maintain the ability to organize tools by providing a tool outline painted on a pegboard (performance skill)
	Performance patterns	Maintain appropriate medication schedule by providing a timer (performance pattern)

Continued

Table C-6 Occupational Therapy Intervention Approaches—cont'd

Approach	Focus of Intervention	Examples
	Context or contexts	Maintain safe and independent access for persons with low vision by providing increased hallway lighting (context)
	Activity demands	Maintain independent gardening for persons with arthritic hands by providing tools and modified grips (activity demand)
	Client factors (body functions, body structures)	Maintain proper digestive system functions by developing a dining program (client factor: body function)
		Maintain upper-extremity muscles necessary for independent wheelchair mobility by developing an after-school-based exercise program (client factor: body structure)
Modify (compensation, adaptation)—an intervention approach directed at "finding ways to revise the current context or activity demands to support performance in the natural setting . . . [includes] compensatory techniques, including enhancing some features to provide cues, or reducing other features to reduce distractibility."[3]	Context or contexts	Modify holiday celebration activities to exclude alcohol to support sobriety (context)
	Activity demands	Modify office equipment (e.g., chair, computer station) to support individual employee body function and performance skill abilities (activity demand)
	Performance patterns	Modify daily routines to provide consistency and predictability to support individual's cognitive ability (performance pattern.)
Prevent (disability prevention)—an intervention approach designed to address clients with or without a disability who are at risk for occupational performance problems. This approach is designed to prevent the occurrence or evolution of barriers to performance in context, or activity variables.[3]	Performance skills	Prevent poor posture when sitting for prolonged periods by providing a chair with proper back support (performance skill)
	Performance patterns	Prevent the use of chemical substances by introducing self-initiated strategies to assist in remaining drug free (performance pattern)

Table C-6   Occupational Therapy Intervention Approaches—cont'd

Approach	Focus of Intervention	Examples
	Context or contexts	Prevent social isolation by suggesting participation in after-work group activities (context)
	Activity demands	Prevent back injury by providing instruction in proper lifting techniques (activity demand)
	Client factors (body functions, body structures)	Prevent increased blood pressure during homemaking activities by learning to monitor blood pressure in a cardiac exercise program (client factor: body function)
		Prevent repetitive stress injury by suggesting that a wrist support splint be worn when typing (client factor: body structure)

Table C-7   Types of Occupational Therapy Interventions

Therapeutic use of self—A practitioner's planned use of his or her personality, insights, perceptions, and judgments as part of the therapeutic process.[6]

Therapeutic use of occupations and activities—Occupations and activities selected for specific clients that meet therapeutic goals. To use occupations/activities therapeutically, contexts, activity demands, and client factors all should be considered in relation to the client's therapeutic goals.

Occupation-based activity	*Purpose*: Allows clients to engage in actual occupations that are part of their own context and match their goals *Examples*: Play on playground equipment during recess Purchase own groceries and prepare a meal Adapt the assembly line to achieve greater safety Put on clothes without assistance
Purposeful activity	*Purpose*: Allows the client to engage in goal-directed behaviors or activities within a therapeutically designed context, leading to an occupation or occupations *Examples*: Practice vegetable slicing Practice drawing a straight line Practice safe ways to get in and out of a bathtub equipped with grab bars Role-play to learn ways to manage anger
Preparatory methods	*Purpose*: Prepares the client for occupational performance; used in preparation for purposeful and occupation-based activities *Examples*: Sensory input to promote optimum response Physical agent modalities Orthotics/splinting (design, fabrication, application) Exercise

Consultation process—A type of intervention in which practitioners use their knowledge and expertise to collaborate with the client. The collaborative process involves identifying the problem, creating possible solutions, trying solutions, and altering them as necessary for greater effectiveness. When providing consultation, the practitioner is not directly responsible for the outcome of the intervention.

Education process—An intervention process that involves the imparting of knowledge and information about occupation and activity and that does not result in the actual performance of the occupation/activity.

Table C-8 Types of Outcomes

Outcome	Description
Occupational performance	The ability to carry out activities of daily life (areas of occupation). Occupational performance can be addressed in two different ways: Improvement—used when a performance deficit is present, often as a result of an injury or disease process. This approach results in increased independence and function in ADL, IADL, education, work, play, leisure, or social participation. Enhancement—used when a performance deficit is not currently present. This approach results in the development of performance skills and performance patterns that augment performance or prevent potential problems from developing in daily life occupations.
Client satisfaction	The client's affective response to his or her perceptions of the process and benefits of receiving occupational therapy services.[4]
Role competence	The ability to effectively meet the demand of roles in which the client engages.
Adaptation	"A change a person makes in his or her response approach when that person encounters and occupational challenge. This change is implemented when the individual's customary response approaches are found inadequate for producing some degree of mastery over the challenge."[2]
Health and wellness	*Health*—"A complete state of physical, mental, and social well-being and not just the absence of diseases and infirmity."[8] *Wellness*—The condition of being in good health, including the appreciation and enjoyment of health. Wellness is more than the lack of disease symptoms; it is a state of mental and physical balance and fitness.
Prevention	Promoting a healthy lifestyle at the individual, group, organizational, community (societal), and governmental or policy level.[1]
Quality of life	A person's dynamic appraisal of his or her life satisfactions (perceptions of progress toward one's goals), self-concept (the composite of beliefs and feelings about oneself), health and functioning (including health status, self-care capabilities, role competence), and socioeconomic factors (e.g., vocation, education, income).[7,10]

ADL, Activities of daily living; *IADL,* instrumental activities of daily living.

Table C-9 Occupational Therapy Practice Framework Process Summary

Evaluation		Intervention		Outcomes
				Engagement in Occupation to Support Participation
Occupational Profile $\longleftrightarrow$	**Analysis of Occupational Performance**	**Intervention Plan**	**Intervention Implementation**	Focus on outcomes as they relate to engagement in occupation to support participation.
Who is the client?	Synthesize information from the occupational profile.	Develop plan that includes objective and measurable goals with timeframe, occupational therapy intervention approach based on theory and evidence, and mechanisms for service delivery.	Determine types of occupational therapy interventions to be used, and carry them out.	**Intervention Review**
Why is the client seeking services?	Observe client's performance in desired occupation/activity.		Monitor client's response according to ongoing assessment and reassessment.	Re-evaluate plan relative to achieving targeted outcomes.
What occupations and activities are successful or are causing problems?	Note the effectiveness of performance skills and patterns, and select assessments to identify factors (context or contexts, activity demands, client factors) that may be influencing performance skills and patterns.	Consider discharge needs and plan.		Modify plan as needed.
What contexts support or inhibit desired outcomes?		Select outcome measures.		Determine need for continuation, discontinuation, or referral.
What is the client's occupational history?	Interpret assessment data to identify facilitators and barriers to performance.	Make recommendation or referral to others as needed.		Select outcome measures.
What are the client's priorities and targeted outcomes?	Develop and refine hypotheses about client's occupational performance strengths and weaknesses.			Measure and use outcomes.
	Collaborate with client to create goals that address targeted outcomes.			
	Delineate areas for intervention based on best practice and evidence.			

$\leftarrow$ Continue to renegotiate intervention plans and targeted outcomes. $\rightarrow$

$\leftarrow$ Ongoing interaction among evaluation, intervention, and outcomes occurs throughout the process. $\rightarrow$

REFERENCES

1. Brownson CA, Scaffa ME: Occupational therapy in the promotion of health and the prevention of disease and disability, *Am J Occup Ther* 55:656-660, 2001.
2. Christiansen CH, Baum CM (eds): *Occupational Therapy: Enabling Function and Well-Being*, Thorofare, NJ, 1997, Slack.
3. Dunn W, McClain LH, Brown C, et al: The ecology of human performance. In Neistadt ME, Crepeau EB (eds): *Willard and Spackman's Occupational Therapy*, ed 9, pp. 525-535, Philadelphia, 1998, Lippincott Williams & Wilkins.
4. Maciejewski M, Kawiecki J, Rockwood T: Satisfaction. In Kane RL (ed): *Understanding Health Care Outcomes Research*, pp. 67-89, Gaithersburg, MD, 1997, Aspen.
5. Neistadt ME, Crepeau EB (eds): *Willard and Spackman's Occupational Therapy*, ed 9, Philadelphia, 1998, Lippincott Williams & Wilkins.
6. Punwar AJ, Peloquin SM: *Occupational Therapy: Principles and Practice*, ed 3, Philadelphia, 2000, Lippincott Williams & Wilkins.
7. Radomski MV: There is more to life than putting on your pants, *Am J Occup Ther* 49:487-490, 1995.
8. World Health Organization: Constitution of the World Health Organization, *Chronicle of the World Health Organization* 1(1):29-40, 1947.
9. World Health Organization: *International Classification of Functioning, Disability and Health (ICF)*, Geneva, Switzerland, 2001, World Health Organization.
10. Zhan L: Quality of life: conceptual and measurement issues, *J Adv Nurs* 17:795-800, 1992.

Resources

PROFESSIONAL ORGANIZATIONS, FOUNDATIONS, AND CERTIFICATION

American Occupational Therapy Association, Inc. (AOTA)
4720 Montgomery Lane
PO Box 31220
Bethesda, MD 20824-1220
Phone: 301-652-2682
TDD: 1-800-377-8555
Fax: 301-652-7711
www.aota.org

American Occupational Therapy Foundation (AOTF)
4720 Montgomery Lane
PO Box 31220
Bethesda, MD 20824-1220
Phone: 301-652-2682
TDD: 800-377-8555
Fax: 301-656-3620
E-mail: aotf@aotf.org
www.aotf.org

Australian Association of Occupational Therapists
OT AUSTRALIA National
6/340 Gore St
Fitzroy, Vic, 3065
Phone: 03 9415-2900
Fax: 03 9416-1421
E-mail: info@ausot.com.au
www.ausot.com.au/

Canadian Association of Occupational Therapists (CAOT)
CTTC Building, Suite 3400
1125 Colonel By Dr
Ottawa, ON K1S 5R1
Canada
Phone: 613-523-CAOT (2268)
Toll-free: 800-434-CAOT (2268)
Fax: 613 523-2552
www.caot.ca/Default.asp

National Board for Certification in Occupational Therapy, Inc. (NBCOT®)
The Eugene B. Casey Building
800 South Frederick Avenue
Suite 200
Gaithersburg, MD 20877-4150
Phone: 301-990-7979
Fax: 301-869-8492
www.nbcot.org

World Federation of Occupational Therapists (WFOT)
PO Box 30
Forrestfield
Western Australia
Australia 6058
Fax: 61 8 9453 9746
E-mail: admin@wfot.org.au
www.wfot.org

RESEARCH AND EDUCATION

American Association of Retired Persons (AARP)
601 E Street NW
Washington, DC 20049
Phone: 1-888-687-2277

Centers for Disease Control and Prevention (CDC)
1600 Clifton Road, N.E.
Atlanta, GA 30333 USA
Phone: (404) 639-3311
Toll-free: 800-CDC-INFO
Public inquiries: (404) 639-3534 / (800) 311-3435
E-mail: cdcinfo@cdc.gov
www.cdc.gov

Centers for Medicare & Medicaid Services
7500 Security Boulevard
Baltimore, MD 21244
Toll-free: 877-267-2323
www.cms.hhs.gov

Department of Education
400 Maryland Avenue, SW
Washington, DC 20202
Toll-free: 1-800-437-0833
www.ed.gov

Department of Health and Human Services
200 Independence Avenue SW
Washington, DC 20201
Phone: 202-619-0257
Toll-free: 1-877-696-6775
www.hhs.gov

National Education Association
www.nea.org

Accreditation A form of regulation that determines whether an organization or program meets a prescribed standard

Accreditation Council for Occupational Therapy Education (ACOTE) The national organization that regulates entry-level education for occupational therapists and for occupational therapy assistants

Active being The view of humans as actively involved in controlling and determining their own behavior

Active listening A manner of communication in which the receiver paraphrases the speaker's words to ensure that he or she understands the intended meaning

Activities of daily living (ADL) Activities involved in taking care of one's own body, including such things as dressing, bathing, grooming, eating, feeding, personal device care, toileting, sexual activity, and sleep/rest

Activity State or condition of being involved (participant); a general class of human actions that is goal-directed

Activity analysis The process in which the steps of an activity and its components are examined to determine the demands on the client

Activity demands The aspects of an activity needed to carry out that activity, such as objects used and their properties, space demands, social demands, sequencing and timing, required actions, required body functions, and required body structures

Activity director The practitioner responsible for planning, implementing, and documenting an ongoing program of activities that meet the needs of the residents

Activity synthesis The process of identifying gaps in performance and bridging those gaps by grading or adapting the activity or the environment in order to provide the "just right challenge" for the client

Acute care The first level on the continuum of care in which a client has a sudden and short-term need for services and is typically seen in a hospital

Adaptation A change in function that promotes survival and self-actualization

Adolescence The period of development between 12 and 20 years of age

Adolf Meyer A Swiss physician committed to a holistic perspective; developed the psychobiological approach to mental illness

Adulthood The period of development after 20 years of age; broken into a young stage (20-40 years of age), middle (40-65 years of age), and late (over 65 years of age)

Advanced beginner A practitioner who is learning to recognize additional cues and beginning to see the client as an individual; still does not see the whole picture

Aging The unique changes that occur over time, such as sensory and physical declines

Aging in place The trend of more elderly people staying at home and living independently or with minimal assistance

Altruism The unselfish concern for the welfare of others

Americans with Disabilities Act of 1990 Legislation that provides civil rights to all individuals with disabilities

American Journal of Occupational Therapy (AJOT) The American Occupational Therapy Association's (AOTA's) official publication that traditionally has served as the main source of research and resource information for the profession

American Occupational Therapy Association (AOTA) Formerly called the National Society for the Promotion of Occupational Therapy; the nationally recognized professional association for occupational therapy practitioners

American Occupational Therapy Foundation (AOTF) A national organization designed to advance the science of occupational therapy and to increase public understanding of the value of occupational therapy

American Occupational Therapy Political Action Committee (AOTPAC) The organization that furthers the legislative aims of the profession by attempting to influence the selection, nomination, election, or appointment of persons to public office

American Student Committee of the Occupational Therapy Association (ASCOTA) Student representatives from all accredited schools who participate in the American Occupational Therapy Association by meeting regularly and providing feedback to the organization

Areas of occupation Various life activities including activities of daily living (ADL), instrumental activities of daily living (IADL), education, work, play, leisure, and social participation

Artistic element The element of clinical reasoning in which the occupational therapy practitioner guides the treatment process and selects the "right action" in the face of uncertainties inherent in the clinical process

Arts and Crafts Movement A late nineteenth-century movement born in reaction to the Industrial Revolution; emphasized craftsmanship and design

Assessment instruments Standardized or nonstandardized measurements used to obtain information about clients

Assessment procedures The clinical techniques and instruments used to determine the strengths and weaknesses of a client for therapeutic purposes

Assistive devices Low- or high-technology aids to improve a person's function

Assistive technology Devices that aid a person in his or her daily life as necessary

Autonomy The freedom to decide and the freedom to act

Axiology component The part of philosophy that is concerned with the study of values

Balanced Budget Act (BBA) of 1997 Legislation intended to reduce Medicare spending, create incentives for development of managed care plans, encourage enrollment in managed care plans, and limit fee-for-service payment and programs

Beneficence A principle that requires that the occupational therapy practitioner contribute to the good health and welfare of the client

Benjamin Rush An American Quaker who was the first physician to institute Moral Treatment practices

Biological sphere Sphere of practice in which clients have medical problems caused by disease, disorder, or trauma

Biomechanical frame of reference A frame of reference derived from theories in kinetics and kinematics; used with individuals who have deficits in the peripheral nervous, musculoskeletal, integumentary (e.g., skin), or cardiopulmonary system

Board certification Certification for the occupational therapist or occupational therapy assistant that incorporates more generalized areas of practice that have an established knowledge base in occupational therapy

Brain plasticity The phenomenon that the brain is capable of change and that through activity one may get improved neurological synapses, improved dendritic growth, or additional pathways

Canadian Model of Occupational Performance A model of practice that emphasizes client-centered care and spirituality

Career development The process of advancing within the service delivery path or transitioning into a role outside of service delivery

Cerebral palsy (CP) A disorder caused by an insult to the brain before during or soon after birth, which manifests in motor abnormalities

Certification The acknowledgement that an individual has the qualifications to be an entry-level practitioner

Childhood Spans early childhood (1-6 years) and later childhood (6-12 years)

Civilian Vocational Rehabilitation Act Act that provided federal funds to states to provide vocational rehabilitation services to civilians with disabilities

Clarification An active listening technique in which the client's thoughts and feelings are summarized or simplified

Client Person served by occupational therapy in a health facility or training center

Client-centered approach An approach in which the client, family, and significant others are active participants throughout the therapeutic process

Client factors Components of activities consisting of body functions and body structures; used to assess functioning, disability, and health

Client-related tasks Routine tasks in which the aide may interact with the client but not as the primary service provider of occupational therapy

Client satisfaction A measure of the client's perception of the process and the benefits received from occupational therapy services

Clinical reasoning The thought process that therapists use to design and carry out intervention; involves complex cognitive and affective skills

Close supervision The need for direct, daily contact with the supervisee

Code of ethics Professional guidelines for making correct or proper choices and decisions for health care practice in the field

Cognitive disability frame of reference A frame of reference based on the premise that cognitive disorders in those with mental health disabilities are caused by neurobiologic defects or deficits related to the biologic functioning of the brain

Competent practitioner A level of clinical reasoning skills in which the practitioner is able to see more facts and to determine the importance of these facts and observations; has a broader understanding of the client's problems and is more likely to individualize treatment; however, flexibility and creativity are still lacking

Concepts Ideas that represent something in the mind of the individual

Conditional reasoning The clinical reasoning strategy in which the occupational therapy practitioner implements intervention and cognitively checks along the way to compare the client's progress in treatment and goals for the future

Confidentiality The expectation that information shared by the client with the occupational therapy practitioner will be kept private and shared only with those directly involved with the intervention

Consultation A type of intervention in which practitioners use their knowledge and expertise to collaborate with the client, caregivers, significant others, or other providers

Context The setting in which the occupation occurs; includes cultural, physical, social, personal, spiritual, temporal, and virtual conditions within and surrounding the client that influence performance

Continuing competence A process in which the occupational therapy practitioner develops and maintains knowledge, performance skills, interpersonal abilities, critical reasoning skills, and ethical reasoning skills necessary to perform his or her professional responsibilities

Continuum of care A way of characterizing health care settings by the level of care required by the client, including the whole spectrum of needs

Developmental delays The general slowing of skills

Developmental frame of reference A frame of reference that postulates that practice in a skill set will enhance brain development and help the child progress through the stages

Diagnosis codes Billing codes that are based on the client's medical condition or the medical justification for needing services

Diagnosis-related groups (DRGs) Groupings of disease categories that Medicare and other third-party payers use as a basis for hospital payment schedules

Dignity The quality or state of being worthy, honored, or esteemed

Direct supervision The supervising occupational therapist is on site and available to provide immediate assistance to the client or supervisee if needed.

Discharge plan The plan developed and implemented to address the resources and supports that may be required upon discontinuation of services

Doctor of Occupational Therapy (OTD) Clinical or practice-based doctoral degree; focuses on practice rather than research

Documentation The process of keeping records on all the aspects of service delivery

Driver rehabilitation specialist An occupational therapy practitioner who evaluates and intervenes in physical, social, cognitive, and psychosocial aspects of functioning that affect driving skills

Education The process of gaining knowledge and information

Education for All Handicapped Children Act of 1975 (PL 94-142) Act that established the right of all children to a free and appropriate education, regardless of handicapping condition

Eleanor Clarke Slagle Known as the mother of occupational therapy; developed the area of habit training and organized the first professional school for occupational therapy practitioners

Emergency procedures Actions to follow in case of an injury or accident in the clinic

Empathy The ability of the occupational therapy practitioner to place himself or herself in the client's position and to understand what he or she is experiencing

Entry-level practitioner A practitioner who is still developing his or her skills and is expected to be held responsible for and accountable in professional activities related to the role

Epistemology component The part of philosophy that investigates critically the nature, origin, and limits of human knowledge

Equality The treatment of all individuals with an attitude of fairness and impartiality and the respecting of each individual's beliefs, values, and lifestyles

Ergonomics The science of fitting jobs to people

Ethical dilemma A situation in which two or more ethical principles collide with one another, making it difficult to determine the best action

Ethical distress Situations that challenge how a practitioner maintains his or her integrity or the integrity of the profession along with the integrity of the profession and examining the "right" behaviors or proper choices and decisions

Ethical element The element of clinical reasoning that takes into account the client's perspective and his or her goals for intervention

Ethics The study and philosophy of human conduct

Evaluation The process of obtaining and interpreting data necessary to understand the individual and design appropriate treatment

Evidence-based practice Basing practice on the best available research evidence

Expert A practitioner who has the clinical reasoning skills to recognize and understand rules of practice, use intuition to know what to do next, and use conditional reasoning

Family-centered care Care that involves working with the family members of the child on goals that are considered important to them

Fidelity Faithfulness

Fieldwork Practical experience applying classroom knowledge to a clinical setting; categorized as Level I (may be observational) or Level II (development of entry-level skills)

Frame of reference (FOR) A system that applies theory and puts principles into practice, providing practitioners with specifics on how to treat specific clients

Freedom An individual's right to exercise choice

Function Action for which a person is fit; the ability to perform

General supervision At least monthly face-to-face contact with the supervisee

George Edward Barton An architect who opened Consolation House for convalescent patients, where occupation was used as a method of treatment

Goal End toward which effort is directed

Grading Changing the process, environment, tools, or materials of the activity to increase or decrease the performance demands on the client

Group More than two people interacting with a common purpose

Group dynamics Refers to the interactions among individuals and how they work together

Habit training A re-education program dedicated to restoring and maintaining health by directing activity to construct new habits and discard ineffective ones

Handicapped Infants and Toddlers Act of 1986 An amendment to the Education for All Handicapped Children Act; includes children from 3 to 5 years of age and initiates new early intervention programs for children from birth to 3 years of age

Health The state of physical, mental, and social well-being

Herbert Hall A physician who adapted the Arts and Crafts Movement for medical purposes

Holistic An approach that deems that each individual should be seen as a complete and unified whole rather than a series of parts or problems to be managed

Hospice Care and services provided to help the client be comfortable during the last stages of a terminal illness

Humanism The belief that the client should be treated as a person, not an object

Ideal self What an individual would like to be if free of the demands of mundane reality

Independence State or condition of being independent (self-reliant)

Individualized education plan (IEP) A plan that charts the problems, goals, and interventions necessary for the child to have success in school

Individuals with Disabilities Education Act (IDEA) of 1991 Legislation that requires school districts to educate students with disabilities in the least restrictive environment

Infancy The period from birth through 1 year of age

Informed consent The knowledgeable and voluntary agreement by which a client undergoes intervention that is in accord with his or her values and preferences

Instrumental activities of daily living (IADLs) Activities, such as meal preparation, money management, care of others, which involve interacting with the environment; often complex; may be considered optional

Interactive reasoning A strategy used by the occupational therapy practitioner when he or she wants to understand the client as a person

Interdisciplinary team A mix of practitioners from different disciplines who maintain their own professional roles and use a cooperative approach that is very interactive and centered on a common problem to solve

Intermediate-level practitioner A practitioner who has increased responsibility and typically pursues specialization in a particular area of practice

Interrater reliability A measure of the likelihood that test scores will be the same no matter who is the examiner

Intervention An approach that involves working with the client through therapy to reach client goals

Interview The primary mechanism for gathering information for the occupational profile; achieved by the occupational therapy practitioner asking the client and significant others questions

Justice The need for all occupational therapy practitioners to abide by the laws that govern the practice and the legal rights of the client

Later adulthood The period of development after 65 years of age

Learned helplessness The phenomenon of less activity and independence in functioning among elderly people that results when older persons are not allowed to engage in activities or when others do everything for them

Least restrictive environment The classroom most similar to a regular classroom in which the student can be successful

Licensure The process by which permission is granted to an individual to engage in a given occupation upon finding that the applicant has attained the minimal degree of competence required to ensure that the public health, safety, and welfare will be reasonably protected

Locus of authority Situations that require a decision about who should be the primary decision maker

Long-term care The level of care needed for clients who are medically stable but have a chronic condition requiring services over time, potentially throughout their lives

Mechanistic The view that sees the human as passive in nature and controlled by the environment in which he or she lives

Media The means by which therapeutic effects are transmitted

Medicare Enacted in 1965; legislation that provides health care assistance for individuals 65 years or older or those who are permanently and totally disabled

Metaphysical component One part of philosophy that addresses questions such as "What is the nature of humankind?"

Methods The steps, sequences, and approaches used to activate the therapeutic effect of a medium

Modality The media and methods used in occupational therapy intervention

Model of Human Occupation A model of practice that views occupation in terms of volition, habituation, performance, and environment

Model of practice A way of organizing that takes the philosophical base of the profession and provides terms to describe practice, tools for evaluation, and a guide for intervention

Morals A view of right and wrong developed as a result of background, values, religious beliefs, and the society in which a person lives

Moral Treatment A movement grounded in the philosophy that all people, even the most challenged, are entitled to consideration and human compassion

Multidisciplinary team A mix of practitioners from multiple disciplines who work together in a common setting but without an interactive relationship

Narrative reasoning The type of clinical reasoning in which storytelling and story creation are used

National Board for Certification in Occupational Therapy (NBCOT®) The organization responsible for administering the national certification examination

National Society for the Promotion of Occupational Therapy Formed on March 15, 1917; marked the birth of the profession of occupational therapy

Non–client-related tasks The preparation of the work area and equipment, clerical tasks, and maintenance activities

Nonmaleficence A principle that instructs the practitioner to not inflict harm to the client

Non-standardized tests Tests that do not provide specific guidelines based upon a normative sample; do not require standardized procedures

Nonverbal communication Communication that includes facial expressions, eye contact, tone of voice, touch, and body language

Normative data Information collected from a representative sample that can then be used by the examiner to make comparisons with his or her clients

Novice A practitioner who is learning the procedural skills (e.g., assessment, diagnostic, and treatment planning procedures) necessary to practice

Observation The means of gathering information about a person or an environment by watching and noticing

Occupation Activity in which one engages that is meaningful and central to one's identity

Occupation as a means The use of a specific occupation to bring about a change in the client's performance

Occupation as an end The desired outcome or product of intervention

Occupation-based activity The performance of occupation-related activities by the client, including activities of daily living, instrumental activities of daily living, work and school tasks, and play or leisure tasks

Occupational adaptation A model of practice that proposes that occupational therapy practitioners examine how they may change the person, environment, or task so the client may engage in occupations

Occupational performance The ability to carry out activities in the areas of occupation

Occupational therapist (OT) An allied health professional who uses occupation, purposeful activity, simulated activities, and preparatory methods to maximize the independence and health of any client who is limited by physical injury or illness, cognitive impairment, psychosocial dysfunction, mental illness, or a developmental or learning disability

Occupational therapy A goal-directed activity that promotes independence in function; the practice of using meaningful occupations and purposeful activities to promote function and participation in life activities

Occupational therapy aide A person who provides services under the supervision of an occupational therapist to clients and therapists and helps maintain the work space

Occupational therapy assistant (OTA) An allied health paraprofessional who, under the direction of an occupational therapist, directs an individual's participation in selected tasks to restore, reinforce, and enhance performance, and promote and maintain health

Occupational therapy practitioner Refers to two different levels of clinicians, an occupational therapist (OT) or an occupational therapy assistant (OTA)

Occupational therapy process The interaction between two active agents involved in the process—the practitioner and the client

Organismic The view that a person's behaviors influence the physical and social environment and that, in turn, the person is affected by changes in the environment

Orthotic device An apparatus used to support, align, prevent, or correct deformities or to improve the function of movable parts of the body

Outcome measures An aspect of program evaluation that evaluates the results of the intervention after the service has been provided

Participatory research Involves the clinician, client, and faculty member in the research process

Patient Person served in a hospital or rehabilitation setting

Perceived self The aspect that others see; what they perceive without the benefit of knowing a person's intentions, motivations, and limitations

Performance patterns The client's habits, routines, and roles

Performance skills Small units of observable action that are linked together in the process of executing a daily life task performance

Person-Environment-Occupation-Performance A model of practice that provides definitions and describes the interactive nature of human beings

Phenomenological That which is determined by the experience of individuals

Phillippe Pinel French physician who advocated humane treatment for mentally ill patients in the late 1700s

Physical agent modalities (PAMs) Preparatory methods used to bring about a response in soft tissue

Play The spontaneous, enjoyable, free from rules, internally motivated activity in which there is no goal or purpose

Political action committees (PACs) The legally sanctioned vehicles through which organizations can engage in political action

Pragmatic reasoning The type of clinical reasoning that takes into consideration factors in the context of the practice setting and in the personal context of the occupational therapy practitioner that may inhibit or facilitate intervention

Preparatory methods Techniques or activities that address the remediation and restoration of problems associated with client factors and body structure, with the long-term purpose of supporting the client's acquisition of performance skills needed to resume his or her roles and daily occupations

Principles Ideas that explain the relationship between two or more concepts

Private for-profit agencies Organizations owned and operated by individuals or a group of investors

Private not-for-profit agencies Organizations that receive special tax exemptions and typically charge a fee for services and maintain a balanced budget to provide services

Private funding sources Businesses that provide funds for medical procedures

Problem-Oriented Medical Record A format that provides a structure to documentation

Procedural reasoning A clinical reasoning strategy used by the occupational therapy practitioner when he or she focuses on the client's disease or disability and determines what will be the most appropriate modalities to use to improve the functional performance

Procedure codes Billing codes that are based on the specific services performed by health care providers

Professional association An organization that exists to protect and promote the profession it represents by (1) providing a communication network and channel for information, (2) regulating itself through the development and enforcement of standards of conduct and performance, and (3) guarding the interests of those within the profession

Professional development Organizing and personally managing a cumulative series of work experiences to add to one's knowledge, motivation, perspectives, skills, and job performance

Professional philosophy A set of values, beliefs, truths, and principles that guide the practitioner's actions

Proficient practitioner A practitioner who views situations as a whole instead of as isolated parts; practical experience allows the proficient practitioner to develop a direction and vision of where the client should be going; able to easily modify the intervention plan if the initial plan does not work

Program evaluation Measuring effectiveness by determining which programs are achieving their goals and objectives, and modifying programs accordingly

Prudence The ability to demonstrate sound judgment, care, and discretion

Psychological sphere A sphere of practice in which client problems manifest as emotional, cognitive, affective, or personality disorders

Public agencies Health care agencies operated by federal, state, or county governments

Public funding sources Agencies at the federal, state, or local level that provide funds for medical procedures

Purposeful activity An activity used in treatment that is goal directed; individual is an active voluntary participant; has both inherent and therapeutic goals

Quality of life A relative measurement of what is meaningful and what provides satisfaction to an individual

Real self A blending of the internal and external worlds involving intention and action plus environmental awareness

Reconstruction aides Civilians who helped rehabilitate soldiers who had been injured in the war so that they could either return to active military duty or be employed in a civilian job

Referral A request for service for a particular client or a change in the degree and direction of service

Reflection A response wherein the purpose is to express in words the feelings and attitudes sensed behind the words of the speaker

Registration The listing of qualified individuals by a professional association or government agency

Regulations Policies describing the implementation and enforcement of laws

Rehabilitation Act of 1973 Act that guaranteed certain rights for people with disabilities, emphasized the need for rehabilitation research, and called for priority service for persons with the most severe disabilities

Rehabilitation Movement The period from 1942 to 1960 in which Veterans Administration hospitals increased in size and number to handle the casualties of war and continued care of veterans

Relationship A connection of different roles to one another

Reliability A measure of how accurately the scores obtained from the test reflect the true performance of the client

Restatement The listener repeats the words of the speaker as they are heard.

Role A pattern of behavior that involves certain rights and duties that an individual is expected, trained, and encouraged to perform in a particular social situation

Role competence The ability to meet the demands of roles

Routine supervision Direct contact at least every 2 weeks with interim supervision as needed

Scientific element One of the three elements of clinical reasoning that demands careful and accurate assessments, analysis, and recording

Screening The process by which the occupational therapy practitioner gathers preliminary information about the client and determines whether further evaluation and occupational therapy intervention are warranted

Self-awareness Knowing one's own true nature; the ability to recognize one's own behavior, emotional responses, and effect created on others

Service competency A useful mechanism by which it is determined that two people performing the same or equivalent procedures will obtain the same or equivalent results

Service management functions Functions that include maintaining a safe and efficient workplace, making daily schedules, documenting treatment, integrating research into practice, billing for services, supervising fieldwork students, marketing and public relations, and performing quality assurance activities

SOAP note The format used for writing the progress note, wherein "S" is subjective information, "O" is objective information, "A" is the assessment, and "P" is the plan

Sociological sphere A sphere of practice wherein clients have problems meeting the expectations of society

Soldier's Rehabilitation Act Act that established a program of vocational rehabilitation for soldiers disabled on active duty

Specialty certification A credential for occupational therapists and occupational therapy assistants that indicates advanced knowledge in a particular area of practice

Splint A device for immobilization, restraint, or support of any part of the body

Standards of practice Guidelines for the delivery of occupational therapy services

Statutes Laws that are enacted by the legislative branch of a government

Structured observation The means of gathering information about a person by watching the client perform a predetermined activity

Subacute care The level in which the client still needs care but does not require an intensive level or specialized service

Supervision A cooperative process in which two or more people participate in a joint effort to establish, maintain, and or elevate a level of competence and performance

Susan Cox Johnson Demonstrated that occupation could be morally uplifting and could improve the mental and physical state of patients and inmates in public hospitals and almshouses

Susan Tracy A nurse involved in the Arts and Crafts Movement and in the training of nurses in the use of occupations

Technology Related Assistance for Individuals with Disabilities Act of 1988 Act that addressed the availability of assistive technology devices and services to individuals with disabilities

Test-retest reliability A measure of the consistency of the results of a given test from one administration to another

Theory A set of ideas that help explain things and how they work

Therapeutic exercise The scientific supervision of exercise for the purpose of preventing muscular atrophy, restoring joint and muscle function, and improving efficiency of cardiovascular and pulmonary function

Therapeutic relationship The interaction between a practitioner and a client in which the occupational therapy practitioner is responsible for facilitating the healing and rehabilitation process

Therapeutic use of occupations and activity The selection of activities and occupations that will meet the therapeutic goals

Therapeutic use of self The art of relating to clients, which involves being aware of oneself and of the client and being in command of what is communicated

Therapy Treatment of an illness or disability

Thomas Kidner An architect who was influential in establishing a presence for occupational therapy in vocational rehabilitation and tuberculosis treatment

Transdisciplinary team A mix of practitioners from different disciplines in which members cross over professional boundaries and share roles and functions

Transition services The coordination or facilitation of services for the purpose of preparing the client for a change

Truthfulness The value demonstrated through behavior that is accountable, honest, and accurate, and that maintains one's professional competence

Universal precautions A set of guidelines designed to prevent the transmission of HIV, HBV, and other blood-borne pathogens to health care providers

Universal stages of loss Stages of death and dying first identified by Elisabeth Kübler-Ross, which include denial, anger, bargaining, depression, and acceptance; can also be applied to individuals experiencing loss due to a disabling condition

Validity Having a true measure of what it claims to measure

Veracity The duty of the health care professional to tell the truth

Vision A statement or ethos of a profession or organization that is developed with the members and constituents over time and that clarifies values, creates a future, and focuses the mission

Wellness The condition of being in good health

William Rush Dunton, Jr. Considered the father of occupational therapy; introduced a regimen of crafts for his patients

William Tuke An English Quaker who opened the York Retreat, which pioneered new methods of treatment of mentally ill patients

World Federation of Occupational Therapists (WFOT) Organization established in 1952 to help occupational therapy practitioners access international information, engage in international exchange, and promote organizations of occupational therapy in schools in countries where none exists

Young adulthood The ages between 20 and 40 years

Photo Credits

Cover page photo: From Croninger, William, University of New England, Biddeford, Maine.

Section 1 opener photo: From Croninger, William, University of New England, Biddeford, Maine.

Chapter 1 opener photo: From Byers-Connon S, Lohman H, Padilla R: *Occupational Therapy with Elders: Strategies for the COTA*, ed 2, St. Louis, 2004, Mosby.

Chapter 2 opener photo: From Case-Smith J: *Occupational Therapy for Children*, ed 5, St. Louis, 2005, Mosby.

Chapter 3 opener photo: From Byers-Connon S, Lohman H, Padilla R: *Occupational Therapy with Elders: Strategies for the COTA*, ed 2, St. Louis, 2004, Mosby.

Chapter 4 opener photo: From Early MB: *Physical Dysfunction Practice Skills for the Occupational Therapy Assistant*, ed 2, St. Louis, 2006, Mosby.

Section 2 opener photo: From Parham LD, Fazio LS: *Play in Occupational Therapy for Children*, St. Louis, 1997, Mosby.

Chapter 5 opener photo: From Sanders MJ: *Ergonomics and the Management of Musculoskeletal Disorders*, ed 2, St. Louis, 2004, Butterworth Heinemann.

Chapter 6 opener photo: From Croninger, William, University of New England, Biddeford, Maine.

Chapter 7 opener photo: From Case-Smith J: *Occupational Therapy for Children*, ed 5, St. Louis, 2005, Mosby.

Chapter 8 opener photo: From Early MB: *Physical Dysfunction Practice Skills for the Occupational Therapy Assistant*, ed 2, St. Louis, 2006, Mosby.

Section 3 opener photo: From Pendleton HM, Schultz-Krohn W: *Pedretti's Occupational Therapy: Practice Skills for Physical Dysfunction*, ed 6, St. Louis, 2006, Mosby.

Chapter 9 opener photo: From Pendleton HM, Schultz-Krohn W: *Pedretti's Occupational Therapy: Practice Skills for Physical Dysfunction*, ed 6, St. Louis, 2006, Mosby.

Chapter 10 opener photo: From O'Brien, Jane, University of New England, Biddeford, Maine.

Chapter 11 opener photo: From Byers-Connon S, Lohman H, Padilla R: *Occupational Therapy with Elders: Strategies for the COTA*, ed 2, St. Louis, 2004, Mosby.

Chapter 12 opener photo: From Campbell SK, Vander Linden DW, Palisano RJ: *Physical Therapy for Children*, ed 4, Philadelphia, 2006, Saunders.

Chapter 13 opener photo: From Pendleton HM, Schultz-Krohn W: *Pedretti's Occupational Therapy: Practice Skills for Physical Dysfunction*, ed 6, St. Louis, 2006, Mosby.

Chapter 14 opener photo: From Lohman H, Padilla R, Byers-Connon S: *Occupational Therapy with Elders: Strategies for the COTA*, St. Louis, 1998, Mosby.

Chapter 15 opener photo: From Campbell SK, Vander Linden DW, Palisano RJ: *Physical Therapy for Children*, ed 4, Philadelphia, 2006, Saunders.

Chapter 16 opener photo: From Byers-Connon S, Lohman H, Padilla R: *Occupational Therapy with Elders: Strategies for the COTA*, ed 2, St. Louis, 2004, Mosby.

Chapter 17 opener photo: From Croninger W, University of New England, Biddeford, Maine.

Index

Page numbers in italics refer to boxes or figures. Page numbers followed by t refer to tables.